THE OFFICIAL PATIENT'S SOURCEBOOK *on* SLEEP APNEA

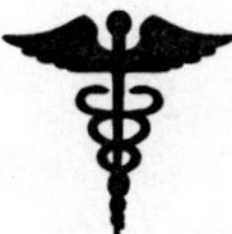

JAMES N. PARKER, M.D.
AND PHILIP M. PARKER, PH.D., EDITORS

ICON Health Publications
ICON Group International, Inc.
4370 La Jolla Village Drive, 4th Floor
San Diego, CA 92122 USA

Printed in the United States of America.

Last digit indicates print number: 10 9 8 7 6 4 5 3 2 1

Publisher, Health Care: Philip Parker, Ph.D.
Editor(s): James Parker, M.D., Philip Parker, Ph.D.

Publisher's note: The ideas, procedures, and suggestions contained in this book are not intended as a substitute for consultation with your physician. All matters regarding your health require medical supervision. As new medical or scientific information becomes available from academic and clinical research, recommended treatments and drug therapies may undergo changes. The authors, editors, and publisher have attempted to make the information in this book up to date and accurate in accord with accepted standards at the time of publication. The authors, editors, and publisher are not responsible for errors or omissions or for consequences from application of the book, and make no warranty, expressed or implied, in regard to the contents of this book. Any practice described in this book should be applied by the reader in accordance with professional standards of care used in regard to the unique circumstances that may apply in each situation, in close consultation with a qualified physician. The reader is advised to always check product information (package inserts) for changes and new information regarding dose and contraindications before taking any drug or pharmacological product. Caution is especially urged when using new or infrequently ordered drugs, herbal remedies, vitamins and supplements, alternative therapies, complementary therapies and medicines, and integrative medical treatments.

Cataloging-in-Publication Data

Parker, James N., 1961-
Parker, Philip M., 1960-

The Official Patient's Sourcebook on Sleep Apnea: A Revised and Updated Directory for the Internet Age/James N. Parker and Philip M. Parker, editors

p. cm.
Includes bibliographical references, glossary and index.
ISBN: 0-497-11058-X
1. Sleep Apnea-Popular works. I. Title.

Disclaimer

Copyright Notice

Dedication

To the healthcare professionals dedicating their time and efforts to the study of sleep apnea.

Acknowledgements

The collective knowledge generated from academic and applied research summarized in various references has been critical in the creation of this sourcebook which is best viewed as a comprehensive compilation and collection of information prepared by various official agencies which directly or indirectly are dedicated to sleep apnea. All of the *Official Patient's Sourcebooks* draw from various agencies and institutions associated with the United States Department of Health and Human Services, and in particular, the Office of the Secretary of Health and Human Services (OS), the Administration for Children and Families (ACF), the Administration on Aging (AOA), the Agency for Healthcare Research and Quality (AHRQ), the Agency for Toxic Substances and Disease Registry (ATSDR), the Centers for Disease Control and Prevention (CDC), the Food and Drug Administration (FDA), the Healthcare Financing Administration (HCFA), the Health Resources and Services Administration (HRSA), the Indian Health Service (IHS), the institutions of the National Institutes of Health (NIH), the Program Support Center (PSC), and the Substance Abuse and Mental Health Services Administration (SAMHSA). In addition to these sources, information gathered from the National Library of Medicine, the United States Patent Office, the European Union, and their related organizations has been invaluable in the creation of this sourcebook. Some of the work represented was financially supported by the Research and Development Committee at INSEAD. This support is gratefully acknowledged. Finally, special thanks are owed to Tiffany Freeman for her excellent editorial support.

About the Editors

James N. Parker, M.D.

Dr. James N. Parker received his Bachelor of Science degree in Psychobiology from the University of California, Riverside and his M.D. from the University of California, San Diego. In addition to authoring numerous research publications, he has lectured at various academic institutions. Dr. Parker is the medical editor for the *Official Patient's Sourcebook* series published by ICON Health Publications.

Philip M. Parker, Ph.D.

Philip M. Parker is the Eli Lilly Chair Professor of Innovation, Business and Society at INSEAD (Fontainebleau, France and Singapore). Dr. Parker has also been Professor at the University of California, San Diego and has taught courses at Harvard University, the Hong Kong University of Science and Technology, the Massachusetts Institute of Technology, Stanford University, and UCLA. Dr. Parker is the associate editor for the *Official Patient's Sourcebook* series published by ICON Health Publications.

About ICON Health Publications

In addition to sleep apnea, *Official Patient's Sourcebooks* are available for the following related topics:

- The Official Patient's Sourcebook on Insomnia
- The Official Patient's Sourcebook on Narcolepsy
- The Official Patient's Sourcebook on Restless Legs Syndrome

To discover more about ICON Health Publications, simply check with your preferred online booksellers, including Barnes&Noble.com and Amazon.com which currently carry all of our titles. Or, feel free to contact us directly for bulk purchases or institutional discounts:

ICON Group International, Inc.
4370 La Jolla Village Drive, Fourth Floor
San Diego, CA 92122 USA
Fax: 858-546-4341
Web site: **www.icongrouponline.com/health**

Table of Contents

INTRODUCTION

Overview

Dr. C. Everett Koop, former U.S. Surgeon General, once said, "The best prescription is knowledge."[1] The Agency for Healthcare Research and Quality (AHRQ) of the National Institutes of Health (NIH) echoes this view and recommends that every patient incorporate education into the treatment process. According to the AHRQ:

> Finding out more about your condition is a good place to start. By contacting groups that support your condition, visiting your local library, and searching on the Internet, you can find good information to help guide your treatment decisions. Some information may be hard to find—especially if you don't know where to look.[2]

As the AHRQ mentions, finding the right information is not an obvious task. Though many physicians and public officials had thought that the emergence of the Internet would do much to assist patients in obtaining reliable information, in March 2001 the National Institutes of Health issued the following warning:

> The number of Web sites offering health-related resources grows every day. Many sites provide valuable information, while others may have information that is unreliable or misleading.[3]

---

[1] Quotation from **http://www.drkoop.com**.

[2] The Agency for Healthcare Research and Quality (AHRQ): **http://www.ahcpr.gov/consumer/diaginfo.htm**.

[3] From the NIH, National Cancer Institute (NCI): **http://cancertrials.nci.nih.gov/beyond/evaluating.html**.

Since the late 1990s, physicians have seen a general increase in patient Internet usage rates. Patients frequently enter their doctor's offices with printed Web pages of home remedies in the guise of latest medical research. This scenario is so common that doctors often spend more time dispelling misleading information than guiding patients through sound therapies. *The Official Patient's Sourcebook on Sleep Apnea* has been created for patients who have decided to make education and research an integral part of the treatment process. The pages that follow will tell you where and how to look for information covering virtually all topics related to sleep apnea, from the essentials to the most advanced areas of research.

The title of this book includes the word "official." This reflects the fact that the sourcebook draws from public, academic, government, and peer-reviewed research. Selected readings from various agencies are reproduced to give you some of the latest official information available to date on sleep apnea.

Given patients' increasing sophistication in using the Internet, abundant references to reliable Internet-based resources are provided throughout this sourcebook. Where possible, guidance is provided on how to obtain free-of-charge, primary research results as well as more detailed information via the Internet. E-book and electronic versions of this sourcebook are fully interactive with each of the Internet sites mentioned (clicking on a hyperlink automatically opens your browser to the site indicated). Hard copy users of this sourcebook can type cited Web addresses directly into their browsers to obtain access to the corresponding sites. Since we are working with ICON Health Publications, hard copy *Sourcebooks* are frequently updated and printed on demand to ensure that the information provided is current.

In addition to extensive references accessible via the Internet, every chapter presents a "Vocabulary Builder." Many health guides offer glossaries of technical or uncommon terms in an appendix. In editing this sourcebook, we have decided to place a smaller glossary within each chapter that covers terms used in that chapter. Given the technical nature of some chapters, you may need to revisit many sections. Building one's vocabulary of medical terms in such a gradual manner has been shown to improve the learning process.

We must emphasize that no sourcebook on sleep apnea should affirm that a specific diagnostic procedure or treatment discussed in a research study, patent, or doctoral dissertation is "correct" or your best option. This sourcebook is no exception. Each patient is unique. Deciding on appropriate options is always up to the patient in consultation with their physician and healthcare providers.

Organization

This sourcebook is organized into three parts. Part I explores basic techniques to researching sleep apnea (e.g. finding guidelines on diagnosis, treatments, and prognosis), followed by a number of topics, including information on how to get in touch with organizations, associations, or other patient networks dedicated to sleep apnea. It also gives you sources of information that can help you find a doctor in your local area specializing in treating sleep apnea. Collectively, the material presented in Part I is a complete primer on basic research topics for patients with sleep apnea.

Part II moves on to advanced research dedicated to sleep apnea. Part II is intended for those willing to invest many hours of hard work and study. It is here that we direct you to the latest scientific and applied research on sleep apnea. When possible, contact names, links via the Internet, and summaries are provided. It is in Part II where the vocabulary process becomes important as authors publishing advanced research frequently use highly specialized language. In general, every attempt is made to recommend "free-to-use" options.

Part III provides appendices of useful background reading for all patients with sleep apnea or related disorders. The appendices are dedicated to more pragmatic issues faced by many patients with sleep apnea. Accessing materials via medical libraries may be the only option for some readers, so a guide is provided for finding local medical libraries which are open to the public. Part III, therefore, focuses on advice that goes beyond the biological and scientific issues facing patients with sleep apnea.

Scope

While this sourcebook covers sleep apnea, your doctor, research publications, and specialists may refer to your condition using a variety of terms. Therefore, you should understand that sleep apnea is often considered a synonym or a condition closely related to the following:

- Central Sleep Apnea
- Nocturnal Upper Airway Occlusion
- Obstructive Sleep Apnea

- Ondine's Curse
- Pediatric Obstructive Sleep Apnea
- Pickwickian Syndrome
- Sleep Apnea Syndrome

In addition to synonyms and related conditions, physicians may refer to sleep apnea using certain coding systems. The International Classification of Diseases, 9th Revision, Clinical Modification (ICD-9-CM) is the most commonly used system of classification for the world's illnesses. Your physician may use this coding system as an administrative or tracking tool. The following classification is commonly used for sleep apnea:[4]

- 780.51 insomnia with sleep apnea
- 780.53 hypersomnia with sleep apnea
- 780.57 other and unspecified sleep apnea

For the purposes of this sourcebook, we have attempted to be as inclusive as possible, looking for official information for all of the synonyms relevant to sleep apnea. You may find it useful to refer to synonyms when accessing databases or interacting with healthcare professionals and medical librarians.

Moving Forward

Since the 1980s, the world has seen a proliferation of healthcare guides covering most illnesses. Some are written by patients or their family members. These generally take a layperson's approach to understanding and coping with an illness or disorder. They can be uplifting, encouraging, and highly supportive. Other guides are authored by physicians or other healthcare providers who have a more clinical outlook. Each of these two styles of guide has its purpose and can be quite useful.

As editors, we have chosen a third route. We have chosen to expose you to as many sources of official and peer-reviewed information as practical, for the purpose of educating you about basic and advanced knowledge as

---

[4] This list is based on the official version of the World Health Organization's 9th Revision, International Classification of Diseases (ICD-9). According to the National Technical Information Service, "ICD-9CM extensions, interpretations, modifications, addenda, or errata other than those approved by the U.S. Public Health Service and the Health Care Financing Administration are not to be considered official and should not be utilized. Continuous maintenance of the ICD-9-CM is the responsibility of the federal government."

recognized by medical science today. You can think of this sourcebook as your personal Internet age reference librarian.

Why "Internet age"? All too often, patients diagnosed with sleep apnea will log on to the Internet, type words into a search engine, and receive several Web site listings which are mostly irrelevant or redundant. These patients are left to wonder where the relevant information is, and how to obtain it. Since only the smallest fraction of information dealing with sleep apnea is even indexed in search engines, a non-systematic approach often leads to frustration and disappointment. With this sourcebook, we hope to direct you to the information you need that you would not likely find using popular Web directories. Beyond Web listings, in many cases we will reproduce brief summaries or abstracts of available reference materials. These abstracts often contain distilled information on topics of discussion.

While we focus on the more scientific aspects of sleep apnea, there is, of course, the emotional side to consider. Later in the sourcebook, we provide a chapter dedicated to helping you find peer groups and associations that can provide additional support beyond research produced by medical science. We hope that the choices we have made give you the most options available in moving forward. In this way, we wish you the best in your efforts to incorporate this educational approach into your treatment plan.

The Editors

PART I: THE ESSENTIALS

ABOUT PART I

Part I has been edited to give you access to what we feel are "the essentials" on sleep apnea. The essentials of a disease typically include the definition or description of the disease, a discussion of who it affects, the signs or symptoms associated with the disease, tests or diagnostic procedures that might be specific to the disease, and treatments for the disease. Your doctor or healthcare provider may have already explained the essentials of sleep apnea to you or even given you a pamphlet or brochure describing sleep apnea. Now you are searching for more in-depth information. As editors, we have decided, nevertheless, to include a discussion on where to find essential information that can complement what your doctor has already told you. In this section we recommend a process, not a particular Web site or reference book. The process ensures that, as you search the Web, you gain background information in such a way as to maximize your understanding.

CHAPTER 1. THE ESSENTIALS ON SLEEP APNEA: GUIDELINES

Overview

Official agencies, as well as federally funded institutions supported by national grants, frequently publish a variety of guidelines on sleep apnea. These are typically called "Fact Sheets" or "Guidelines." They can take the form of a brochure, information kit, pamphlet, or flyer. Often they are only a few pages in length. The great advantage of guidelines over other sources is that they are often written with the patient in mind. Since new guidelines on sleep apnea can appear at any moment and be published by a number of sources, the best approach to finding guidelines is to systematically scan the Internet-based services that post them.

The National Institutes of Health (NIH)[5]

The National Institutes of Health (NIH) is the first place to search for relatively current patient guidelines and fact sheets on sleep apnea. Originally founded in 1887, the NIH is one of the world's foremost medical research centers and the federal focal point for medical research in the United States. At any given time, the NIH supports some 35,000 research grants at universities, medical schools, and other research and training institutions, both nationally and internationally. The rosters of those who have conducted research or who have received NIH support over the years include the world's most illustrious scientists and physicians. Among them are 97 scientists who have won the Nobel Prize for achievement in medicine.

---

[5] Adapted from the NIH: **http://www.nih.gov/about/NIHoverview.html**.

There is no guarantee that any one Institute will have a guideline on a specific disease, though the National Institutes of Health collectively publish over 600 guidelines for both common and rare diseases. The best way to access NIH guidelines is via the Internet. Although the NIH is organized into many different Institutes and Offices, the following is a list of key Web sites where you are most likely to find NIH clinical guidelines and publications dealing with sleep apnea and associated conditions:

- Office of the Director (OD); guidelines consolidated across agencies available at **http://www.nih.gov/health/consumer/conkey.htm**
- National Library of Medicine (NLM); extensive encyclopedia (A.D.A.M., Inc.) with guidelines available at **http://www.nlm.nih.gov/medlineplus/healthtopics.html**
- National Heart, Lung, and Blood Institute (NHLBI); guidelines at **http://www.nhlbi.nih.gov/guidelines/index.htm**

Among these, the National Heart, Lung, and Blood Institute (NHLBI) is particularly noteworthy. The NHLBI provides leadership for a national program in diseases of the heart, blood vessels, lung, and blood; blood resources; and sleep disorders.[6] Since October 1997, the NHLBI has also had administrative responsibility for the NIH Woman's Health Initiative. The Institute plans, conducts, fosters, and supports an integrated and coordinated program of basic research, clinical investigations and trials, observational studies, and demonstration and education projects. Research is related to the causes, prevention, diagnosis, and treatment of heart, blood vessel, lung, and blood diseases; and sleep disorders. The NHLBI plans and directs research in development and evaluation of interventions and devices related to prevention, treatment, and rehabilitation of patients suffering from such diseases and disorders. It also supports research on clinical use of blood and all aspects of the management of blood resources. Research is conducted in the Institute's own laboratories and by scientific institutions and individuals supported by research grants and contracts. For health professionals and the public, the NHLBI conducts educational activities, including development and dissemination of materials in the above areas, with an emphasis on prevention.

Within the NHLBI, the National Center on Sleep Disorders Research (NCSDR) was established in 1993 to combat a serious public health concern.[7]

---

[6] This paragraph has been adapted from the NHLBI: **http://www.nhlbi.nih.gov/about/org/mission.htm**. "Adapted" signifies that a passage is reproduced exactly or slightly edited for this book.

[7] This paragraph has been adapted from the NCSDR: **http://www.nhlbisupport.com/sleep/about/about.htm**.

About 70 million Americans suffer from sleep problems; among them, nearly 60 percent have a chronic disorder. Each year, sleep disorders, sleep deprivation, and sleepiness add an estimated $15.9 billion to the national healthcare bill. Additional costs to society for related health problems, lost worker productivity, and accidents have not been calculated. Sleep disorders and disturbances of sleep comprise a broad range of problems, including sleep apnea, narcolepsy, insomnia, parasomnia, jet-lag syndrome, and disturbed biological and circadian rhythms. The Center seeks to fulfill its goal of improving the health of Americans by serving four key functions: research, training, technology transfer, and coordination.

- **Research**: Sleep disorders span many medical fields, requiring multidisciplinary approaches not only to treatment, but also to basic research. The Center works with neuroscientists, cellular and molecular biologists, geneticists, physiologists, neuropsychiatrists, immunologists, pulmonary specialists, cardiologists, epidemiologists, behavioral scientists, and other experts. Ongoing research is supported by the NIH and other Federal agencies.
- **Training**: Training researchers in sleep disorders is rigorous and time-consuming. The Center seeks to support and promote formal training programs on the doctoral and postdoctoral levels. It also plans to expand existing career development paths and create new training programs for scientists in sleep disorders research.
- **Technology Transfer**: The Center seeks to ensure that research results lead to health benefits. It works towards this goal by educating health care professionals about sleep disorders and research findings, encouraging medical schools to add sleep disorders to their curricula, working with leading experts to develop clinical guidelines, and sponsoring continuing medical education programs.
- **Coordination**: The Center coordinates the Federal Government's efforts on sleep disorders and works closely with other public, private, and nonprofit groups. The Center works to share information among these groups and encourage their cooperation, especially in crosscutting areas. It also seeks to improve communication among scientists, policymakers, and health care professionals.

The following patient guideline was recently published by the NHLBI and the NCSDR on sleep apnea.

What Is Sleep Apnea?[8]

Sleep apnea is a common disorder that can be very serious.

In sleep apnea, your breathing stops or gets very shallow while you are sleeping. Each pause typically lasts 10-20 seconds or more. These pauses can occur 20 to 30 times or more an hour.

The most common type of sleep apnea is obstructive sleep apnea. During sleep, enough air cannot flow into your lungs through your mouth and nose even though you try to breathe. When this happens, the amount of oxygen in your blood may drop. Normal breaths then start again with a loud snort or choking sound.

Your sleep is not restful because:

- These brief episodes of increased airway resistance (and breathing pauses) occur many times.
- You may have many brief drops in your oxygen levels of the blood.
- You move out of deep sleep and into light sleep several times during the night, resulting in poor sleep quality.

When your sleep is upset throughout the night, you can be very sleepy during the day.

- People with sleep apnea often have loud snoring. However, not everyone who snores has sleep apnea. Some people with sleep apnea don't know they snore.
- Sleep apnea happens more often in people who are overweight, but even thin people can have it.
- Most people don't know they have sleep apnea. They don't know that they are having problems breathing while they are sleeping.
- A family member and/or bed partner may notice the signs of sleep apnea first.

Untreated sleep apnea can increase the chance of having high blood pressure and even a heart attack or stroke. Untreated sleep apnea can also increase the risk of diabetes and the risk for work-related accidents and driving accidents.

---

[8] Adapted from the National Heart, Lung, and Blood Institute (NHLBI): **http://www.nhlbi.nih.gov/health/dci/Diseases/SleepApnea/SleepApnea_WhatIs.html**.

What Causes Sleep Apnea?

Sleep apnea happens when enough air cannot move into your lungs while you are sleeping.

Obstructive Sleep Apnea

When you are awake and normally during sleep, your throat muscles keep your throat open and air flows into your lungs. However, in obstructive sleep apnea, the throat briefly collapses, causing pauses in your breathing. With pauses in breathing, your oxygen level in your blood may drop. This happens when:

- Your throat muscles and tongue relax more than is normal.
- Your tonsils and adenoids are large.
- You are overweight. The extra soft tissue in your throat makes it harder to keep the throat area open.
- The shape of your head and neck (bony structure) results in somewhat smaller airway size in the mouth and throat area.

With the throat frequently fully or partly blocked during sleep, enough air cannot flow into your lungs, even though efforts to breathe continue. Your breathing may become hard and noisy and may even stop for short periods of time (apneas).

Central Apnea

Central apnea is a rare type of sleep apnea that happens when the area of your brain that controls your breathing doesn't send the correct signals to the breathing muscles. There is then no effort to breathe at all for brief periods. Snoring does not typically occur in central apnea.

Who Gets Obstructive Sleep Apnea?

Anyone can have obstructive sleep apnea.

It is estimated that more than 12 million Americans have obstructive sleep apnea. More than half the people who have sleep apnea are overweight, and most snore heavily.

Adults most likely to have sleep apnea:

- Snore loudly.
- Are overweight.
- Have high blood pressure.
- Have decreased size of the airways in their nose, throat, or mouth. This can be caused by the shape of these structures or by medical conditions causing congestion in these areas, such as hay fever or other allergies.
- Have a family history of sleep apnea.

Sleep apnea is more common in men. One out of 25 middle-aged men and 1 out of 50 middle-aged women have sleep apnea that causes them to be very sleepy during the day. Sleep apnea is more common in African Americans, Hispanics, and Pacific Islanders. If someone in your family has sleep apnea, you are more likely to develop sleep apnea than someone without a family history of the condition.

Obstructive sleep apnea can also occur in children who snore. If your child snores, you should discuss it with your child's doctor or health care provider.

What Are the Signs and Symptoms of Sleep Apnea?

The most common signs of sleep apnea are:

- Loud snoring
- Choking or gasping during sleep
- Fighting sleepiness during the day (even at work or while driving)

Your family members may notice the symptoms before you do. You will likely not otherwise be aware that you have problems breathing while asleep.

Others signs of sleep apnea may include:

- Morning headaches
- Memory or learning problems
- Feeling irritable
- Not being able to concentrate on your work
- Mood swings or personality changes, perhaps feeling depressed

- Dry throat upon awaking
- Frequent urination at night

How Is Sleep Apnea Diagnosed?

Some of the ways to help doctors diagnose sleep apnea include:

- A medical history that includes asking you and your family questions about how you sleep and how you function during the day
- Checking your mouth, nose, and throat for extra or large tissues, for example tonsils, uvula (the tissue that hangs from the middle of the back of the mouth), and soft palate (roof of your mouth in the back of your throat)
- A sleep recording of what happens with your breathing

Polysomnogram (PSG) Sleep Recording

A sleep recording is a test that is often done in a sleep center or sleep laboratory, which may be part of a hospital. You may stay overnight in the sleep center, although sleep studies are sometimes done in the home. The most common sleep recording used to find out if you have sleep apnea is called a polysomnogram (poly-SOM-no-gram) or PSG. This test records:

- Brain activity
- Eye movement
- Muscle activity
- Breathing and heart rate
- How much air moves in and out of your lungs while you are sleeping
- The percent of oxygen in your blood

A PSG is painless. You will go to sleep as usual. The staff at the sleep center will monitor your sleep throughout the night. The results of your PSG will be analyzed by a sleep medicine specialist to see if you have sleep apnea, how severe it is, and what treatment may be recommended.

In certain circumstances, the PSG can be done at home. A home monitor can be used to record heart rate, how air moves in and out of your lungs, the amount of oxygen in your blood, and your breathing effort. For this test, a technician will come to your home and help you apply the monitor you will wear overnight. You will go to sleep as usual, and the technician will come back the next morning to get the monitor and send the results to your doctor.

Once all your tests are completed, the sleep medicine specialist will review the results and work with you and your family to develop a treatment plan. In some cases, you may also need to see another physician for evaluation of:

- Lung problems (pulmonologist)
- Problems with the brain or nerves (neurologist)
- Heart or blood pressure problems (cardiology)
- Ear, nose, or throat problems (ENT)
- Psychologist or psychiatrist

How Is Sleep Apnea Treated?

Treatment is aimed at restoring regular nighttime breathing and relieving symptoms such as very loud snoring and daytime sleepiness.

If you have mild sleep apnea, some changes in daily activities or habits may be all that are needed:

- Avoid alcohol, smoking, and medications that make you sleepy. They will make it harder for your throat to stay open while you sleep.
- Lose weight if you are overweight. Even a little weight loss can improve your symptoms.
- Sleep on your side instead of your back. Sleeping on your side may help keep your throat open.

People with moderate or severe sleep apnea will need to make these changes as well. They also will need other treatments such as:

Continuous Positive Airway Pressure (CPAP)

CPAP is the most common treatment for sleep apnea. For this treatment, you will wear a mask over your nose during sleep that blows air into your throat at a pressure level that is right for you. The increased airway pressure acts to keep the throat open while you sleep. The air pressure is adjusted so that it is just enough to stop these airways from briefly getting too small during sleep.

Sleep apnea will return if CPAP is stopped or if it is not used correctly. Usually, a technician comes to your home to bring the CPAP equipment. The technician will set up the CPAP machine and make adjustments based on your doctor's orders.

CPAP treatment may cause side effects in some people. Some side effects are:

- Dry or stuffy nose
- Irritation of the skin on your face
- Bloating of your stomach
- Sore eyes
- Headaches

If you are having trouble with CPAP side effects, work with your sleep medicine specialist and technician. Together you can do things to reduce these side effects, such as:

- Using a nasal spray to relieve a dry, stuffy, or runny nose
- Adjusting the CPAP settings
- Adjusting the size/fit of the mask
- Adding moisture to the air as it flows through the mask
- Using a CPAP machine that can automatically adjust the amount of air pressure to the level that is required to keep the airway open
- Using a CPAP machine that will start with a low air pressure and slowly increase the air pressure as you fall asleep

People with severe sleep apnea symptoms generally feel much better once they begin treatment with CPAP. When using CPAP, it is very important that you follow up with your doctor. If you are having side effects, talk to your doctor.

Mouthpiece

A mouthpiece (oral appliance) may be helpful in some people with mild sleep apnea. Some doctors may also recommend this if you snore loudly but do not have sleep apnea.

A custom-fit plastic mouthpiece will be made by a dentist or orthodontist. An orthodontist is a specialist in correcting teeth or jaw problems. The mouthpiece will adjust your lower jaw and your tongue to help keep the airway in your throat open while you are sleeping. Air can then flow easily into your lungs because there is less resistance to breathing.

Possible side effects of the mouthpiece include damage to your:

- Teeth
- Gums
- Jaw

Follow up with your dentist or orthodontist to check for any side effects and to be sure that your mouthpiece fits.

Surgery

Some people with sleep apnea may benefit from surgery. The type of surgery depends on the cause of the sleep apnea:

- Surgery to remove the tonsils and adenoids if they are blocking the airway. This surgery is especially helpful for children.
- Uvulopalatopharyngoplasty (UPPP) is a surgery that removes the tonsils, uvula (the tissue that hangs from the middle of the back of the roof of the mouth), and part of your soft palate (roof of your mouth in the back of your throat). This surgery is only effective for some people with sleep apnea.
- Laser-assisted uvulopalatoplasty (LAUP) is a surgery that can stop snoring but is probably not helpful in treating sleep apnea. A laser device is used to remove the uvula and part of the soft palate. Because the main symptom of sleep apnea-snoring-is stopped, it is important to have a sleep study before having this surgery.
- Tracheostomy is a surgery used in severe sleep apnea. A small hole is made in the windpipe and a tube is inserted. Air will flow through the tube and into the lungs. This surgery is very successful but is needed only in patients not responding to all other possible treatments.

Other possible surgeries for some people with sleep apnea include:

- Rebuilding the lower jaw
- Surgery of the nose
- Surgery to treat obesity

Currently, there are no medications for the treatment of sleep apnea.

Living with Sleep Apnea

- Getting treatment for sleep apnea and following your doctor's advice can help you and your family members.
- Getting treatment for sleep apnea can help snoring and improve your sleep.
- Treating sleep apnea helps you feel rested during the day.
- Many people will benefit by making changes, such as stopping smoking and losing weight.
- Some will need to wear a mask at night that will help keep the throat open and improve breathing.
- A few will need to have surgery to remove tonsils and adenoids, part of the uvula (the tissue that hangs from the middle of the back of the roof of the mouth), and/or the soft palate (roof of your mouth in the back of your throat) that may block the airway.
- Regular and ongoing follow up with your sleep medicine specialist who will check if your treatment is working and if you are having any side effects.

For Family and Friends, What Can You Do to Help?

Often, people with sleep apnea do not know they have it. They are not aware that their breathing stops and starts many times while they are sleeping.

Family members or bed partners are usually the first ones to notice that the person snores and stops breathing while sleeping. It is important for people with sleep apnea to get medical help. They are at higher risk for car crashes and work-related accidents and other medical problems due to their sleepiness.

People with sleep apnea may fall asleep during the day, even when:

- Driving a car
- Working
- Talking on the phone

Sleep apnea can be very serious. It is important that people with sleep apnea see their doctor to treat and control this disorder. Treatment may improve the person's overall health and happiness, and the quality of sleep both for the person and the entire family.

For More Information

Information about sleep disorders research can be obtained from the NCSDR. In addition, the NHLBI Information Center can provide you with sleep education materials as well as other publications relating to heart, lung, and blood diseases.

National Center on Sleep Disorders Research
Two Rockledge Centre Suite 7024
6701 Rockledge Drive MSC 7920
Bethesda, MD 20892-7920
(301) 435-0199
(301) 480-3451 (fax)
The mission of the NCSDR is to support research, training, and education about sleep disorders. The center is located within the National Heart, Lung, and Blood Institute (NHLBI) of the National Institutes of Health. The NHLBI supports a variety of research and training programs focusing on cardiopulmonary disorders in sleep, designed to fill critical gaps in the understanding of the causes, diagnosis, treatment, and prevention of sleep-disordered breathing.

NHLBI Information Center
P.O. Box 30105
Bethesda, MD 20824-0105
(301) 592-8573
(301) 592-8563 (fax)

More Guideline Sources

The guideline above on sleep apnea is only one example of the kind of material that you can find online and free of charge. The remainder of this chapter will direct you to other sources which either publish or can help you find additional guidelines on topics related to sleep apnea. Many of the guidelines listed below address topics that may be of particular relevance to your specific situation or of special interest to only some patients with sleep apnea. Due to space limitations these sources are listed in a concise manner. Do not hesitate to consult the following sources by either using the Internet hyperlink provided, or, in cases where the contact information is provided, contacting the publisher or author directly.

Topic Pages: MEDLINEplus

For patients wishing to go beyond guidelines published by specific Institutes of the NIH, the National Library of Medicine has created a vast and patient-oriented healthcare information portal called MEDLINEplus. Within this Internet-based system are "health topic pages." You can think of a health topic page as a guide to patient guides. To access this system, log on to **http://www.nlm.nih.gov/medlineplus/healthtopics.html**. From there you can either search using the alphabetical index or browse by broad topic areas. Recently, MEDLINEplus listed the following as being relevant to sleep apnea:

Congenital Heart Disease
http://www.nlm.nih.gov/medlineplus/congenitalheartdisease.html

Heart Failure
http://www.nlm.nih.gov/medlineplus/heartfailure.html

Infant and Newborn Care
http://www.nlm.nih.gov/medlineplus/infantandnewborncare.html

Metabolic Disorders
http://www.nlm.nih.gov/medlineplus/metabolicdisorders.html

Occupational Health
http://www.nlm.nih.gov/medlineplus/occupationalhealth.html

Sleep Apnea
http://www.nlm.nih.gov/medlineplus/sleepapnea.html

Sleep Disorders
http://www.nlm.nih.gov/medlineplus/sleepdisorders.html

Sudden Infant Death Syndrome
http://www.nlm.nih.gov/medlineplus/suddeninfantdeathsyndrome.html

Toilet Training and Bedwetting
http://www.nlm.nih.gov/medlineplus/toilettrainingandbedwetting.html

Tooth Disorders
http://www.nlm.nih.gov/medlineplus/toothdisorders.html

Within the health topic page dedicated to sleep apnea, the following was recently recommended to patients:

- Treatment

  Can Anti-Snoring Claims Be Cause for Alarm?
  Source: Federal Trade Commission
  http://www.ftc.gov/bcp/conline/pubs/alerts/snorealrt.htm

  Choosing a Continuous Positive Airway Pressure (CPAP)
  Source: American Sleep Apnea Association
  http://www.sleepapnea.org/cpap.htm

  Choosing a Mask and Headgear
  Source: American Sleep Apnea Association
  http://www.sleepapnea.org/mask.htm

  Continuous Positive Airway Pressure (CPAP)
  Source: American Academy of Otolaryngology--Head and Neck Surgery
  http://www.entnet.org/healthinfo/snoring/cpap.cfm

  Laser Assisted Uvula Palatoplasty (LAUP)
  Source: American Academy of Otolaryngology--Head and Neck Surgery
  http://www.entnet.org/healthinfo/snoring/laup.cfm

  Lessening the Effects of Sleep Apnea
  Source: American Association for Respiratory Care
  http://www.aarc.org/patient_education/tips/apnea.html

- Children

  Apnea and Your Child
  Source: Nemours Foundation
  http://kidshealth.org/parent/general/sleep/apnea.html

  Having Your Child Evaluated for Obstructive Sleep Apnea
  Source: American Sleep Apnea Association
  http://www.sleepapnea.org/child.html

- From the National Institutes of Health

  Sleep Apnea
  Source: National Center on Sleep Disorders Research
  http://www.nhlbi.nih.gov/health/public/sleep/sleepapn.pdf

Sleep Apnea
Source: National Institute of Neurological Disorders and Stroke
http://www.ninds.nih.gov/health_and_medical/disorders/sleep_apnea.htm

- Latest News

Oral Appliance Adjustments Helpful for Sleep Apnea
Source: 06/03/2004, Reuters Health
http://www.nlm.nih.gov//www.nlm.nih.gov/medlineplus/news/fullstory_18149.html

Sleep Apnea Treatment Improves Heart Risks
Source: 06/16/2004, Reuters Health
http://www.nlm.nih.gov//www.nlm.nih.gov/medlineplus/news/fullstory_18410.html

- Organizations

American Sleep Apnea Association
http://www.sleepapnea.org/

National Center on Sleep Disorders Research
http://www.nhlbi.nih.gov/about/ncsdr/

National Heart, Lung, and Blood Institute
http://www.nhlbi.nih.gov/

National Institute of Neurological Disorders and Stroke
http://www.ninds.nih.gov/

National Sleep Foundation
http://www.sleepfoundation.org/

- Research

Breathing Problems during Sleep and Daytime Behavior Problems
Source: Nemours Foundation
http://kidshealth.org/research/sleep_behavior.html

'White Coat Hypertension' Common Among Sleep Apnea Patients
Source: American College of Chest Physicians
http://www.chestnet.org/about/press/archives/2004/march/0304_1.php

You may also choose to use the search utility provided by MEDLINEplus at the following Web address: **http://www.nlm.nih.gov/medlineplus/**. Simply type a keyword into the search box and click "Search." This utility is similar to the NIH search utility, with the exception that it only includes materials that are linked within the MEDLINEplus system (mostly patient-oriented information). It also has the disadvantage of generating unstructured results. We recommend, therefore, that you use this method only if you have a very targeted search.

The Combined Health Information Database (CHID)

CHID Online is a reference tool that maintains a database directory of thousands of journal articles and patient education guidelines on sleep apnea and related conditions. One of the advantages of CHID over other sources is that it offers summaries that describe the guidelines available, including contact information and pricing. CHID's general Web site is **http://chid.nih.gov/**. To search this database, go to **http://chid.nih.gov/detail/detail.html**. In particular, you can use the advanced search options to look up pamphlets, reports, brochures, and information kits. The following was recently posted in this archive:

- **Pediatric Obstructive Sleep Apnea**

  Source: Alexandria, VA: American Academy of Otolaryngology-Head and Neck Surgery. 2003.

  Contact: Available from American Academy of Otolaryngology-Head and Neck Surgery. One Prince St., Alexandria, VA 22314-3357. (703) 836-4444. TTY: (703) 519-1585. Web site: www.entnet.org/kidsent. PRICE: Available free online.

  Summary: Sleep disordered breathing (SDB) can lead to a number of health-related problems in children, such as snoring, sleep deprivation, abnormal urine production, slowed growth, and the learning problems attention deficit disorder and attention deficit hyperactivity disorder. This fact sheet provides background information on pediatric obstructive **sleep apnea,** including its consequences, diagnosis, and treatment.

The National Guideline Clearinghouse™

The National Guideline Clearinghouse™ offers hundreds of evidence-based clinical practice guidelines published in the United States and other countries. You can search their site located at **http://www.guideline.gov** by using the keyword "sleep apnea" or synonyms. The following was recently posted:

- **Clinical practice guideline: diagnosis and management of childhood obstructive sleep apnea syndrome**

  Source: American Academy of Pediatrics - Medical Specialty Society; 2002 April; 9 pages

  http://www.guideline.gov/summary/summary.aspx?doc_id=3205&nbr=2431&string=sleep+AND+apnea

- **Practice parameters for the use of auto-titrating continuous positive airway pressure devices for titrating pressures and treating adult patients with obstructive sleep apnea syndrome**

  Source: American Academy of Sleep Medicine - Professional Association; 2002 March 15; 5 pages

  http://www.guideline.gov/summary/summary.aspx?doc_id=3181&nbr=2407&string=sleep+AND+apnea

- **Practice parameters for the use of portable monitoring devices in the investigation of suspected obstructive sleep apnea in adults.**

  Source: American Academy of Sleep Medicine - Professional Association; 2003 November 1; 7 pages

  http://www.guideline.gov/summary/summary.aspx?doc_id=4369&nbr=3291&string=sleep+AND+apnea

Healthfinder™

Healthfinder™ is an additional source sponsored by the U.S. Department of Health and Human Services which offers links to hundreds of other sites that contain healthcare information. This Web site is located at **http://www.healthfinder.gov**. Again, keyword searches can be used to find guidelines. The following was recently found in this database:

- **Facts About Sleep Apnea**

  Summary: This brochure discusses sleep apnea and how it is treated.

  Source: National Center on Sleep Disorders Research, National Heart, Lung, and Blood Institute

  http://www.healthfinder.gov/scripts/recordpass.asp?RecordType=0&RecordID=411

- **Snoring & Apnea**

  Summary: This consumer health informtion document discusses snoring, obstructive sleep apnea and the advantages of oral appliance therapy to treat sleep apnea.

  Source: Academy of Dental Sleep Medicine

  http://www.healthfinder.gov/scripts/recordpass.asp?RecordType=0&RecordID=4404

The NIH Search Utility

After browsing the references listed at the beginning of this chapter, you may want to explore the NIH search utility. This allows you to search for documents on over 100 selected Web sites that comprise the NIH-WEB-SPACE. Each of these servers is "crawled" and indexed on an ongoing basis. Your search will produce a list of various documents, all of which will relate in some way to sleep apnea. The drawbacks of this approach are that the information is not organized by theme and that the references are often a mix of information for professionals and patients. Nevertheless, a large number of the listed Web sites provide useful background information. We can only recommend this route, therefore, for relatively rare or specific disorders, or when using highly targeted searches. To use the NIH search utility, visit the following Web page: **http://search.nih.gov/index.html**.

Additional Web Sources

A number of Web sites that often link to government sites are available to the public. These can also point you in the direction of essential information. The following is a representative sample:

- AOL: **http://search.aol.com/cat.adp?id=168&layer=&from=subcats**
- Family Village: **http://www.familyvillage.wisc.edu/specific.htm**
- Google: **http://directory.google.com/Top/Health/Conditions_and_Diseases/**
- Med Help International: **http://www.medhelp.org/HealthTopics/A.html**
- Open Directory Project: **http://dmoz.org/Health/Conditions_and_Diseases/**
- Yahoo.com: **http://dir.yahoo.com/Health/Diseases_and_Conditions/**
- WebMD®Health: **http://my.webmd.com/health_topics**

Vocabulary Builder

The material in this chapter may have contained a number of unfamiliar words. The following Vocabulary Builder introduces you to terms used in this chapter that have not been covered in the previous chapter:

Adjustment: The dynamic process wherein the thoughts, feelings, behavior, and biophysiological mechanisms of the individual continually change to adjust to the environment. [NIH]

Airway: A device for securing unobstructed passage of air into and out of the lungs during general anesthesia. [NIH]

Apnea: Cessation of breathing. [NIH]

Circadian: Repeated more or less daily, i. e. on a 23- to 25-hour cycle. [NIH]

Lag: The time elapsing between application of a stimulus and the resulting reaction. [NIH]

Monitor: An apparatus which automatically records such physiological signs as respiration, pulse, and blood pressure in an anesthetized patient or one undergoing surgical or other procedures. [NIH]

Narcolepsy: A condition of unknown cause characterized by a periodic uncontrollable tendency to fall asleep. [NIH]

Nerve: A cordlike structure of nervous tissue that connects parts of the nervous system with other tissues of the body and conveys nervous impulses to, or away from, these tissues. [NIH]

Pediatrics: The branch of medical science concerned with children and their diseases. [NIH]

Specialist: In medicine, one who concentrates on 1 special branch of medical science. [NIH]

Uvula: Uvula palatinae; specifically, the tongue-like process which projects from the middle of the posterior edge of the soft palate. [NIH]

Windpipe: A rigid tube, 10 cm long, extending from the cricoid cartilage to the upper border of the fifth thoracic vertebra. [NIH]

CHAPTER 2. SEEKING GUIDANCE

Overview

Some patients are comforted by the knowledge that a number of organizations dedicate their resources to helping people with sleep apnea. These associations can become invaluable sources of information and advice. Many associations offer aftercare support, financial assistance, and other important services. Furthermore, healthcare research has shown that support groups often help people to better cope with their conditions.[9] In addition to support groups, your physician can be a valuable source of guidance and support. Therefore, finding a physician that can work with your unique situation is a very important aspect of your care.

In this chapter, we direct you to resources that can help you find patient organizations and medical specialists. We begin by describing how to find associations and peer groups that can help you better understand and cope with sleep apnea. The chapter ends with a discussion on how to find a doctor that is right for you.

Associations and Sleep Apnea

As mentioned by the Agency for Healthcare Research and Quality, sometimes the emotional side of an illness can be as taxing as the physical side.[10] You may have fears or feel overwhelmed by your situation. Everyone has different ways of dealing with disease or physical injury. Your attitude, your expectations, and how well you cope with your condition can all

---

[9] Churches, synagogues, and other houses of worship might also have groups that can offer you the social support you need.

[10] This section has been adapted from **http://www.ahcpr.gov/consumer/diaginf5.htm**.

influence your well-being. This is true for both minor conditions and serious illnesses. For example, a study on female breast cancer survivors revealed that women who participated in support groups lived longer and experienced better quality of life when compared with women who did not participate. In the support group, women learned coping skills and had the opportunity to share their feelings with other women in the same situation.

In addition to associations or groups that your doctor might recommend, we suggest that you consider the following list (if there is a fee for an association, you may want to check with your insurance provider to find out if the cost will be covered):

- **American Sleep Apnea Association**

  Telephone: (202) 293-3650

  Fax: (202) 293-3656

  Email: asaa@nicom.com

  Web Site: http://www.sleepapnea.org

  Background: The American **Sleep Apnea** Association (ASAA) is a not-for-profit, health service organization dedicated to reducing injuries, disabilities, and potentially life-threatening complications that may be caused by **sleep apnea,** a condition characterized by breathing difficulties while sleeping. **Sleep apnea** may occur during childhood and/or adulthood, may be genetic, and/or may occur due to or in association with a number of different underlying disorders. Established in 1990, the Association works to improve the well-being of affected individuals and family members; promotes early diagnosis and appropriate treatment of **sleep apnea** through innovative efforts to educate the general public and health care professionals; and supports basic research into the causes and treatments of the disorder. The Association also fosters the nationwide ASAA A.W.A.K.E. Network, a network of self-help groups that provide additional information and support to individuals affected by **sleep apnea.** The American **Sleep Apnea** Association provides educational materials including a videotape, brochures, a regular newsletter, and guidelines to help individuals start local support groups.

Finding Associations

There are a several Internet directories that provide lists of medical associations with information on or resources relating to sleep apnea. By consulting all of associations listed in this chapter, you will have nearly exhausted all sources for patient associations concerned with sleep apnea.

The National Health Information Center (NHIC)

The National Health Information Center (NHIC) offers a free referral service to help people find organizations that provide information about sleep apnea. For more information, see the NHIC's Web site at **http://www.health.gov/NHIC/** or contact an information specialist by calling 1-800-336-4797.

DIRLINE

A comprehensive source of information on associations is the DIRLINE database maintained by the National Library of Medicine. The database comprises some 10,000 records of organizations, research centers, and government institutes and associations which primarily focus on health and biomedicine. DIRLINE is available via the Internet at the following Web site: **http://dirline.nlm.nih.gov/**. Simply type in "sleep apnea" (or a synonym) or the name of a topic, and the site will list information contained in the database on all relevant organizations.

The Combined Health Information Database

Another comprehensive source of information on healthcare associations is the Combined Health Information Database. Using the "Detailed Search" option, you will need to limit your search to "Organizations" and "sleep apnea". Type the following hyperlink into your Web browser: **http://chid.nih.gov/detail/detail.html**. To find associations, use the drop boxes at the bottom of the search page where "You may refine your search by." For publication date, select "All Years." Then, select your preferred language and the format option "Organization Resource Sheet." By making these selections and typing in "sleep apnea" (or synonyms) into the "For these words:" box, you will only receive results on organizations dealing with sleep apnea. You should check back periodically with this database since it is updated every 3 months.

The National Organization for Rare Disorders, Inc.

The National Organization for Rare Disorders, Inc. has prepared a Web site that provides, at no charge, lists of associations organized by specific diseases. You can access this database at the following Web site:

http://www.rarediseases.org/search/orgsearch.html. Type "sleep apnea" (or a synonym) in the search box, and click "Submit Query."

Online Support Groups

In addition to support groups, commercial Internet service providers offer forums and chat rooms for people with different illnesses and conditions. WebMD®, for example, offers such a service at its Web site: **http://boards.webmd.com/roundtable**. These online self-help communities can help you connect with a network of people whose concerns are similar to yours. Online support groups are places where people can talk informally. If you read about a novel approach, consult with your doctor or other healthcare providers, as the treatments or discoveries you hear about may not be scientifically proven to be safe and effective.

Finding Doctors

One of the most important aspects of your treatment will be the relationship between you and your doctor or specialist. All patients with sleep apnea must go through the process of selecting a physician. While this process will vary from person to person, the Agency for Healthcare Research and Quality makes a number of suggestions, including the following:[11]

- If you are in a managed care plan, check the plan's list of doctors first.
- Ask doctors or other health professionals who work with doctors, such as hospital nurses, for referrals.
- Call a hospital's doctor referral service, but keep in mind that these services usually refer you to doctors on staff at that particular hospital. The services do not have information on the quality of care that these doctors provide.
- Some local medical societies offer lists of member doctors. Again, these lists do not have information on the quality of care that these doctors provide.

Additional steps you can take to locate doctors include the following:

- Check with the associations listed earlier in this chapter.

---

[11] This section has been adapted from the AHRQ: **www.ahrq.gov/consumer/qntascii/qntdr.htm**.

- Information on doctors in some states is available on the Internet at **http://www.docboard.org**. This Web site is run by "Administrators in Medicine," a group of state medical board directors.
- The American Board of Medical Specialties can tell you if your doctor is board certified. "Certified" means that the doctor has completed a training program in a specialty and has passed an exam, or "board," to assess his or her knowledge, skills, and experience to provide quality patient care in that specialty. Primary care doctors may also be certified as specialists. The AMBS Web site is located at **http://www.abms.org/newsearch.asp**.[12] You can also contact the ABMS by phone at 1-866-ASK-ABMS.
- You can call the American Medical Association (AMA) at 800-665-2882 for information on training, specialties, and board certification for many licensed doctors in the United States. This information also can be found in "Physician Select" at the AMA's Web site: **http://www.ama-assn.org/aps/amahg.htm**.

If the previous sources did not meet your needs, you may want to log on to the Web site of the National Organization for Rare Disorders (NORD) at **http://www.rarediseases.org/**. NORD maintains a database of doctors with expertise in various rare diseases. The Metabolic Information Network (MIN), 800-945-2188, also maintains a database of physicians with expertise in various metabolic diseases.

Selecting Your Doctor[13]

When you have compiled a list of prospective doctors, call each of their offices. First, ask if the doctor accepts your health insurance plan and if he or she is taking new patients. If the doctor is not covered by your plan, ask yourself if you are prepared to pay the extra costs. The next step is to schedule a visit with your chosen physician. During the first visit you will have the opportunity to evaluate your doctor and to find out if you feel comfortable with him or her. Ask yourself, did the doctor:

- Give me a chance to ask questions about sleep apnea?
- Really listen to my questions?

---

[12] While board certification is a good measure of a doctor's knowledge, it is possible to receive quality care from doctors who are not board certified.

[13] This section has been adapted from the AHRQ: **www.ahrq.gov/consumer/qntascii/qntdr.htm**.

- Answer in terms I understood?
- Show respect for me?
- Ask me questions?
- Make me feel comfortable?
- Address the health problem(s) I came with?
- Ask me my preferences about different kinds of treatments for sleep apnea?
- Spend enough time with me?

Trust your instincts when deciding if the doctor is right for you. But remember, it might take time for the relationship to develop. It takes more than one visit for you and your doctor to get to know each other.

Working with Your Doctor[14]

Research has shown that patients who have good relationships with their doctors tend to be more satisfied with their care and have better results. Here are some tips to help you and your doctor become partners:

- You know important things about your symptoms and your health history. Tell your doctor what you think he or she needs to know.
- It is important to tell your doctor personal information, even if it makes you feel embarrassed or uncomfortable.
- Bring a "health history" list with you (and keep it up to date).
- Always bring any medications you are currently taking with you to the appointment, or you can bring a list of your medications including dosage and frequency information. Talk about any allergies or reactions you have had to your medications.
- Tell your doctor about any natural or alternative medicines you are taking.
- Bring other medical information, such as x-ray films, test results, and medical records.
- Ask questions. If you don't, your doctor will assume that you understood everything that was said.

[14] This section has been adapted from the AHRQ: **www.ahrq.gov/consumer/qntascii/qntdr.htm**.

- Write down your questions before your visit. List the most important ones first to make sure that they are addressed.
- Consider bringing a friend with you to the appointment to help you ask questions. This person can also help you understand and/or remember the answers.
- Ask your doctor to draw pictures if you think that this would help you understand.
- Take notes. Some doctors do not mind if you bring a tape recorder to help you remember things, but always ask first.
- Let your doctor know if you need more time. If there is not time that day, perhaps you can speak to a nurse or physician assistant on staff or schedule a telephone appointment.
- Take information home. Ask for written instructions. Your doctor may also have brochures and audio and videotapes that can help you.
- After leaving the doctor's office, take responsibility for your care. If you have questions, call. If your symptoms get worse or if you have problems with your medication, call. If you had tests and do not hear from your doctor, call for your test results. If your doctor recommended that you have certain tests, schedule an appointment to get them done. If your doctor said you should see an additional specialist, make an appointment.

By following these steps, you will enhance the relationship you will have with your physician.

Broader Health-Related Resources

In addition to the references above, the NIH has set up guidance Web sites that can help patients find healthcare professionals. These include:[15]

- Caregivers:
http://www.nlm.nih.gov/medlineplus/caregivers.html
- Choosing a Doctor or Healthcare Service:
http://www.nlm.nih.gov/medlineplus/choosingadoctororhealthcareservice.html
- Hospitals and Health Facilities:
http://www.nlm.nih.gov/medlineplus/healthfacilities.html

---

[15] You can access this information at **http://www.nlm.nih.gov/medlineplus/healthsystem.html**.

PART II: ADDITIONAL RESOURCES AND ADVANCED MATERIAL

ABOUT PART II

In Part II, we introduce you to additional resources and advanced research on sleep apnea. All too often, patients who conduct their own research are overwhelmed by the difficulty in finding and organizing information. The purpose of the following chapters is to provide you an organized and structured format to help you find additional information resources on sleep apnea. In Part II, as in Part I, our objective is not to interpret the latest advances on sleep apnea or render an opinion. Rather, our goal is to give you access to original research and to increase your awareness of sources you may not have already considered. In this way, you will come across the advanced materials often referred to in pamphlets, books, or other general works. Once again, some of this material is technical in nature, so consultation with a professional familiar with sleep apnea is suggested.

CHAPTER 3. STUDIES ON SLEEP APNEA

Overview

Every year, academic studies are published on sleep apnea or related conditions. Broadly speaking, there are two types of studies. The first are peer reviewed. Generally, the content of these studies has been reviewed by scientists or physicians. Peer-reviewed studies are typically published in scientific journals and are usually available at medical libraries. The second type of studies is non-peer reviewed. These works include summary articles that do not use or report scientific results. These often appear in the popular press, newsletters, or similar periodicals.

In this chapter, we will show you how to locate peer-reviewed references and studies on sleep apnea. We will begin by discussing research that has been summarized and is free to view by the public via the Internet. We then show you how to generate a bibliography on sleep apnea and teach you how to keep current on new studies as they are published or undertaken by the scientific community.

The Combined Health Information Database

The Combined Health Information Database summarizes studies across numerous federal agencies. To limit your investigation to research studies and sleep apnea, you will need to use the advanced search options. First, go to **http://chid.nih.gov/index.html**. From there, select the "Detailed Search" option (or go directly to that page with the following hyperlink: **http://chid.nih.gov/detail/detail.html**). The trick in extracting studies is found in the drop boxes at the bottom of the search page where "You may refine your search by." Select the dates and language you prefer, and the format option "Journal Article." At the top of the search form, select the number of records you would like to see (we recommend 100) and check the box to display "whole records." We recommend that you type in "sleep apnea" (or synonyms) into the "For these words:" box. Consider using the option "anywhere in record" to make your search as broad as possible. If you want to limit the search to only a particular field, such as the title of the journal, then select this option in the "Search in these fields" drop box. The following is a sample of what you can expect from this type of search:

- **Maxillomandibular Advancement Surgery for Obstructive Sleep Apnea Syndrome**

  Source: JADA. Journal of the American Dental Association. 133(11): 1489-1497. November 2002.

  Contact: Available from American Dental Association. ADA Publishing Co, Inc., 211 East Chicago Avenue, Chicago, IL 60611. (312) 440-2867. Website: www.ada.org.

  Summary: Although maxillomandibular advancement (MMA) surgery is highly successful, the indications for and staging of MMA in the treatment of obstructive **sleep apnea** syndrome (OSAS) have not been settled upon. In this article, the author presents a retrospective review of several published case series with inclusion criteria of 20 or more patients who underwent MMA and received documented preoperative and postoperative diagnostic polysomnography. Protocols of MMA as a primary versus secondary operation, with and without adjunctive procedures in a site-specific approach, are compared and discussed. As an extrapharyngeal operation that enlarges and stabilizes the entire velo-orohypopharyngeal airway, MMA, which can be safely combined with adjunctive nonpharyngeal procedures, may circumvent the staging dilemmas associated with multiple, less successful, segmental, invasive, pharyngeal procedures. In accordance with current goals and guidelines governing OSAS surgery, MMA does not need to be limited to severe OSAS cases as a last resort after other procedures have failed but, rather, is also indicated as an initial operation for velo-orohypopharyngeal narrowing. The author concludes that the diagnosis and management of OSAS requires a multidisciplinary team approach, including a working relationship between the dentist and sleep physician. General dentists and dental specialists who participate in the management of snoring and OSAS cases should have some knowledge of basic sleep medicine. 5 figures. 1 table. 55 references.

- **Heart in Uremia: Role of Hypertension, Hypotension, and Sleep Apnea**

  Source: American Journal of Kidney Diseases. 38(4 Supplement 1): S38-S46. October 2001.

  Contact: Available from W.B. Saunders Company. Periodicals Department, 6277 Sea Harbor Drive, Orlando, FL 32887-4800. (800) 654-2452 or (407) 345-4000.

  Summary: Cardiovascular disease is the leading cause of morbidity (illness) and mortality (death) in patients with end stage renal (kidney) disease (ESRD). The causes of this morbidity and mortality include those usually found in the general population, those related to the uremic status, and those related to dialysis treatment. This article focuses on the specific roles of hypertension (high blood pressure), hypotension (low blood pressure), anemia (low levels of hemoglobin, the oxygen carrying parts of the blood), hypoalbuminemia (low levels of protein in the blood), malnutrition, dyslipidemia (unhealthy levels of fats in the blood), reactive C protein, calcium-phosphate product, dialysis modalities (hemodialysis versus peritoneal dialysis), and hyperhomocysteinemia. The authors put special emphasis on hyperparathyroidism as a traditional toxin. The emergent role of **sleep apnea** has been confirmed in animal models as well as in humans studied using polysomnography. There are difficulties in diagnosing coronary disease, because angiography has some risks, is expensive, and should be reserved for patients having symptoms of heart failure, patients with diabetes mellitus, or patients entering a transplantation list. This allows patients with coronary disease to undergo revascularization (adding blood vessels) through coronary artery bypass (preferably) or percutaneous transluminal angioplasty. Patients for whom surgery is not appropriate should be treated using more traditional medical procedures. 2 figures. 1 table. 36 references.

- **Treating Obstructive Sleep Apnea and Snoring: Assessment of an Anterior Mandibular Positioning Device**

  Source: JADA. Journal of the American Dental Association. 131(6): 765-771. June 2000.

  Contact: Available from American Dental Association. ADA Publishing Co, Inc., 211 East Chicago Avenue, Chicago, IL 60611.

  Summary: Dental devices have been used to help manage snoring and obstructive **sleep apnea,** or OSA. This article reports on patients' compliance with and complications of long term use of an anterior mandibular positioning, or AMP, device. The device used was a custom made, two piece, full coverage, adjustable acrylic appliance, used nightly. The appliance advanced the mandible by 75 percent of the patient's maximum protrusive distance. The study sample included 65 consecutive patients with mild to moderate obstructive **sleep apnea** and snoring. Long term use (three years or more) of the AMP device in these patients was 51 percent (27 of 53 patients). Of the 53 responding patients, 40 percent reported jaw or facial muscle pain, 40 percent had occlusal changes, 38 percent reported tooth pain, 30 percent reported jaw joint pain, and 30 percent experienced xerostomia. Of the 27 long term AMP users, 22 rated themselves as being very satisfied and four as somewhat satisfied; one person was neither satisfied nor dissatisfied with the appliance. The authors conclude that with use of the AMP device, 40 percent of patients will develop some minor complications of jaw, mouth, or tooth pain, and approximately 26 percent of long term users might experience a painless but irreversible change in their occlusion. Annual follow up office visits with the dentist appear necessary for early detection of these changes. 4 figures. 23 references.

- **Sleep Apnea in End-Stage Renal Disease**

  Source: Seminars in Dialysis. 4(1): 52-58. January-March 1991.

  Summary: Information regarding the prevalence and diagnosis of sleep disorders in patients with renal disease is limited, but interest in such abnormalities has increased over the last several years. This article reviews the literature on **sleep apnea** in end-stage renal disease (ESRD). Topics include diagnosis, the prevalence of **sleep apnea** in ESRD, etiological considerations, and treatment interventions. The author stresses that effective diagnosis and treatment of **sleep apnea** are required by physicians if we are to continue to make headway in improving the quality of life for ESRD patients. 1 figure. 2 tables. 58 references.

- **Obstructive Sleep Apnea: Its Relevance in the Care of Diabetic Patients**

  Source: Clinical Diabetes. 20(3): 126-132. Summer 2002.

  Contact: Available from American Diabetes Association. 1701 North Beauregard Street, Alexandria, VA 22311. (800) 232-3472. Website: www.diabetes.org.

  Summary: Obstructive **sleep apnea** (OSA) is a common and frequently unrecognized disorders. OSA is often found in patients with obesity, diabetes, and cardiovascular disease, and there is growing evidence that **sleep apnea** is independently associated with increased cardiovascular morbidity (related disease or complications). This article reviews the presentation, diagnosis, and treatment of OSA and its related health risks. The authors discuss the proposed associations between OSA and diabetes and insulin resistance. The authors conclude that diabetes and OSA are common disorders that often coexist in the setting of shared risk factors and perhaps a similar metabolic environment. Currently, emphasis is being placed on identifying and treating modifiable cardiovascular risk factors, such as tobacco abuse, obesity, hyperglycemia, hypertension, and dyslipidemia. The authors stress that there is growing evidence that OSA should be added to this list. 2 tables. 68 references.

- **Nocturnal Polyuria in Type 2 Diabetes: A Symptom of Obstructive Sleep Apnea**

  Source: Diabetes Educator. 28(3): 424-434. May-June 2002.

  Contact: Available from American Association of Diabetes Educators. 100 West Monroe Street, 4th Floor, Chicago, IL 60603-1901. (312) 424-2426.

  Summary: Polyuria (excessive urination) and nocturia (getting up at night to urinate) in individuals with type 2 diabetes may be due to obstructive **sleep apnea** (OSA), a recently recognized etiology (cause) of excess nighttime urine production. This article reports on an exploratory study that examined the relationships among glucose control, OSA, and nocturnal urine production. A sample of community-dwelling older adults (20 nondiabetic subjects and 10 poorly controlled type 2 diabetes subjects) was recruited based on self-report of nocturia more than twice per night. Participants were monitored on a metabolic research unit for 24 hours to track intake and output, collect blood and urine samples, and conduct an overnight polysomnography sleep study. None of the subjects had fasting serum glucose levels above the renal threshold. OSA was found in 65 percent of subjects. Those with moderate or severe OSA had significantly greater overnight urine production than subjects without OSA. Subjects with type 2 diabetes and moderate or severe OSA had the highest nocturnal urine production. The authors conclude that the high incidence of undetected OSA in subjects with type 2 diabetes with nocturia suggests that nocturia, OSA, and type 2 diabetes frequently coexist and may be interrelated. The article concludes with a list of resources, including Internet, books, pamphlets, and professional contacts, for readers who want to obtain more information. 2 figures. 3 tables. 42 references.

- **Improvement of Sleep Apnea in Patients with Chronic Renal Failure Who Undergo Nocturnal Hemodialysis**

  Source: New England Journal of Medicine. 344(2): 102-107. January 11, 2001.

Summary: Sleep apnea (defined as the absence of airflow for longer than 10 seconds; it usually interrupts sleep) is common in patients with chronic renal failure (CRF) and is not improved by either conventional hemodialysis of peritoneal dialysis. With nocturnal hemodialysis, patients undergo hemodialysis seven nights per week at home, while sleeping. This article reports on a study undertaken to investigate the role of nocturnal hemodialysis in correcting **sleep apnea** in patients with CRF. Fourteen patients who were undergoing conventional hemodialysis for four hours on each of three days per week underwent overnight polysomnography (a measurement of sleep). The patients were then switched to nocturnal hemodialysis for eight hours during each of six or seven nights a week. They underwent polysomnography again 6 to 15 months later on one night when they were undergoing nocturnal hemodialysis and on another night when they were not. The mean serum creatinine concentration (a measurement of kidney or replacement kidney function) was significantly lower during the period when the patients were undergoing nocturnal hemodialysis than during the period when they were undergoing conventional hemodialysis. The conversion from conventional hemodialysis to nocturnal hemodialysis was associated with a reduction in the frequency of apnea and hypopnea from 25 (plus or minus 25) to 8 (plus or minus 8) episodes per hour of sleep. This reduction occurred predominantly in seven patients with **sleep apnea,** in whom the frequency of episodes fell from 46 (plus or minus 19) to 9 (plus or minus 9) episodes per hour, accompanied by increases in the minimal oxygen saturation, transcutaneous partial pressure of carbon dioxide, and serum bicarbonate concentration. During the period when these seven patients were undergoing nocturnal hemodialysis, the apnea hypopnea index measured on nights when they were not undergoing nocturnal hemodialysis was greater than that on nights when they were undergoing nocturnal hemodialysis, but it still remained lower than it had been during the period when they were undergoing conventional hemodialysis. The authors conclude that nocturnal hemodialysis corrects **sleep apnea** associated with chronic renal failure. 2 figures. 4 tables. 22 references.

- **Obstructive Sleep Apnea: A Case Report**

  Source: Journal of the Tennessee Dental Association. 82(3): 48-51. Fall 2002.

  Contact: Available from Journal of the Tennessee Dental Association. 2104 Sunset Place, Nashville, TN 37212. E-mail: tda@tenndental.org.

  Summary: Sleep-disordered breathing is a spectrum of relatively common medical problems ranging from apnea to hypopnea to upper airway resistance syndrome. Apnea is the temporary cessation of airflow during sleep for 10 seconds or more, despite continued ventilatory effort. Hypopnea is a reduction of 25 percent in airflow followed by arousal or desaturation of two percent or more. Upper airway resistance syndrome (UARS) involves frequent arousals in response to increased respiratory effect as a result of upper airway narrowing without overt apnea or hypopnea. This article reviews obstructive **sleep apnea** (OSA), a problem showing up in 4 percent of American males and 2 percent of American females. The authors stress that the role of dentistry in diagnosing and treating OSA is significant given the profession's knowledge of cephalometric radiography, oral appliances, and orthognathic surgery. Topics include epidemiology, symptoms, diagnostic tests, classification, and treatment options. The case report describes a 32 year old white male whose chief complaints were inability to sleep, snoring, daytime hypersomnolence, lack of energy, inability to sustain exercise, and obesity. 7 figures. 10 references.

- **Dental Side Effects of an Oral Device To Treat Snoring and Obstructive Sleep Apnea**

  Source: Sleep. 22(2): 237-240. March 15, 1999.

  Contact: Available from American Sleep Disorders Association. 6301 Bandel Road, Suite 101, Rochester, MN 55901. (507) 529-0804.

  Summary: Snoring and obstructive **sleep apnea** (OSA) are common and related conditions with major social and health implication. These conditions can be treated successfully with dental devices that reposition the mandible (lower jaw). Despite wide use, side effects of these devices have not yet been systematically evaluated. This article reports on a study undertaken to evaluate the side effects of a mandibular advancement splint (MAS). The research consisted of a questionnaire survey and dental examination of a consecutive case series of patients treated with the MAS. Attempts were made to contact all 191 patients treated over a 5 year period in a dental outpatient clinic; all patients had snored loudly and habitually with or without OSA prior to treatment. Of 191 patients treated, 132 agreed to complete the questionnaire and 106 underwent examination. Of the 132 interviewed, patient and partner report indicated that the device was well tolerated and controlled snoring satisfactorily in 100 patients after 31 (plus or minus 18) months of use. Dental side effects were reported in 107 patients, although these were mostly minor, and only 10 patients ceased using the device because of them. Side effects included excessive salivation (40 patients), xerostomia (30 patients), temporomandibular joint pain (35 patients), dental discomfort (35 patients), myofacial discomfort (33 patients), and bite changes (16 patients). Of 106 patients examined, 30 had increased maximal opening and 76 had no change compared with pretreatment records. Temporomandibular joint noises were found in 9 patients, and occlusal changes in 15. None of these effects could be related to degree of opening or protrusion produced by the MAS. The authors conclude that dental side effects occur in a significant proportion of patients using the MAS. In most cases, these are minor and their importance must be balanced against the efficacy of the MAS in treating snoring and OSA. 1 appendix. 2 figures. 9 references. (AA-M).

- **Dentistry's Role in the Management of Obstructive Sleep Apnea**

  Source: Journal of the Greater Houston Dental Society. 71(4): 29-30. November 1999.

  Contact: Available from Greater Houston Dental Society. One Greenway Plaza, Suite 110, Houston, TX 77046. (713) 961-4337. Fax (713) 961-3617. E-mail: ghds@flash.net. Website: www.ghds.com.

  Summary: Snoring may be one symptom of a potentially life threatening sleep related disorder known as obstructive **sleep apnea** (OSA). This article describes how the dental community is actively playing a role in understanding, managing, and treating OSA. OSA occurs when the pharyngeal airways, which include the tongue, palate, and pharynx, collapse during sleep. The authors outline the signs and symptoms, complications of the condition, diagnosis, treatment, use of oral appliances, and the effects of oral appliance therapy. Dentists may participate in the management of OSA patients by understanding OSA, recognizing the signs and symptoms, developing a relationship with the patient's physician or sleep specialist, and having resources and referrals available for patients. Diagnosis is based on the clinical signs and symptoms, physical examination, as well as head, neck, and oral examinations. Age and obesity are two significant predictors of OSA. The two most commonly used types of oral appliances used during sleep are the tongue retaining device and the mandibular (lower jaw) repositioning splint. 6 references.

- **Sleep Apnea in Alzheimer's Patients and the Healthy Elderly**

  Source: Scholarly Inquiry for Nursing Practice: An International Journal. 1(3): 221-235. 1987.

  Summary: The incidence of **sleep apnea** was explored in 80 elderly subjects. Through the use of several criteria, **sleep apnea** was found more frequently in Alzheimer's patients (n equals 24) than in healthy controls (n equals 56). Alzheimer's patients were also found to have a significantly higher proportion of apnea related to non-rapid eye movement than to rapid eye movement sleep. Apnea-positive Alzheimer's patients also had significantly more awake time during the course of the night. A significant positive correlation between apnea index and severity of dementia, as measured by the Blessed Dementia Rating Scale, was found for apnea-positive Alzheimer's patients (r equals 0.57, p less than.01) as well as for the entire sample of Alzheimer's patients (r equals 0.41, p less than.05). Neuropathological implications are discussed, as well as the implications for nursing practice. 37 references. (AA).

- **Snoring and Obstructive Sleep Apnea From a Dental Perspective**

  Source: CDA Journal. Journal of the California Dental Association. 26(8): 557-565. August 1998.

  Contact: Available from California Dental Association (CDA). 1201 K Street, Sacramento, CA 95814. (916) 443-0505.

  Summary: This article considers the problems of snoring and obstructive **sleep apnea** from a dental perspective. The author stresses the proper diagnosis and treatment of sleep related disorders are best handled via a team approach. This team may include a general dentist treating in conjunction with other sleep specialists. The author provides a dental overview of sleep related breathing disorders, including key definitions, an outline of a diagnostic protocol, a discussion of the factors involved in decision making, and a summary of the wide variety of treatment modalities. Treatment methods discussed include general behavioral measures, surgical approaches (tracheotomy, nasal reconstruction, uvulopalatopharyngoplasty, and orthognathic procedures), and dental appliances. The author concludes with recommendations for the dentist who wishes to play a role in both the recognition and treatment of sleep disorders. These include revising the standard medical questionnaires to include questions on sleep disorders and snoring, revising how the intraoral examination is done (to incorporate evaluation of the oropharyngeal airway, the tongue, the mandible, and the nasal airway), and working closely with other health care professionals. 2 tables. 36 references. (AA-M).

- **Diagnosing and Comanaging Patients with Obstructive Sleep Apnea Syndrome**

  Source: JADA. Journal of the American Dental Association. 131(8): 1178-1184. August 2000.

  Contact: Available from American Dental Association. ADA Publishing Co, Inc., 211 East Chicago Avenue, Chicago, IL 60611.

Summary: This article discusses the diagnosis and management of patients with obstructive **sleep apnea** syndrome (OSAS), a common, but underdiagnosed, disorder that can be fatal. The disorder is characterized by repetitive episodes of complete or partial upper airway obstruction leading to absent or diminished airflow into the lungs. These episodes usually last 10 to 30 seconds and result in loud snoring, a decrease in oxygen saturation, and chronic daytime sleepiness and fatigue. The obstruction is caused by the soft palate, base of the tongue or both collapsing against the pharyngeal walls because of decreased muscle tone during sleep. Potentially fatal systemic illnesses frequently associated with this disorder include hypertension, pulmonary (lung) hypertension, heart failure, nocturnal cardiac dysrhythmias, myocardial infarction (heart attack), and ischemic stroke. The classic signs and symptoms of OSAS may be recognizable by dental practitioners. Common findings in the medical history include daytime sleepiness, snoring, hypertension, and type 2 diabetes mellitus. Common clinical findings include male gender, obesity, increased neck circumference, excessive fat deposition in the palate, tongue (macroglossia) and pharynx, a long soft palate, a small recessive mandible and maxilla, and calcified carotid artery atheromas on parnoramic and lateral cephalometric radiographs. After confirmation of the diagnosis by a physician, dentists can participate in management of the disorder by fabricating mandibular advancement appliances and performing surgical procedures that prevent recurrent airway obstruction. 6 figures. 43 references.

- **Sleep Apnea in End Stage Renal Disease**

  Source: ANNA Journal. American Nephrology Nurses Association Journal. 24(6): 645-654. December 1997.

  Contact: Available from American Nephrology Nurses Association. Box 56, East Holly Avenue, Pitman, NJ 08071. (609) 256-2320.

  Summary: This article familiarizes nephrology nurses with the **sleep apnea** syndrome, a disorder that is characterized by repetitive episodes of the cessation of breathing (apneas) or diminished airflow (hypopneas) that occur during sleep, and is usually, although not always, associated with a reduction in the oxygen saturation of the blood. The author reviews risk factors, clinical features, diagnostic strategies, and treatments. The author also discusses recent research linking **sleep apnea** with end-stage renal disease (ESRD). In diagnosing **sleep apnea** syndrome, the total number of apneas and hypopneas that occur during a sleep period are usually added together and then divided by the number of hours spent sleeping to obtain a respiratory disturbance index (RDI). While disrupted sleep and daytime sleepiness are significant problems, cardiopulmonary abnormalities are also important complications associated with **sleep apnea.** Risk factors for **sleep apnea** include obesity, craniofacial abnormalities, male gender, certain medical illnesses, lifestyle factors (use of alcohol and central nervous system depressants, smoking, exposure to allergens), and cardiovascular diseases. The author reviews nine studies of ESRD and **sleep apnea,** all of which demonstrated that **sleep apnea** has a prominent presence in ESRD, that both hemodialysis and peritoneal dialysis patients are vulnerable to it, and that dialysis itself seems to have little effect on its clinical expression. These studies showed that the incidence of **sleep apnea** is most likely much higher in this group than in the general population, but they did not succeed in determining the exact prevalence of **sleep apnea** in chronic renal failure because of subject selection bias and small sample sizes. The author concludes that patients with ESRD who have symptoms related to sleep-wake problems should be evaluated. Treatment of a sleeping disorder thus revealed is likely to have a drastic impact on the quality of life experienced by these patients. 4 figures. 2 tables. 26 references. (AA-M).

- **Practice Parameters for the Treatment of Snoring and Obstructive Sleep Apnea with Oral Appliances: An American Sleep Disorders Association Report**

  Source: Sleep. 186(6): 511-513. 1995.

  Contact: Available from American Sleep Disorders Association. Standards of Practice Committee, 1610 14th Street, N.W., Suite 300, Rochester, MN 55901-2200. (507) 287-6006.

  Summary: This article presents clinical guidelines, reviewed and approved by the Board of Directors of the American Sleep Disorders Association (ASDA), that provide recommendations for the use of oral appliances for the treatment of snoring and obstructive **sleep apnea** (OSA). The authors note that the U.S. FDA has approved some of the available oral appliances for the treatment of snoring, with and without OSA, even though limited data from controlled studies supporting the effectiveness and safety of these devices have been published. After a background section briefly describing the problems and morbidity associated with snoring and OSA, the article presents recommendations in the following areas: diagnosis, treatment objectives, indications, follow-up, and appliance fitting. A brief conclusion addresses recommendations for future research. 1 table. 3 references.

- **Treating Obstructive Sleep Apnea: Can An Intraoral Prosthesis Help?**

  Source: JADA. Journal of the American Dental Association. 126(4): 461-466. April 1995.

Summary: This article reports on a study of the effectiveness of an intraoral airway maintenance prosthesis used to treat obstructive **sleep apnea** syndrome (OSAS). The author presents a review of the relevant literature, and then describes the materials and methods used in the study of five men who were diagnosed with OSAS. The author goes into some detail in his discussion of the cephalometric technique. The prosthesis, which can be constructed and modified easily by a dentist, significantly reduced the number of apneas per night and the syndrome's severity in the subjects studied. 4 figures. 1 table. 13 references. (AA-M).

- **Obstructive Sleep Apnea Surgery: Genioglossus Advancement Revisited**

  Source: Journal of Oral and Maxillofacial Surgery. 59(10): 1181-1184. October 2001.

  Contact: Available from W.B. Saunders Company. Periodicals Department, P.O. Box 629239, Orlando, FL 32862-8239. (800) 654-2452.

  Summary: This article reports on a study that evaluated the accuracy of a genioglossus advancement (GA) technique (rectangular window) to incorporate the genial tubercle or genioglossus muscle complex (GGC) in patients with obstructive **sleep apnea.** The prospective study consisted of 38 consecutive patients who underwent GA. All 38 pairs of genial tubercles were captured. Thirty-one patients had both bellies of the genioglossus muscle incorporated. Two patients had a complete belly and a partial (greater than 50 percent) belly of the muscle captured. Five patients had only a portion of both muscle bellies included. The incomplete incorporation of the muscles in the bone flap was caused by the limited lateral extension of the osteotomy beyond the genial tubercles. The causes of the limited lateral osteotomy extension included crowding of the lower incisors as well as the presence of elongated or medially angulated canine roots. The results of this study show that the rectangular osteotomy technique accurately captures the genial tubercles and enables an adequate amount of the genioglossus muscle to be incorporated and advanced. 6 figures. 15 references.

- **Glossoptosis (Posterior Displacement of the Tongue) During Sleep: A Frequent Cause of Sleep Apnea in Pediatric Patients Referred for Dynamic Sleep Fluoroscopy**

  Source: AJR (American Journal of Roentgenology). 175(6): 1557-1559. December 2000.

Contact: Available from American Roentgen Ray Society. 44211 Slatestone Court, Leesburg, VA 20147-5109. (800) 438-2777 or (703) 729-3353. Fax (703) 729-4839. Email: subscribe@arrs.org.

Summary: This article reports on a study undertaken to evaluate the frequency of glossoptosis (posterior displacement of the tongue) as a cause of **sleep apnea** in pediatric patients referred for fluoroscopic sleep studies. The authors reviewed seventy consecutive dynamic fluoroscopic sleep studies performed to evaluate **sleep apnea.** All patients had been sedated and examined with lateral fluoroscopy during sleep. Anatomic changes in the airway were correlated with episodes of oxygen desaturation (lower levels of oxygen in the blood). Cases of glossoptosis, in which the tongue moved posteriorly during sleep and abutted the posterior pharynx (airway), resulting in airway obstruction and oxygen desaturation, were identified. Of the 70 sleep studies reviewed, glossoptosis was the cause of airway obstruction in 17 patients (24 percent). Mean age in these 17 patients was 3 years (range, 5 days to 13 years). Seven of the 17 children were younger than 1 year old. Only three patients had no underlying medical problems. Four patients had macroglossia (Down syndrome, n = 3; duplicated tongue, n = 1) as a cause and three patients had micro or retrognathia (small or receding jaw). Six patients had neuromuscular abnormalities. The authors conclude that glossoptosis was a cause of airway obstruction in 25 percent of pediatric patients referred for fluoroscopic sleep studies. Attention to this anatomic region is important when evaluating children with **sleep apnea.** 2 figures. 19 references.

- **Sleep Apnea: A Serious Disorder**

  Source: Access. 9(7): 32-36. August 1995.

  Contact: Available from American Dental Hygienists' Association (ADHA). 444 North Michigan Avenue, Chicago, IL 60611. (800) 243-2342 or (312) 440-8900; Fax (312) 440-8929; E-mail: adha@ix.netcom.com; http://www.adha.org.

  Summary: This article, from a journal for dental hygienists, reviews the problem of **sleep apnea** and its precursor, snoring. Topics covered include the epidemiology of **sleep apnea;** obstructive **sleep apnea** (OSA); the symptoms of snoring and **sleep apnea;** the consequences of an OSA episode; central **sleep apnea** (CSA); the association of **sleep apnea** and hypertension; treatment options, including nonsurgical, nonpharmalogical interventions, pharmacological interventions, and surgical interventions; and the oral health care professional's responsibility with regard to **sleep apnea.** One sidebar describes the appliances that have received FDA clearance for the treatment of snoring. 18 references.

Federally Funded Research on Sleep Apnea

The U.S. Government supports a variety of research studies relating to sleep apnea and associated conditions. These studies are tracked by the Office of Extramural Research at the National Institutes of Health.[16] CRISP (Computerized Retrieval of Information on Scientific Projects) is a searchable database of federally funded biomedical research projects conducted at universities, hospitals, and other institutions. Visit CRISP at **http://crisp.cit.nih.gov/crisp/crisp_query.generate_screen**. You can perform targeted searches by various criteria including geography, date, as well as topics related to sleep apnea and related conditions.

For most of the studies, the agencies reporting into CRISP provide summaries or abstracts. As opposed to clinical trial research using patients, many federally funded studies use animals or simulated models to explore sleep apnea and related conditions. In some cases, therefore, it may be difficult to understand how some basic or fundamental research could eventually translate into medical practice. The following sample is typical of the type of information found when searching the CRISP database for sleep apnea:

- **Project Title: ABSOLUTE NEAR INFRARED BRAIN OXIMETER**

  Principal Investigator & Institution: Michalos, Antonios;; Iss, Inc. 1602 Newton Dr Champaign, Il 61822

  Timing: Fiscal Year 2003; Project Start 12-SEP-2000; Project End 31-MAY-2005

  Summary: (provided by applicant): Our goals in Phase I have been completed and showed the feasibility of our approach. We applied Near-Infrared Spectroscopy (NIRS), a non-invasive method and an affordable, portable, bedside technique for the diagnosis of the degree of the hypoxic insult in the brain, in **sleep apnea,** during daytime napping. It has been suggested that chronic, recurrent hypoxia during sleep leads to brain injury, which causes neuropsychological deficits and decline of cognitive

---

16 Healthcare projects are funded by the National Institutes of Health (NIH), Substance Abuse and Mental Health Services (SAMHSA), Health Resources and Services Administration (HRSA), Food and Drug Administration (FDA), Centers for Disease Control and Prevention (CDCP), Agency for Healthcare Research and Quality (AHRQ), and Office of Assistant Secretary of Health (OASH).

function. Cerebrovascular accidents, including fatal strokes are not uncommon. Conventional polysomnography, a relatively expensive test, detects **sleep apnea** at various sleep stages and determines arterial oxygen saturation. However, current clinical methods do not provide information on brain oxygenation, which is important especially in subjects with preexisting anatomical or functional vascular pathology. NIRS enables continuous real-time measurements of changes in the hemoglobin oxygenation and blood volume, thus providing information on tissue oxygenation and hemodynamics. In Phase II we propose the development of a tool and the application of NIRS to determine cerebral hemodynamics during sleep, in association to overnight polysomnographic sleep studies. Our goal is the development of reliable, cost efficient instrumentation for early detection of cerebral hemodynamic abnormalities in **sleep apnea,** for the prevention of hypoxic cerebral morbidity and mortality.

Website: http://crisp.cit.nih.gov/crisp/Crisp_Query.Generate_Screen

- **Project Title: ACTIVATION OF TONGUE MUSCLES IN OBSTRUCTIVE SLEEP APNEA**

  Principal Investigator & Institution: Durand, Dominique M.; Professor; Biomedical Engineering; Case Western Reserve University 10900 Euclid Ave Cleveland, Oh 44106

  Timing: Fiscal Year 2002; Project Start 01-FEB-2001; Project End 31-DEC-2004

  Summary: adapted from applicant's abstract) This project aims to develop an experimental therapy for **obstructive sleep apnea** (OSA) using electrical stimulation of the hypoglossal nerve. The PI proposes to use a multi-channel stimulation technique for selective activation of portions of the hypoglossal nerve to activate individual tongue muscles selectively. Such stimulation might increase control over the tongue muscles and improve efficiency for electrical stimulation to remove pharyngeal obstruction. There are 3 aims to be tested in dogs. Aim 1 will determine the maximum muscle selectivity that can be obtained with a multi-contact electrode on the hypoglossal nerve. Aim 2 will evaluate the mechanical dilation of the airways due to selective stimulation. Aim 3 will determine the optimum electrode geometries and stimulation paradigms for airway dilation in chronic dogs. It is anticipated that the experimental delineation and validation of these methods will lead to a design of a neuroprosthetic device for the treatment of OSA.

  Website: http://crisp.cit.nih.gov/crisp/Crisp_Query.Generate_Screen

- **Project Title: ADVANCED AT-HOME SCREENING DEVICE FOR SLEEP APNEA**

  Principal Investigator & Institution: Cooke, Arthur V.;; Active Signal Technologies, Inc. 13025 Beaver Dam Rd Cockeysville, Md 21030

  Timing: Fiscal Year 2002; Project Start 15-JUN-1999; Project End 31-AUG-2004

  Summary: Active Signal Technologies proposes to further develop its self applied, electrodeless home monitoring device for **sleep apnea** with the ultimate goal of making clinical diagnosis available to a much larger population of sleep disorder patients than currently possible. Preliminary results from Phase I have shown that much of the diagnostically rich airflow information captured in the sleep lab with a nasal mask and pneumotachograph can be replicated using an unobtrusive external tracheal contact sensor. Because this flow data has such important ramifications, the present proposal is being directed primarily to optimizing the sensor to work uniformly across a wide variety of cervical morphometries, and building real-time signal processing routines to separate snore, obstruction sounds, etc, from the broadband "hiss" of pure air movement in the trachea. This specific focus recognizes the broad application potential of the breathing sensor, not only as a critical component for the home monitoring device and as an alternative to a mask in the sleep lab but also throughout the field of respiratory care. In addition, the sensor captures far more acoustic information than just quantitative tidal volume and qualitative flow patterns, and hence can be used to characterize obstruction, respiratory effort, etc. PROPOSED COMMERCIAL APPLICATIONS: With approximately 10 million people suffering from **obstructive sleep apnea** alone yet <250,000 being tested per year in sleep clinics, the AAMS has a huge potential market. The AAMS priced at $1000 provides the patient with a cost-effective, accurate screening option in the comfort of his or her home.

  Website: http://crisp.cit.nih.gov/crisp/Crisp_Query.Generate_Screen

- **Project Title: AGE,GENDER, SEROTONIN AND RESPIRATORY CONTROL**

  Principal Investigator & Institution: Behan, Mary; Professor; Comparative Biosciences; University of Wisconsin Madison 750 University Ave Madison, Wi 53706

  Timing: Fiscal Year 2002; Project Start 15-AUG-2001; Project End 31-JUL-2006

  Summary: Serotonin (5HT) plays a major role in breathing and the control of upper airway function. The proposed research will test the hypothesis that, with increasing age, there is a gender- specific decrease in serotonergic modulation of respiratory motoneurons. Because of gender-related differences, aging males may be uniquely susceptible to breathing disorders such as **obstructive sleep apnea.** Our preliminary data indicate that 5HT immunoreactivity in the hypoglossal nucleus decreases with age in male rats, but increases with age in female rats. Furthermore, long term facilitation, a 5HT-dependent increase in respiratory motor output following intermittent hypoxia, decreases to older male rats, but increases to older female rats. This is the first description of age-associated change in serotonergic modulation of respiratory control, and the first description of sexual dimorphism in age-related changes in any aspect of the serotonergic nervous system. The proposed research will test the hypothesis that gonadal hormones have a neuroprotective role in the maintenance of serotonergic modulation of respiratory motoneurons in female rats with increasing age, and can potentially reverse or delay the age-associated changes that occur in male rats. Five specific aims are proposed, each corresponding to a testable hypothesis. First, we will use neurochemical and anatomical assays to detect age- and gender- related changes in key elements of the serotonergic neuromodulatory system (5HT, 5HT receptors, and the serotonin reuptake transport protein) in hypoglossal and phrenic motor nuclei. Secondly, we propose to determine if there are functional consequences of aging and gender on respiratory responses to hypoxia in awake rats. Thirdly, we will test the hypothesis that serotonin-dependent components of the hypoxic ventilatory response are decreased selectively with aging in male rats. Finally, we propose to investigate the influence of neutering and hormone replacement therapy (estrogen, progesterone, testosterone) on our anatomical and physiological indices of serotonergic modulation of respiration in male and female rats. To our knowledge, this is the first proposal to study age and gender effects on any form of plasticity in respiratory control. An understanding of these mechanisms may lead to therapeutic strategies for intervention in age-related breathing disorders that affect both men and women such as **obstructive sleep apnea.**

Website: http://crisp.cit.nih.gov/crisp/Crisp_Query.Generate_Screen

- **Project Title: AGING, EPISODIC HYPOXIA, AND VAGAL CARDIAC PROJECTIONS**

  Principal Investigator & Institution: Cheng, Zixi; Pediatrics; University of Louisville Jouett Hall, Belknap Campus Louisville, Ky 40292

  Timing: Fiscal Year 2003; Project Start 01-JUN-2003; Project End 31-MAY-2008

Summary: (provided by applicant): Aging and the syndrome of **obstructive sleep apnea,** which is characterized by chronic intermittent hypoxia (CIH), are commonly associated with increased incidence and severity of hypertension, orthostatic intolerance, and cardiovascular diseases. However, our understanding of the neural mechanisms underlying these dysfunctions is impeded by a lack of structural information on autonomic nerve terminals and the circuitry within the cardiac tissues. Vagal projections to the heart originate from a sensory ganglion, i.e., the nodose ganglion, and the motor neuron pools in the brainstem, i.e., the nucleus ambiguus (NA) and the dorsal motor nucleus of the vagus (DmnX). The overall goal of the present application is to determine the functional deficits of the vagal control of the heart induced by aging, CIH, or both, and to identify the damage to the cardiac neural circuitry, specifically to the vagal axonal projections to the heart. Vagal control of particular cardiac functions will be measured in young (3months), middle age (12months) and aged (24 months) Fischer 344 rats. The vagal cardiac axons and terminals, and glutamatergic transmission within the NA and DmnX will be examined qualitatively and quantitatively using a battery of techniques that will include anterograde neural tracing, stereological counting, confocal microscopy, Neurolucida digitization, and dual immunohistochemistry. These anatomical findings will be assessed in conjunction with physiological responses to enhance our understanding of structure-function relationships. Aim 1 will assess aging-associated attenuation of baroreflex and vagal control of the heart, and the associated structural changes of vagal projections to the heart and aortic arch. Aim 2 will evaluate CIH-induced reduction of baroreflex sensitivity and vagal controls and the parallel vagal cardiac axon degeneration. Aim2 will also determine whether aging and CIH interact to induce more severe functional and anatomical damage to the vagal cardiac axons. Aim 3 will study changes in glutamatergic transmission within the caudal brainstem complex (NTS, NA, DmnX) during aging and following CIH. Collectively, the proposed experiments will advance our knowledge of brain-heart interactions and provide unique insights into the remodeling of vagal outflow to cardiac tissues during aging and following CIH.

Website: http://crisp.cit.nih.gov/crisp/Crisp_Query.Generate_Screen

- **Project Title: ALZHEIMER CAREGIVER COPING: MENTAL AND PHYSICAL HEALTH**

  Principal Investigator & Institution: Grant, Igor; Professor & Executive Vice Chairman; Psychiatry; University of California San Diego La Jolla, Ca 920930934

Timing: Fiscal Year 2002; Project Start 30-SEP-1997; Project End 31-AUG-2006

Summary: The experiences of elderly caregivers of Alzheimer relatives (CG) can be viewed as a model of chronic human stress in aging. Our work in the past funding cycle has been guided by the notion that such stress is accompanied by increased sympathoadrenalmedullary (SAM) activation whose cardiovascular and molecular responses may be amplified by superimposed stressors such as excessive care demands relative to respite received ("vulnerable CG"). The results to date indicate heightened basal circulating epinephrine (E) in vulnerable CG, altered L-selectin cell adhesion molecule (CAM) expression, down- regulation of beta-adrenergic receptors of lymphocytes, but no systematic changes in heart rate or blood pressure variability. Vulnerable CG who received a two week respite intervention demonstrated lessened circulating E in response to stressors compared to wait-listed CG, but there were no systematic treatment-related changes in other variables. Pilot data revealed: 1) increased expression of procoagulation factors (especially D-Dimer) which correlated with amount of sleep disturbance and level of catecholamines; 2) Vulnerable CG had less total sleep time and more awakenings than nonvulnerable CG. In the proposed research we wish to refine our understanding of the molecular changes underlying chronic and acute stress in elderly caregiving. The basic theory is that the chronic stress of caregiving yields a state of relative SAM arousal reflected in greater resting and stressor-related releases of catecholamines. As outcome variables of chronic and acute stressors related to caregiving, we shall focus on coagulation factors and cellular adhesion molecules, each of which has been associated with heightened risk of cardiovascular morbidity and mortality. The general hypothesis is that elderly caregivers, versus noncaregiving controls (NC) will have greater SAM arousal and greater expression of coagulation and adhesion molecules. It is posited further that those caregivers who have background medical risks (history of cardiovascular disease or hypertension), and who experienced superimposed stressors, such as excessive caregiving demands, or other negative life events, will be selectively vulnerable to these physiological changes. Disturbed sleep environment is posited to be one of the pathways whereby caregiving stressors are translated into SAM arousal and molecular changes. The study design calls for recruitment of 120 elderly caregivers (CG) and 60 noncaregiving controls (NC). Laboratory-derived speech stressor tasks will be used to probe differences in SAM responsivity to speech stressors between CG and NC, as well as CG at several levels of "mismatch" between caregiving demand and respite received. At-home polysomnography and actigraphy will monitor sleep disruption, sleep disorders (e.g., sleep apnea), and circadian activity variation. In the longitudinal phase, subjects will be re-evaluated annually to determine if hypothesized recovery of SAM arousability occurs in those CG who have placed their spouse, or whose spouse has died. The results of this research should bring us closer to understanding the physiological and molecular mechanisms underlying increased morbidity in elderly persons under chronic stress.

Website: http://crisp.cit.nih.gov/crisp/Crisp_Query.Generate_Screen

- **Project Title: ANDROGENS & SLEEP: APNEA EPIDEMIOLOGY & PATHOPHYSIOLOGY**

  Principal Investigator & Institution: Fogel, Robert B.;; Brigham and Women's Hospital 75 Francis Street Boston, Ma 02115

  Timing: Fiscal Year 2002; Project Start 01-AUG-2000; Project End 31-JUL-2005

  Summary: (Adapted from the applicant's abstract) **Obstructive sleep apnea** (OSA) is a common disorder with important consequences for afflicted individuals. This disorder is characterized by recurrent pharyngeal collapse during sleep with subsequent repetitive arousals, along with substantial hypoxia and hypercapnia. Associated consequences include daytime somnolence, decreased performance on cognitive and vigilance testing and decreased quality of life. In addition, there is also increasing evidence that OSA may lead to adverse cardiovascular outcomes such as hypertension, arrhythmias, myocardial infarction and stroke. The pathophysiology of **sleep apnea** is dependent upon a complex interaction between upper airway anatomy, pharyngeal dilator muscle function and ventilatory control mechanisms, and the effects of state related changes in these variables. Substantial literature indicates that this disorder is much more common in men than in women, and that androgens in both men and women can exacerbate the disorder. However, neither the true extent of the effect of androgens on **sleep apnea** incidence and severity, nor the mechanisms by which androgens predispose to apnea have been well delineated to this point. With the proposed Mentored Patient-Oriented Research Career Development Award, the applicant will build upon his prior experiences investigating the role of androgens in the pathophysiology of **sleep apnea.** Based upon very positive experiences in the laboratory to date, the applicant is firmly committed to a career in academic pulmonary and critical care medicine, focused primarily on clinical research. The laboratory of Dr. David P. White at the Brigham and Women's Hospital will provide a rich intellectual environment.

  Website: http://crisp.cit.nih.gov/crisp/Crisp_Query.Generate_Screen

- **Project Title: APPLES: APNEA POSITIVE PRESSURE LONG-TERM EFFICACY STUDY**

  Principal Investigator & Institution: Dement, William C.; L W & J Q Berry Professor of Psychiatry; Psychiatry and Behavioral Sci; Stanford University Stanford, Ca 94305

  Timing: Fiscal Year 2002; Project Start 30-SEP-2002; Project End 31-JUL-2007

  Summary: (provided by applicant): Nasal continuous positive airway pressure (CPAP) therapy is in widespread use as the primary treatment for the **obstructive sleep apnea** syndrome (OSAS), a sleep-related breathing disorder affecting more than 15 million Americans. The therapeutic effectiveness of CPAP in providing significant, stable, and long-term neurocognitive or other functional benefits to patients with OSAS has not been systematically investigated. The revised proposed study is a randomized, blinded, sham-controlled, multi-center trial of CPAP therapy. The principal aims of the study are: 1) to assess the long-term effectiveness of CPAP therapy on neurocognitive function, mood, sleepiness, and quality of life by administering tests of these indices to subjects randomly assigned to active or sham CPAP; 2) to identify specific neurocognitive deficits associated with OSAS in a large, heterogeneous subject population; 3) to determine which deficits in neurocognitive function in OSAS subjects are reversible and most sensitive to the effects of CPAP; 4) to develop a composite multivariate outcome measure from the results of this study that can be used to assess the clinical effectiveness of CPAP in improving neurocognitive function, mood, sleepiness, and quality of life; and 5) to use functional magnetic resonance imaging to compare cortical activation before and after CPAP therapy, and to assess whether this change is associated with improvement in specific neurocognitive task performance. The primary endpoint of this proposed study is the effect of 6 months of CPAP treatment on neurocognitive function. A total of 1050 subjects (525 per treatment group) will be enrolled from the patient populations at five sites (Stanford; U of Arizona; Harvard; St. Luke's Hospital, MO; St. Mary's Hospital, WA). This study will advance our knowledge of the major, most debilitating, clinically relevant OSAS-associated conditions, and, by scientifically establishing the effectiveness of CPAP therapy, should greatly improve access for the countless victims now denied treatment.

  Website: http://crisp.cit.nih.gov/crisp/Crisp_Query.Generate_Screen

- **Project Title: ASTHMA CLINICAL RESEARCH NETWORK**

  Principal Investigator & Institution: Wasserman, Stephen I.; Professor of Medicine; Medicine; University of California San Diego La Jolla, Ca 920930934

  Timing: Fiscal Year 2003; Project Start 15-SEP-2003; Project End 31-JUL-2008

  Summary: (provided by applicant): A consortium of investigators at the University of California, San Diego with extensive experience in, and a commitment to, clinical research collaborations in the area of asthma, are proposing two multi-center clinical trials for the NIH-sponsored Asthma Clinical Research Network. The UCSD consortium is led by Drs. Stephen Wasserman and Joe Ramsdell. Study 1 will be undertaken in stable steroid dependent asthmatic adults. It will examine the effect of etanercept, an inhibitor of TNF-alpha, in an 18-week, double-blind, placebo-controlled clinical trial in this population. The primary outcome to be evaluated will be the ability of this agent to permit significant reduction in inhaled steroid dosage without exacerbation. Study 2 will also employ a double-blind, placebo-controlled design. This trial will evaluate the ability of CPAP to improve nocturnal asthma, in a population of overweight, adult patients with moderate-to-severe asthma, who also suffer from sleep disordered breathing. Patients for these, and other Network trials, will be recruited from the Medicine, Pulmonary and Allergy clinics of UCSD, the San Diego VA, the San Diego US Naval Hospital, and Kaiser- Permanente. The available population is large, multi-racial and multi-ethnic, reflecting the San Diego environment. We are also proposing an educational program, under the direction of Dr. Andrew Ries, which will utilize the extensive resources available at UCSD.

  Website: http://crisp.cit.nih.gov/crisp/Crisp_Query.Generate_Screen

- **Project Title: BDNF IN PLASTICITY OF CHEMOAFFERENT PATHWAY**

  Principal Investigator & Institution: Katz, David M.;; Case Western Reserve University 10900 Euclid Ave Cleveland, Oh 44106

  Timing: Fiscal Year 2002; Project Start 01-FEB-2002; Project End 31-DEC-2006

  Summary: (provided by applicant): The aim of the proposed research is to define the role of Brain-Derived Neurotrophic Factor (BDNF) in activity-dependent plasticity in the developing chemoafferent pathway. Chemoafferent neurons are the link between peripheral chemoreceptors and the brainstem, and thereby play a pivotal role in cardiorespiratory homeostasis. At birth, chemoafferent reflexes are immature, and perturbations in oxygen availability can derange postnatal development of cardiorespiratory responses to acute hypoxia. However, mechanisms that underlie chemoreflex development and plasticity are largely undefined. This proposal is based on our recent discoveries that 1) Chemoafferent neurons in the newborn rat nodose-petrosal ganglion complex (NPG) express high levels of BDNF messenger RNA and protein, 2) BDNF protein is released from NPG neurons in response to patterned electrical stimulation in vitro, and 3) BDNF acutely inhibits glutamatergic AMPA receptors in second-order relay neurons in the nucleus tractus solitarius (nTS), the primary site of chemoafferent projections to the brainstem. Together, these data indicate a new role for BDNF as a modulator of excitatory synaptic transmission between primary chemoafferent neurons and second-order relay neurons in nTS. In view of increasing evidence that BDNF plays a critical role in long-term synaptic plasticity elsewhere in the brain, we hypothesize that BDNF plays a similar role at chemoafferent synapses in nTS. Moreover, based on our preliminary data, we hypothesize that BDNF signaling in nTS is regulated by changes in oxygen availability, and thereby contributes to derangements in chemoreflex function following chronic sustained or intermittent hypoxia. Therefore, the proposed research is designed to further define mechanisms of BDNF expression and release in chemoafferent neurons after birth, including the role of chronic sustained and intermittent hypoxia, in vivo and in vitro. In addition, we will characterize postsynaptic effects of BDNF on developing nTS neurons, including regulation of transmitter receptor expression and dendritic growth. Moreover, we will determine the role of BDNF in functional plasticity in vivo by analyzing development of peripheral chemoreflexes in transgenic mice in which BDNF signaling is disrupted selectively after birth. By defining mechanisms of activity-dependent plasticity in the PG and nTS, the proposed research may shed light on cellular and molecular mechanisms relevant to understanding and improved management of hypoventilation and apnea syndromes in neonates and infants, as well as mechanisms that contribute to altered cardiorespiratory control in adult **obstructive sleep apnea** and chronic obstructive pulmonary disease. Moreover, it is hoped that elucidating development of this system will, in turn, create a model of neurotrophin function applicable to the nervous system as a whole.

Website: http://crisp.cit.nih.gov/crisp/Crisp_Query.Generate_Screen

- **Project Title: BEHAVIORAL EFFECT OF OBSTRUCTIVE SLEEP APNEA IN CHILDREN**

  Principal Investigator & Institution: Chervin, Ronald D.; Associate Professor and Director; Neurology; University of Michigan at Ann Arbor 3003 South State, Room 1040 Ann Arbor, Mi 481091274

  Timing: Fiscal Year 2002; Project Start 01-AUG-1999; Project End 31-JUL-2004

  Summary: Adenotonsillectomy (AT) remains one of the most common surgical procedures performed in children, but indications for AT have changed in recent years. Surgeons now perform AT in many instances for suspected obstructive sleep-disordered breathing (SDB), and sometimes for daytime behaviors that may be a consequence of SDB, especially inattention and hyperactivity. However, whether SDB causes these and other disruptive behaviors, the precise nature of these behaviors, and what types or levels of SDB may be of concern are not well known. Without such knowledge, pediatricians and otolaryngologists do not often make use of objective preoperative testing that could help to assess for SDB or abnormal behavior. The main goals of the research described in this proposal are to (1) better define whether inattention and hyperactivity are frequent among children who undergo AT, (2) identify measures and levels of SDB that are indicative of these behaviors, (3) test whether improvement in SDB after AT is associated with improvement in behavior, and (4) investigate the hypothesis that SDB is a cause of inattention, hyperactivity, and related behaviors in some children. Subjects will be 5 through 12 year-old children recruited after they have been scheduled by their physicians for AT (n = 200) or hernia repair (n = 75 controls). A battery of well-validated behavioral assessment tools, cognitive tests, and structured psychiatric interviews will be used before surgery to define what behaviors are more prominent in the children scheduled for AT rather than hernia repair. All children will undergo preoperative polysomnography which will include, for the first time in such a series, equipment that can detect subtle forms of SDB which may be particularly prevalent in children. Results will allow determination of what polysomnographic findings are associated with well-defined adverse behavioral outcomes. Finally, preoperative and postoperative testing in these subjects will provide a controlled non-randomized trial of AT for SDB, demonstrate whether SDB-associated abnormal behaviors improve after AT, and provide strong evidence for whether SDB is a cause of these behaviors.

  Website: http://crisp.cit.nih.gov/crisp/Crisp_Query.Generate_Screen

- **Project Title: CARDIOVASCULAR RESPONSES TO CHRONIC INTERMITTENT HYPOXIA**

  Principal Investigator & Institution: Mifflin, Steven W.; Professor; Pharmacology; University of Texas Hlth Sci Ctr San Ant 7703 Floyd Curl Dr San Antonio, Tx 78229

  Timing: Fiscal Year 2002; Project Start 30-SEP-2000; Project End 31-AUG-2004

  Summary: Chronic intermittent hypoxia (CIH) is a widely used model for the repetitive bouts of hypoxemia that occur during sleep in **sleep apnea** patients. During such apneic periods, hypoxia activates chemoreceptors that evoke reflex increases in arterial pressure. In humans with **sleep apnea** and animals exposed to CIH the repetitive periods of hypoxia during sleep result in tonically increased arterial pressure during waking hours, likely the result of elevated levels of sympathetic nerve activity and an enhanced response to acute hypoxia. The goal of the present project is to investigate the central pathways and mechanisms that underlie this persistent increase in sympathetic nerve activity. It is hypothesized that CIH leads to alterations in ligand gated excitatory and/or inhibitory amino acid receptors in noradrenergic (A2) neurons in the nucleus of the solitary tract (NTS) so that their discharge is increased compared to before CIH. These neurons transmit this enhanced discharge to sympatho-excitatory neuron in the paraventricular nucleus (PVN) of the hypothalamus. PVN neurons receiving the catecholaminergic input include neurons that release corticotropin releasing factor (CRF) as a transmitter. The CRF releasing PVN neurons mediate, at least in part, the enhanced sympathetic discharge observed following CIH via projections to the RVLM and by stimulating corticosterone release. Both in vivo and in vitro approaches will be used and microinjection, electro-physiological and molecular studies are proposed to characterize the synaptic integration of chemoreceptor inputs and the molecular regulation of the neurotransmitter receptors that mediate these integrative processes. The specific aims are designed to assess: 1) The integration of arterial chemoreceptor inputs within the NTS following CIH; 2) The integration of A2, noradrenergic inputs within the PVN following CIH; and 3) The functional activation of the CRF system within the PVN following CIH.

  Website: http://crisp.cit.nih.gov/crisp/Crisp_Query.Generate_Screen

- **Project Title: CARDIOVASCULAR STRESS OF SLEEP APNEA AND HEART FAILURE**

  Principal Investigator & Institution: Schwartz, Alan R.; Associate Professor of Medicine; Medicine; Johns Hopkins University 3400 N Charles St Baltimore, Md 21218

Timing: Fiscal Year 2002; Project Start 30-SEP-2002; Project End 31-JUL-2006

Summary: (provided by applicant): **Sleep apnea** is a common disorder associated with an increased risk of cardiovascular disease, and is particularly prevalent in heart failure patients. The cardiovascular risk of **sleep apnea** is likely to be amplified in the presence of heart failure since each disorder can aggravate the other. This proposal examines the interrelationship between **sleep apnea** and heart failure, and the mechanisms leading to cardiovascular stress when the two interact. Our proposal is predicated on the notion that **sleep apnea** increases cardiovascular stress, and further worsens left ventricular function in heart failure patients. Our major hypothesis is that a reciprocal interaction exists between **sleep apnea** and heart failure, wherein sleep-related disturbances in key mediators lead to acute and chronic increases in cardiovascular stress and worsening left ventricular function. To test this hypothesis, experiments are proposed in humans and murine models of **sleep apnea** and heart failure. In Specific Aims 1 and 2, heart failure patients will be intensively studied nocturnally to elucidate the mechanisms by which **sleep apnea** and its associated arousals and hypoxemic episodes increase cardiovascular stress acutely and perpetuate cardiovascular stress chronically. In Specific Aims 3 and 4, studies in novel murine models of chronic intermittent and sleep-induced hypoxia will examine the mechanisms in which **sleep apnea** and heart failure interact at the cardiac and central nervous system level. This potentially harmful interaction will be explored by assessing responses in: (a) novel mediators of cardiovascular stress (reactive oxygen species, cytokines, leptin, and insulin), (b) an important biomarker of acute and chronic cardiovascular stress (B-type natriuretic peptide, BNP), (c) cardiac tissue, and in (d) cardiac and CNS gene expression. The research plan will elucidate new mechanisms causing excess cardiovascular morbidity and mortality in heart failure, as well as provide new approaches to detect, monitor and treat **sleep apnea** in heart failure patients.

Website: http://crisp.cit.nih.gov/crisp/Crisp_Query.Generate_Screen

- **Project Title: CAUSES OF SLEEP-INDUCED BREATHING INSTABILITIES**

  Principal Investigator & Institution: Dempsey, Jerome A.; Professor; Population Health Sciences; University of Wisconsin Madison 750 University Ave Madison, Wi 53706

  Timing: Fiscal Year 2002; Project Start 01-APR-1999; Project End 31-MAR-2004

Summary: During sleep and with the loss of the "wakefulness" drive to pump and upper airway respiratory muscles, the control of breathing becomes highly dependent upon and vulnerable to reflexive feedback inputs from chemoreceptors and mechanoreceptors. Accordingly, sleep-induced breathing instabilities are common and have a significant prevalence even in the general population. Sleep unmasks a highly sensitive hypocapnic-induced apneic threshold, but we do not know what role this mechanism plays in various types of sleep-disordered breathing, because we do not know its sites of action, its changes in sensitivity in the presence of powerful background influences such as CNS hypoxia, chronic hypocapnia/hypercapnia, changing sleep states, or changing stimuli to breathe which might be specific to sleep. We will use sleeping humans and dogs, the latter with extra corporeal perfusion of isolated carotid chemoreceptors-to quantify the effect of these influences on both the apneic threshold and on the important stabilizing mechanism of short term potentiation of ventilatory output. This dog model with isolation of carotid chemoreceptors will also be used to address the question of central versus peripheral hypoxic effects on periodic breathing in sleep. A second dog model as well as human patients with chronic heart failure will be studied to address the mechanisms of Cheyne-Stokes respiration, with specific emphasis on the effects of the added stimulus to hyperventilation originating from the lungs of the patient in congestive heart failure. Finally, we will use dogs and humans-with and without innervated lungs-to address the role of non-chemical, mechanoreceptor inhibitory feedback effects during sleep on upper airway and pump muscles; a) influences from high frequency low amplitude pressure oscillations in the upper airway; b) the effects of amplitude, timing and duration of normocapnic mechanical ventilation on the resetting of inherent respiratory rhythm and on the "short-term inhibition" of respiratory motor output following cessation of phasic inhibitory sensory input. These latter studies conduced in sleep are important to testing the sensitivity of respiratory control mechanisms to mechanical feedback-a problem which remains relatively unexplored, especially in the human.

Website: http://crisp.cit.nih.gov/crisp/Crisp_Query.Generate_Screen

- **Project Title: CHEMORECEPTORS AND HYPERTENSION AND SLEEP APNEA**

  Principal Investigator & Institution: Loredo, Jose S.; Medicine; University of California San Diego La Jolla, Ca 920930934

  Timing: Fiscal Year 2002; Project Start 01-AUG-1999; Project End 31-JUL-2004

Summary: The career development plan for this award will consist of two components: A research project and a didactic program. The research project aims to characterize the function of peripheral chemoreceptors and their relation to the sympathetic nervous system (SNS) and blood pressure (BP) in hypertensive patients with **obstructive sleep apnea** (OSA). Previous work has suggested that apneic hypertensives have high tonic chemoreceptor activity, and depressed chemoreceptor sensitivity. The project's hypothesis is that high tonic chemoreceptor activity contributes to the development of maintenance of hypertension and high SNS tone in OSA patients. To test this hypothesis it is necessary to study four groups of patients: hypertensives and normotensives , with and without **sleep apnea.** The specific goals of this randomized double blind cross over study include 1) Characterization of tonic chemoreceptor activity by measuring ventilation at room air and during chemoreceptor blockade with 100% O2. 2) Characterization of chemoreceptor sensitivity by measuring ventilation during hypoxia. 3) Characterization of SNS activity at baseline and its response to chemoreceptor blockade or stimulation. 4) Determination of the effect of 7 days nocturnal supplemental O2 on BP, SNS, and chemoreceptor function. If the hypothesis is correct, that high tonic chemoreceptor activity is associated with hypertension and high SNS activity in OSA patients, then treatment with supplemental oxygen may decrease BP and normalize SNS function. A short term implication is that patients with mild to moderate OSA unable to tolerate continuous posit8ive airway pressure, may benefit from nocturnal O2 alone. The didactic program will supplement the clinical research training background of the applicant. The program includes courses in epidemiology, biostatistics, and sleep medicine. Further didactic instruction will include courses and symposia on advanced statistics, clinical trials design and ethical conduct of clinical research. This training will provide the basis of an MPH degree and a solid theoretical background for future conduct of quality clinical research.

Website: http://crisp.cit.nih.gov/crisp/Crisp_Query.Generate_Screen

- **Project Title: CHOLINERGIC ASPECTS OF THE CAROTID BODY IN SLEEP APNEA**

  Principal Investigator & Institution: O'donnell, Christopher P.; Associate Professor of Medicine; Medicine; Johns Hopkins University 3400 N Charles St Baltimore, Md 21218

  Timing: Fiscal Year 2002; Project Start 30-SEP-2000; Project End 31-AUG-2004

Summary: The prevalence of **Obstructive Sleep Apnea** (OSA) is increasing dramatically in the U.S. representing a serious health risk. The primary consequence of airway obstruction during sleep is to cause hypoxemia which stimulates the carotid body, leading to increased respiratory drive until arousal from sleep restores upper airway patency. This project proposes to determine the mechanisms by which the carotid body senses and responds to the repetitive intermittent periods of hypoxemia in OSA. Based on the critically important role of acetylcholine as an excitatory neurotransmitter in the carotid body's chemotransduction of hypoxia, it is hypothesized 1) that the repetitive intermittent hypoxia of OSA alters cholinergic transduction pathways in the carotid body, and 2) that the sensitivity of the carotid body is determined genetically. Specific Aim 1 will examine the impact of repetitive intermittent hypoxia during sleep on carotid body function in a novel, murine model of sleep disordered breathing. Specific Aim 2 will investigate the pattern of acetylcholine and other neurotransmitter release from the carotid body, as well as recording carotid sinus nerve activity, in response to repetitive intermittent hypoxia. Specific Aim 3 will use immunohistochemical and patch clamp analyses to determine if neuronal nicotinic acetylcholine receptors (nAChRs) can account for differential hypoxic responsiveness between mouse strains with differential hypoxic responsiveness and determine whether repetitive intermittent hypoxia upregulates expression of subtypes of nAChRs.

Website: http://crisp.cit.nih.gov/crisp/Crisp_Query.Generate_Screen

- **Project Title: COGNITIVE BENEFITS OF TREATING SLEEP APNEA IN DEMENTIA**

  Principal Investigator & Institution: Ancoli-Israel, Sonia; Professor; Psychiatry; University of California San Diego La Jolla, Ca 920930934

  Timing: Fiscal Year 2002; Project Start 01-MAY-1989; Project End 31-JAN-2006

  Summary: (adapted from Investigator's abstract) Studies have shown that there is a strong relationship between sleep disordered breathing (SDB) and dementia and patients with Alzheimer's Disease having a high rate of SDB. This application will examine whether treating SDB with nasal CPAP in patients with AD will result in improvement in cognitive functioning. The specific aims are to assess whether patients with mild AD will tolerate CPAP and be compliant with the treatment; to examine the effect of CPAP treatment on SDB; to examine the effects of CPAP treatment on cognitive functioning in patients with mild AD and SDB; to examine whether improvement is greater after 6 weeks of CPAP treatment than after 3 weeks. Because caregivers are often disturbed by the patient's poor sleep, the effect of treatment on the caregiver will also be evaluated. The secondary aim is to evaluate whether caregivers feel that their own sleep improves as the patient's sleep improves. Patients will be randomized to a CPAP treatment group or sham CPAP group. After 3 weeks, the sham group will also be switched to CPAP. Measures of neuropsychological performance will be obtained at baseline and after 3 and 6 weeks of treatment.

Website: http://crisp.cit.nih.gov/crisp/Crisp_Query.Generate_Screen

- **Project Title: COMPUTATIONAL STUDIES OF THE RESPIRATORY BRAINSTEM**

  Principal Investigator & Institution: Lindsey, Bruce G.; Professor; Physiology and Biophysics; University of South Florida 4202 E Fowler Ave Tampa, Fl 33620

  Timing: Fiscal Year 2002; Project Start 30-SEP-2002; Project End 31-AUG-2007

  Summary: (provided by applicant): Understanding the control of breathing is an important goal in integrative biology and medicine. Sleep disorders in newborns and adults that disrupt breathing have been implicated in the development of pulmonary and systemic hypertension and other disorders and risks. The goal of this collaborative project is to develop a unified model of the brainstem respiratory network and to identify potential sites where abnormalities can disrupt breathing and its control. Detailed biophysical and large-scale simulations will guide associated in vivo and in vitro neurophysiological and pharmacological experiments to test model-based hypotheses on sub-cellular, cellular, network and systems level mechanisms that transform the respiratory network during the transitions between eupnea and hyperventilation apnea, from eupnea to gasping, and during sleep and waking. Experimental feedback will be used to iteratively tune the model. The project has five aims: 1. Develop a comprehensive computational model of the ventrolateral medullary "core" respiratory network and use it as a tool for interactive modeling/experimental studies on the neural control of breathing. 2. Evaluate interactions among the medullary central pattern generator (CPG), the pontine respiratory group, the nuclei of the solitary tract, and the raphe nuclei. 3. Elucidate mechanisms underlying network reconfiguration and the respiratory motor patterns associated with transient changes in chemical drive and gasping. 4. Identify inputs to the pontine-medullary respiratory network that can produce the respiratory motor patterns observed during the sleep-wake cycle and that can cause **sleep apnea.** These inputs or their absence are ultimately responsible for sleep disorders. 5. Test biophysical, cellular, and network mechanisms for a) rate and synchrony "coding" and network stability. This project will bring together researchers from universities in five states. Members of the group have a common interest in the control of breathing, complementary areas of expertise, large and growing experimental databases, and long-standing collegial relationships. The project will be a catalyst for the development and sharing of advanced multi-array recording technologies and computational methods, modeling and simulation tools, and large data sets.

Website: http://crisp.cit.nih.gov/crisp/Crisp_Query.Generate_Screen

- **Project Title: CONTROL OF BREATHING DURING PHYSIOLOGIC CONDITIONS**

  Principal Investigator & Institution: Forster, Hubert V.; Professor; Physiology; Medical College of Wisconsin Po Box26509 Milwaukee, Wi 532260509

  Timing: Fiscal Year 2002; Project Start 01-JUN-1986; Project End 31-MAY-2005

  Summary: Several theories on the neural control of breathing that were based on data from reduced preparations were not supported by our recent findings in awake and asleep goats on the effects of rostral medullary neuronal dysfunction and/or carotid body denervation (CBD). Some findings mimicked the altered breathing found in **obstructive sleep apnea** (OSA) and congenital central hypoventilation syndrome (CCHS). The mechanisms that mediated these effects are not established, but one likely mechanism is through intracranial chemoreceptors for years thought to exist only near the ventral medullary surface (including the retrotrapezoid nucleus RTN)). However, findings in reduced preparations of chemoreceptors at widespread brain sites have raised questions related to the location and role of chemoreceptors that affect breathing in awake and asleep states and whether brain chemoreceptor sensitivity is altered by CBD. One recently identified site of chemoreception is the medullary raphe nuclei (MRN) whose role in the control of breathing during awake and asleep states remains speculative. Accordingly, to study chemosensitivity and the role of the RTN and MRN in the control of breathing, we will implant microtubules into these nuclei of goats to: a) create a focal acidosis by dialysis of mock cerebrospinal fluid with different PCO2's, or b) induce neuronal dysfunction through injection of glutamate or serotonin receptor antagonists or agonists, or a neurotoxin. Major hypotheses are: 1) focal acidosis (equivalent to that breathing 7 percent inspired CO2, delta brain pH approximately -.05) in the RTN will increase breathing in awake, but not asleep states, while acidosis in the MRN will increase breathing in asleep, but not awake states, 2) at RTN sites where focal acidosis increases breathing, neuronal dysfunction will attenuate whole body CO2 sensitivity, but not alter rest and exercise breathing, 3) neuronal dysfunction in the MRN will attenuate CO2 sensitivity and rest and exercise breathing, 4) during the first 10 days after CBD, the effect of RTN and MRN focal acidosis will be attenuated but 15 plus days after CBD, the effect of focal acidosis will be accentuated. and 5) at most RTN and MRN sites, the acute effects of neurotoxic lesions will be hypoventilation (rest and exercise) and attenuated CO2 sensitivity; the acute effects of these lesions will be greater in CBD than in intact goats, but recovery after lesioning will be greater in intact than in CBD goats. Our unique studies are important because hypotheses generated largely from reduced preparations will be tested in awake and asleep states to enhance the understanding of medullary chemoreceptor contribution to the control of breathing and how abnormalities in this contribution may underlie diseases such as OSA, CCHS, and the Sudden Infant Death Syndrome.

Website: http://crisp.cit.nih.gov/crisp/Crisp_Query.Generate_Screen

- **Project Title: CONTROL OF BREATHING IN RECOVERY FROM APNEA**

  Principal Investigator & Institution: Thach, Bradley T.; Professor; Pediatrics; Washington University Lindell and Skinker Blvd St. Louis, Mo 63130

  Timing: Fiscal Year 2002; Project Start 30-SEP-1977; Project End 31-MAY-2004

  Summary: The Sudden Infant Death Syndrome (SIDS) remains a leading cause of infant deaths inspite of recent highly successful public health interventions designed to reduce SIDS risks (The U.S. "Back to Sleep" campaign, "BTS"). We propose to study several physiologic and neuro-developmental mechanisms potentially involved in the etiology of SIDS, as well as, pertinent environmental factors. The research will focus on three areas. In the first of these, we plan to study the physiology of recovery from severe hypoxia by gasping (autoresuscitation, AR). These studies will determine if the previously documented developmentally acquired defect in AR, originally described in SWR mice, is present in other inbred strains and species and, furthermore, if underlying mechanisms causing AR failure are similar to those in SWR mice. Additionally, the effects of increased environmental temperature on AR will be evaluated. Also, Home apnea monitor recordings of infants dying suddenly and unexpectedly while being monitored will be studied to determine if there is evidence of attempted AR and if so, potential reasons for its failure. The second part of our studies will be directed to prospectively obtaining data on the case history, death scene and postmortem examination of infant's dying with the diagnoses of SIDS, accidental suffocation and "cause of death undetermined" in the St. Louis metropolitan area. The aim is to determine how many of these deaths are preventable by public acceptance of current "BTS" guidelines and how many might be prevented by future additions or changes in the recommendations to child caretakers. In connection with this study, we will perform special death scene investigations in certain SIDS and accidental suffocation deaths combined with laboratory death scene reconstruction studies in order to determine if additional simple guidelines for parents and child equipment manufactures can be formulated in order to prevent infant deaths. Finally, we will study development of the infant's ability to avoid potentially suffocating environments during sleep, and determine the potential role of the infant's past experience on this development.

Website: http://crisp.cit.nih.gov/crisp/Crisp_Query.Generate_Screen

- **Project Title: CONTROL-RESPIRATORY MODULATION OF SYMPATHETIC ACTIVITY**

  Principal Investigator & Institution: Dick, Thomas E.; Associate Professor; Medicine; Case Western Reserve University 10900 Euclid Ave Cleveland, Oh 44106

  Timing: Fiscal Year 2002; Project Start 01-SEP-2000; Project End 31-JUL-2004

  Summary: (Applicant's abstract): **Sleep apnea syndrome** is prevalent (3-5 percent of the adult population) and associated with significant morbidity including hypertension. The increased blood pressure appears to result from an up-regulation of basal sympathetic nerve activity (SNA). Treatment reverses this up-regulation. We theorize that the up-regulation of SNA results from both short- and long-term sequelae of episodic hypoxemia associated with **sleep apnea.** The respiratory and cardiovascular systems are coordinated in the maintenance of homeostasis. Respiratory modulation of SNA is an aspect of this coordination. Not only is SNA modulated with the respiratory cycle but also this modulation increases during and following brief periods of hypoxemia. The neural substrate for this coordination is undefined. Recent studies have focused on neuronal interaction between medullary respiratory-modulated and pre-motor sympathetic neurons of the rostral ventrolateral medulla (RVLM). However, neurons in the dorsolateral (dl) pontine Kolliker-Fuse (KF) nucleus are the only brainstem neurons other than the those in the NTS that project to the RVLM and that are activated by hypoxia. We hypothesize that a direct pontomedullary interaction between respiratory-modulated neurons of the KF nucleus and neurons in RVLM contributes to the respiratory modulation of sympathetic activity and that this interaction underlies the enhanced respiratory modulation of sympathetic activity during and following hypoxia. To test this hypothesis, we propose a series of neurophysiologic experiments addressing the following specific aims: 1) to determine if inhibition of dl pontine activity blocks the transient and sustained increases in respiratory modulation of SNA during and following hypoxia, 2) to determine if activation of dl pons enhances respiratory modulation of SNA, and 3) to determine if respiratory-modulated KF neurons project to and excite RVLM neurons and if these KF neurons are activated during and after hypoxia. We will investigate the neural substrate controlling respiration and blood pressure, the transient and sustained consequences of brief hypoxemia on this control, and the modulation of this control by morbidity, i.e., the development of hypertension. We propose experiments in normo- and hypertensive rats as well as in cats to evaluate the dl pontine influence on SNA, the changes in this influence with transient hypoxemia and hypertension. These proposed studies examine the mechanism of up-regulation of sympathetic nerve activity that is associated with **sleep apnea.**

Website: http://crisp.cit.nih.gov/crisp/Crisp_Query.Generate_Screen

- **Project Title: CORE--BIOSTATISTICS AND RECRUITMENT**

  Principal Investigator & Institution: Maislin, Greg;; University of Pennsylvania 3451 Walnut Street Philadelphia, Pa 19104

  Timing: Fiscal Year 2003; Project Start 15-SEP-2003; Project End 31-AUG-2008

  Summary: The Biostatistical and Recruitment Core (formally, Human Assessment and Biostatistics Core) will continue to play an integral role as part of the Special Center of Research in Neurobiology of Sleep and **Sleep Apnea.**. The Core's specific aims (functions) are: 1) to meet the biostatistical needs of the two human study projects and two animal projects providing innovative solutions to data analysis challenges arising from these projects (all projects); 2) to provide centralized statistical programming and data management resources to the human projects (Projects by Weaver and Kuna and; 3) to apply existing methods and to make substantial contributions to the development of optimal statistical methods related to defining phenotypic characteristics associated with genetic control of homeostatic sleep regulation (Projects by Weaver and Kuna; 4) to support database management infrastructure development for the human and animal (all projects); 5) to promote the sound use of statistical principles and experimental design by all SCOR investigators (all projects); and 6) to provide the recruitment infrastructure enabling recruitment of apnea patients (Project by Weaver) and twins (Project by Kuna), the latter to be facilitated through a partnership with an existing twin cohort (PennTwins, E. Coccaro). Core C (Biostatistical and Recruitment Core) is comprised of a very experienced team of biostatisticians, statistical programmers, database managers, and clinical recruitment personnel. There exists a long history of collaboration among Core C staff and between Core C staff and SCOR investigators. The Core Leader of Core C has been SCOR biostatistician since its inception in 1988 and Core Leader since 1990. He has an extensive record of collaboration with SCOR investigators as well as original research in the field of sleep. The Core Leader (Senior Biostatistician) will be assisted by an Associate Biostatistician whose focus will be on providing biostatistical support to the animal studies and who is experienced in applying the mixed effects statistical models appropriate for the experimental designs proposed for these projects. Core C also includes a senior SAS TM statistical programmer with a longtime association with the Core who specializes in the development of analysis systems for implementation of complex statistical models that utilize data from multiple sources, an experienced database manager/statistical programmer with expertise in Access database development, and a data clerk. In addition, the Core Leader will be assisted by an experienced senior clinical study recruiter who will direct the human studies recruitment function, provide liaison with the PennTwins Cohort, and who will be assisted by additional recruitment staff. The experience, scientific interest, and long history of collaboration with SCOR investigators make the Biostatistical and Recruitment Core well-positioned to provide state-of-the-art statistical, database management, and human studies recruitment support to the projects while contributing to the advancement of statistical methods necessary to address the specific aims of the projects.

Website: http://crisp.cit.nih.gov/crisp/Crisp_Query.Generate_Screen

- **Project Title: CYCLICAL HYPOXIA--SUSCEPTIBILITY TO NEURONAL INJURY**

Principal Investigator & Institution: Haddad, Gabriel G.; Pediatrics; Yeshiva University 500 W 185Th St New York, Ny 10033

Timing: Fiscal Year 2002; Project Start 30-SEP-2000; Project End 31-AUG-2004

Summary: In considering how neurons and glia in the central nervous system respond, adapt or get injured when exposed to short and long term hypoxia using cellular and molecular techniques, it has now become clear that the responses to hypoxia and the mechanisms that underlie these responses are dependent on a number of factors, such as severity of hypoxia, history of previous hypoxic exposure, and ontogeny. One of the important consequences of obstructive sleep apnea/hypoventilation syndrome (OSHA) in both children and adults is a cyclical hypoxia with a major O2 desaturations that can occur with every cycle. This cyclical hypoxia generally occurs throughout the night and can repeat itself tens to hundreds of times. The effects of this cyclical hypoxia on behavior and neural function are ill defined. Although there has been a substantial amount of work to delineate the molecular mechanisms of O2 sensing, there are still many important questions that are unanswered. Because cortical neurons have been shown to be vulnerable to hypoxic exposure, the work will focus on the neocortex. Since 1) repetitive hypoxia in OSAH can be severe and can occur over prolonged periods of months and years and 2) the impact of cyclical hypoxia may depend on the level of CNS maturation, the investigators have formulated the following 3 specific hypothesis: 1) in-vivo cyclical hypoxia renders neurons more susceptible to injury, as evidenced by poor ionic homeostasis and mitochondrial dysfunction, especially when stressed subsequently with hypoxia: 2) in-vivo cyclical hypoxia alters gene expression and renders neurons more susceptible to programmed cell death, and 3) in vivo- cyclical hypoxia has a more profound impact on the inherent electrophysiologic properties of neurons, their metabolism, and their susceptibility to injury and cell death when exposure occurs in early life, as compared to that in the mature rodent. This work may shed light on mechanisms of a variety of diseases, including OSAH, apnea of infancy, postnatal cardiorespiratory diseases that reduce O2 delivery, myocardial infarcts, and cerebrovascular accidents and stroke.

Website: http://crisp.cit.nih.gov/crisp/Crisp_Query.Generate_Screen

- **Project Title: DEPRESSION, SLEEP DISORDERS AND CORONARY HEART DISEASE**

  Principal Investigator & Institution: Carney, Robert M.; Professor of Medical Psychology; Psychiatry; Washington University Lindell and Skinker Blvd St. Louis, Mo 63130

  Timing: Fiscal Year 2002; Project Start 30-SEP-2000; Project End 31-JUL-2004

  Summary: Description (adapted from the investigator's abstract): Clinical depression is a risk factor for mortality and morbidity after acute myocardial infarction (MI), yet little is known about the underlying mechanisms that account for this. The purpose of this study is to examine a potential mechanism, cardiovascular response to disordered sleep. Three months after an MI, 75 patients who meet the DSM-IV criteria for major depression will be selected and matched for gender, age, BMI to patients without depression. Polysomnography will be performed to determine the frequency and severity of cardiac responses to sleep disordered breathing and sleep architecture measures. The following hypotheses will be tested: 1) patients with depression have greater cardiac response to episodes of **sleep apnea** than non-depressed patients; 2) patients with depression without sleep disordered breathing have shorter REM latency, increased REM density, reduced slow wave sleep and worse sleep efficiency; 3) increased cardiac response to sleep disordered breathing, a shorter REM latency, increased REM density, decreased slow wave sleep are associated with electro cardio-graphic abnormalities predictive of cardiac events in post MI patients.

Website: http://crisp.cit.nih.gov/crisp/Crisp_Query.Generate_Screen

- **Project Title: DIASTOLIC DYSFUNCTION & ATRIAL FIBRILLATION IN ELDERLY**

  Principal Investigator & Institution: Tsang, Teresa S.;; Mayo Clinic Coll of Medicine, Rochester 200 1St St Sw Rochester, Mn 55905

  Timing: Fiscal Year 2003; Project Start 30-SEP-2003; Project End 31-AUG-2008

  Summary: (provided by applicant): Nonvalvular atrial fibrillation (AF) is an age-related public health problem associated with marked morbidity and mortality. We propose to prospectively examine the structural, hemodynamic, and neurohormonal/ inflammatory factors associated with first AF and investigate whether **sleep apnea** independently predicts AF. In Aim 1, we will confirm that diastolic function and left atrial (LA) volume are predictive of AF, incremental to clinical and other echocardiographic variables. We hypothesize that diastolic dysfunction and increased LA volume independently predict nonvalvular AF. In Aim 2, the distribution and correlates of changes in diastolic function and LA volume will be described, and we will determine whether serial measurements of these parameters provide incremental information on risk of AF. In Aim 3, we plan to explore how neurohormonal activation, specifically atrial natriuretic peptide (ANP) release, and the inflammatory marker, C-reactive protein (CRP), are associated with LA size, diastolic function, and AF development. We hypothesize that there is an independent role for ANP, but not for CRP, in the prediction of AF, after clinical and echocardiographic parameters have been considered. In Aim 4, we will assess relationships between arterial stiffness, diastolic function and LA volume, and determine whether arterial stiffness independently predicts AF. In Aim 5, we will evaluate **sleep apnea** as an independent predictor of AF development, after accounting for other clinical and echocardiographic risk factors. We plan to recruit 800 adults at significant risk for nonvalvular AF on the basis of age > 65 years and the presence of two or more known AF risk factors (hypertension, diabetes, history of coronary artery disease, and history of congestive heart failure). Prior history of AF, embolic stroke, organic valvular disease and congenital heart disease are the major exclusion criteria. All participants must be able to provide informed consent. Echocardiography, electrocardiogram (ECG), ANP, CRP, noninvasive arterial stiffness assessments (pulse wave velocity and augmentation index) will be obtained at baseline and annually thereafter. The Berlin Sleep Questionnaire to assess risk of **sleep apnea** will be completed by all participants at baseline and annually. A subgroup of 200 participants will undergo sleep studies, using a portable recording system, for detection of **sleep apnea.** Ascertainment of AF involves regular ECG surveillance, and patient report of AF with ECG confirmation. Identification of the cascade of factors contributing to AF development will have important implications in primary prevention of this major public health problem.

Website: http://crisp.cit.nih.gov/crisp/Crisp_Query.Generate_Screen

- **Project Title: DIFFERENTIAL VULNERABILITY TO MORBIDITIES OF SLEEP APNEA**

  Principal Investigator & Institution: Veasey, Sigrid C.; Professor; Medicine; University of Pennsylvania 3451 Walnut Street Philadelphia, Pa 19104

  Timing: Fiscal Year 2002; Project Start 30-SEP-2000; Project End 31-JUL-2004

  Summary: (Adapted from the applicant's abstract) **Obstructive sleep apnea** (OSA) affects over 2% of the adult population in the United states and is associated with significant neurobehavioral and cardiovascular morbidities. The morbidities of OSA relate at least in part to sleep fragmentation and intermittent hypoxia, both consequences of sleep-related collapse of the upper airway. In humans with OSA, there is significant variance in the manifestation of both the neurobehavioral and cardiovascular consequences. This variance in morbidity is only partially explained by the severity of disease. These investigators believe that vulnerability tot he morbidities of OSA is, in part, genetically-determined. For this proposal, they will focus on the substantial neurobehavioral consequences of **sleep apnea.** To begin to determine the genetic mechanisms contributing to the differential vulnerabilities, they will look separately at sleep fragmentation and chronic intermittent hypoxia (CIH) responses in inbred strains of mice. They will first expand the phenotypical response to sleep disruption to include, not only electroencephalographic changes, but also to characterize the neurobehavioral responses: sleepiness, changes in motor activity, learning, short and long term memory, vigilance and recovery for each of these parameters following exposure to sleep fragmentation or CIH. Responses to CIH will be characterized in the same manner. A high throughput screening algorithm will be validated against the full phenotypic responses to detect not only mutant sleep responses but mutant neurobehavioral responses characteristic of OSA. Therefore, this work provides an essential foundation for determining gene function in the susceptibility of sleepiness, impaired cognation and behavioral responses caused by **obstructive sleep apnea.** (End of Abstract.)

Website: http://crisp.cit.nih.gov/crisp/Crisp_Query.Generate_Screen

- **Project Title: EFFECT OF SLEEP DEPRIVATION ON INFLAMMATORY MARKERS**

  Principal Investigator & Institution: Wright, Kenneth P.; Associate Neuroscientist; Integrative Physiology; University of Colorado at Boulder Boulder, Co 80309

  Timing: Fiscal Year 2003; Project Start 01-JUN-2003; Project End 31-MAY-2005

  Summary: (provided by applicant): Heart disease, vascular disease and respiratory sleep disturbance are common and complex disorders with interactions among the cardiovascular, immune, neuroendocrine, sleep and circadian systems. Because inflammation in response to acute and chronic stress responsible for tissue damage associated with disease, recent efforts to understand mechanisms underlying these disorders have lead to studies that investigated inflammatory markers. These research efforts have revealed that high plasma levels of several novel inflammatory markers-cell adhesion molecules and pro-inflammatory cytokines-predict cardiovascular morbidity and mortality. High plasma levels of these markers are also reported to be associated with the severity of **sleep apnea.** A variety of stressors have been reported to initiate the inflammatory response, however, whether the stress of sleep deprivation also produces higher levels of these novel inflammatory markers is unknown. The current grant application takes an integrative physiological approach to understanding health consequences of sleep deprivation by forming new collaborations between experts in vascular physiology, neuronimmunophysiology, neuroendocrinology and sleep and circadian physiology. We are requesting funds to analyze existing biological specimens that were collected under controlled laboratory conditions from healthy women and men who underwent baseline sleep and wakefulness recording and 40 hours of total sleep deprivation. We propose to test the following specific hypothesis: 0 that acute total sleep deprivation will increase circulating levels of proinflammatory cell adhesion molecules; and ii) that acute total sleep deprivation will increase circulating levels of pro-inflammatory cytokines. We also propose to measure stress hormones to determine the relationship between changes in inflammatory cell adhesion molecules, cytokines and stress hormones during sleep deprivation and during baseline sleep. Because sleep loss is an independent risk factor for heart disease and chronic sleep loss is a consequence of **sleep apnea,** the results of the proposed study could have important implications for understanding the molecular mechanisms underlying these disorders and their association with sleep loss. This work could also have a significant impact on our understanding of the health consequences of sleep loss, which would have implications for public health and safety.

Website: http://crisp.cit.nih.gov/crisp/Crisp_Query.Generate_Screen

- **Project Title: EFFECTS OF SLEEP APNEA ON METABOLIC FUNCTION**

  Principal Investigator & Institution: Punjabi, Naresh M.; Assistant Professor; Medicine; Johns Hopkins University 3400 N Charles St Baltimore, Md 21218

  Timing: Fiscal Year 2003; Project Start 30-SEP-2003; Project End 31-JUL-2007

  Summary: (provided by applicant): **Sleep apnea** is a chronic condition associated with an increased risk of hypertension and cardiovascular disease. Recent data suggest that **sleep apnea** is also associated with metabolic dysfunction that is characterized by glucose intolerance and insulin resistance. Although several studies indicate that the association between **sleep apnea** and metabolic dysfunction is independent of confounders including obesity, it remains to be determined whether the association is causal. Moreover, whether intermittent hypoxemia and/or sleep fragmentation are in the putative causal pathway is unknown. The major objective of our proposal is to determine whether **sleep apnea** produces metabolic dysfunction and delineate the underlying mechanisms. Our primary hypothesis is that intermittent hypoxemia and recurrent arousals from sleep lead to acute and chronic changes in metabolic function. In Specific Aim 1, we will examine whether nighttime and daytime profiles of metabolic function differ between patients with **sleep apnea** and control subjects matched on age, race, gender, and obesity. We hypothesize that, compared to control subjects, patients with **sleep apnea** will demonstrate: a) marked abnormalities in nighttime profiles of glucose, insulin, and insulin secretion rate; b) impairment in daytime glucose tolerance, insulin sensitivity, and glucose effectiveness; and c) an increase in sympathetic activity and serum levels of leptin, cortisol, IL-6, and TNF-ct that are independently correlated with the severity of intermittent hypoxemia and frequency of arousals. In Specific Aim 2, we will examine whether experimental sleep fragmentation and **sleep apnea** (sleep fragmentation with intermittent hypoxemia) alter metabolic dysfunction in normal subjects. We hypothesize that: a) sleep fragmentation in normal individuals will alter nighttime profiles of glucose, insulin, and insulin secretion rate and worsen daytime measures of glucose tolerance, insulin resistance, and glucose effectiveness; b) intermittent hypoxemia in association with sleep fragmentation will potentiate the adverse effects of sleep fragmentation alone; and c) experimental sleep fragmentation and **sleep apnea** will increase sympathetic activity and serum levels of cortisol, leptin, TNF-alpha and IL-6 in association with impaired glucose homeostasis. Novel experimental paradigms have been developed to determine the independent roles of sleep fragmentation and **sleep apnea** on metabolic function. Given the epidemic of obesity and diabetes, understanding the role of **sleep apnea** as a risk factor for metabolic dysfunction has public health significance in terms of prevention and treatment of diabetes, hypertension, and cardiovascular disease.

Website: http://crisp.cit.nih.gov/crisp/Crisp_Query.Generate_Screen

- **Project Title: EFFECTS OF TREATING OBSTRUCTIVE SLEEP APNEA IN EPILEPSY**

  Principal Investigator & Institution: Malow, Beth A.; Associate Professor; Neurology; University of Michigan at Ann Arbor 3003 South State, Room 1040 Ann Arbor, Mi 481091274

  Timing: Fiscal Year 2002; Project Start 15-SEP-2002; Project End 31-JUL-2003

  Summary: (provided by applicant): Epilepsy affects approximately 2.5 million Americans, resulting in substantial disability. Because up to 30% of patients with epilepsy continue to have seizures despite appropriate treatment with antiepileptic medications, additional interventions to improve seizure control are needed. One approach to improving seizure control is to treat coexisting sleep disorders, such as **obstructive sleep apnea. Obstructive sleep apnea** (OSA) may exacerbate seizures via sleep fragmentation, sleep deprivation, or other pathophysiological processes that have not yet been determined. The investigators recently documented that OSA is common in epilepsy patients with seizures refractory to medical treatment. In addition, preliminary data in the form of retrospective case series by the investigators and others have suggested that treatment of OSA may improve seizure control. However, no prospective studies have been done to verify these findings. Proof that treating OSA is effective in reducing seizure frequency will require a multicenter Randomized Clinical Trial (RCT). This large RCT will test the hypothesis that treatment of OSA in patients with epilepsy refractory to medical treatment will reduce seizure frequency. In addition, the RCT will assess the impact of treating OSA on health-related quality of life and on daytime sleepiness, common concerns in epilepsy patients that are often attributable to antiepileptic medications or to frequent seizures rather than to a coexisting sleep disorder. The proposed aims of the Pilot Clinical Trial (PCT) are to determine critical information for the design of the RCT to allow for the testing of the above hypotheses in the RCT. In the PCT subjects 18 years and older with 4 or more seizures per month who meet survey criteria for OSA and other study criteria will be recruited at 3 different sites from epilepsy patients seen in clinical settings. A total of 60 subjects will be observed longitudinally through PSG confirmation and treatment of OSA and randomized to either therapeutic continuous positive airway pressure (CPAP) or sub-therapeutic (placebo or sham) CPAP in order to determine tolerability. Rates of adherence to therapeutic and sham CPAP and dropout rates due to antiepileptic drug changes during the treatment phase will be estimated. Specifically, the proposed PCT will: 1. Evaluate screening ranges on the **Sleep Apnea** scale of the Sleep Disorders Questionnaire (DA/SDQ), a survey instrument that is used to determine whether subjects are eligible for inclusion into the RCT. 2. Determine the necessity of performing two nights of PSG in patients with epilepsy. A second night of study increases the cost and may decrease recruitment in the RCT, but may be important to include given the night-to-night variability in the PSG and the potential for seizure occurrence during recordings. The working hypothesis is that one night of PSG will be sufficient for the RCT. 3. Determine rates of adherence to therapeutic and sham CPAP, dropout rates due to antiepileptic drug changes, and response rates will provide valuable data for planning the RCT. 4. Develop quality control measures to ensure accurate and consistent data collection among sites in the RCT, including aspects related to remote data entry and standardization of performance and interpretation of PSG studies across sites.

Website: http://crisp.cit.nih.gov/crisp/Crisp_Query.Generate_Screen

- **Project Title: EVALUATION OF DIAGNOSTIC TESTS FOR PEDIATRIC SLEEP APNEA**

  Principal Investigator & Institution: Rosen, Carol L.; Associate Professor; Pediatrics; Case Western Reserve University 10900 Euclid Ave Cleveland, Oh 44106

  Timing: Fiscal Year 2002; Project Start 01-AUG-2000; Project End 31-JUL-2005

  Summary: The candidate is an experienced academic clinician, trained in pediatric pulmonology and sleep medicine, who plans to re-train in clinical epidemiology. This award is expected to help transition the candidate's focus from physiological testing to clinical epidemiology. The candidate's career goals are to develop an independent research career concentrating on the identification, diagnosis, treatment, and outcomes assessment of **obstructive sleep apnea** (OSA) in children. The specific objective of the research proposal is the rigorous systematic assessment (reliability, accuracy, and cost effectiveness) of a diagnostic strategy for OSA in children that relies on clinical predictors and simplified home (unattended) monitoring. The candidate proposes a five-year training program with an experienced team of faculty mentors from strong research departments. This plan describes activities (advanced degree coursework, independent study, patient based clinical research) focused on developing skills in clinical epidemiology with immediate applications to the diagnosis of sleep disordered breathing in children. Specific activities in the plan include research training in statistical methods, experience with data analysis in large databases, supervised experience in preparation of grant proposals for individual research support, and training in the responsible conduct of research. The proposed research addresses important knowledge gaps about diagnostic testing for OSA in children and provides important new data for rational and cost-effective application of technology to an under-recognized health condition of children. Furthermore, clarification of the role of diagnostic testing and outcome assessment in pediatric OSA will be crucial for future randomized controlled trials of treatment efficacy; mechanistic studies, and population based studies of pediatric sleep disorder breathing. Finally, the proposal will provide a key training opportunity to foster the candidate's career development as a clinical epidemiologist with a commitment to patient based research in pediatric sleep medicine and pulmonology.

  Website: http://crisp.cit.nih.gov/crisp/Crisp_Query.Generate_Screen

- **Project Title: FAMILIAL AGGREGATION AND NATURAL HISTORY OF SLEEP APNEA**

  Principal Investigator & Institution: Redline, Susan S.; Professor of Pediatrics, Medicine & Epid; Medicine; Case Western Reserve University 10900 Euclid Ave Cleveland, Oh 44106

  Timing: Fiscal Year 2002; Project Start 01-AUG-1990; Project End 31-MAR-2006

  Summary: In this genetic-epidemiological study of **Obstructive Sleep Apnea** (OSA), we propose further investigation of the genetic and etiologic bases for OSA and OSA-associated co-morbidities in a unique, racially diverse family cohort (n= 2200) who have previously undergone overnight sleep studies. Cohort members from structurally informative families for OSA (n=700), most of whom will have had a genome scan performed prior to the study's inception, will undergo additional physiological and biochemical measurements and longitudinal follow-up to derive detailed phenotypic characterization of OSA and related cardiovascular disease (CVD) risk factors and subclinical disease. Newly available technology will be used to quantify specific and sensitive indices of obstructive breathing parameters and sleep fragmentation. These will provide more precise estimates of the OSA phenotype. Subjects also will undergo a biochemical profile and evaluations of vascular function, including assessment of novel CVD risk factors that may be related to OSA based on: i. common genes (e.g., that influence fat distribution); and/or ii. their role as indices of OSA disease severity (e.g., reflecting hypoxic or adrenergic tissue responses). Studies include: In-laboratory determination of sleep-related hypoxemia, arousal, airflow limitation and respiratory effort; b. In-laboratory assessment of biochemical markers, anthropometry, and physiological functions (many measured both in the evening and morning surrounding the sleep study); c. In-home re-assessment of the apnea hypopnea index (AHI), using comparable technology to what was used in the first 10 years of the study. Rigorous analyses, using a variance components-segregation analysis framework, will be used to: i. derive new phenotypes for OSA with estimates of heritability; ii. Assess genetic linkages for these phenotypes; iii. Determine metabolic and vascular responses to OSA-related nocturnal stresses; iv. Model longitudinal changes in the AHI. We will dissect the sharing or non-sharing of the genetic and non-genetic determinants of phenotypes potentially on a causal pathway leading to OSA. Additional longitudinal follow-up of this cohort will identify determinants of OSA progression, the co-variation of OSA with other risk factors, and its natural history. These studies will provide new data that will address the genetics and pathophysiology of OSA and associated traits. Such data are needed to address critical questions regarding the treatment and prevention of a disorder with a huge public health impact related to its high prevalence and associated co-morbidity (CVD, hypertension, sleepiness, impaired quality of life, accidents).

Website: http://crisp.cit.nih.gov/crisp/Crisp_Query.Generate_Screen

- **Project Title: GENETICS AND INTERMITTENT MYOCARDIAL HYPOXIA**

  Principal Investigator & Institution: Baker, John E.; Professor; Surgery; Medical College of Wisconsin Po Box26509 Milwaukee, Wi 532260509

  Timing: Fiscal Year 2002; Project Start 30-SEP-2000; Project End 31-AUG-2004

  Summary: The overall objective is to localize the gene(s) responsible for susceptibility to myocardial ischemia caused by intermittent hypoxia and characterize the physiology in a novel model system. Patients with **obstructive sleep apnea** have an increased cardiovascular morbidity and mortality. Diseases such as hypertension, hyperlipidemia and diabetes mellitus have an underlying genetic basis and represent risk factors for ischemic heart disease. However, the genetic components(s) underlying the impact of intermittent hypoxia on susceptibility to myocardial ischemia are unknown. It is hypothesized that genetic factors are responsible for increased susceptibility to myocardial ischemia caused by intermittent hypoxia in Dahl S rats compared with Brown Norway rats. This hypothesis will be tested by crossing the Brown Norway with Dahl S rat. The isolated heart model and coronary vessels will be used to facilitate discrete, well-controlled investigations of susceptibility to ischemia with and without prior intermittent hypoxia. A total genome scan will be performed to map quantitative trait loci (QTLs) involved in adaption to intermittent hypoxia and susceptibility to myocardial ischemia. Phenotypic difference between parents and the congenic derivatives resulting form ischemia and reperfusion will be characterized. The specific aims are to: 1) Determine the phenotypic differences of isolated hearts and coronary vessels from the parental strains by studying the responses to: ischemia alone and adaptation to intermittent hypoxia prior to ischemia; 2) Map the gene(s) responsible for adaption in intermittent hypoxia and susceptibility to myocardial ischemia using a total genome scan approach; 3) Develop congenic strains in response to: ischemia alone and adaptation to intermittent hypoxia prior to ischemia; and 4) Use microarray technology to study the expression of genes within the heart adapted to intermittent hypoxia. This project may provide detailed information regarding the genetic basis for adaption to intermittent hypoxia and susceptibility to myocardial ischemia in a genetic model system, which may prove useful for detailed physiological, biochemical and pharmacological assessment.

Website: http://crisp.cit.nih.gov/crisp/Crisp_Query.Generate_Screen

- **Project Title: HYPOTHALAMIC CONTROL OF ENERGY EXPENDITURE AND BREATHING**

  Principal Investigator & Institution: Mack, Serdia O.; Physiology and Biophysics; Howard University Washington, Dc 20059

  Timing: Fiscal Year 2004; Project Start 01-SEP-2004; Project End 31-AUG-2008

  Summary: (provided by applicant): Obesity results from an imbalance between energy intake and energy expenditure and often is associated with respiratory disorders including **obstructive sleep apnea,** hypoventilation, and hypoxemia. The consequences of obesity-related respiratory disease range from excessive daytime sleepiness to severe cardiopulmonary disorders. The mechanisms that are responsible for obesity-associated disorders remain to be clarified; however, it is likely that changes in neural input to regions of the brain that control the activity of upper airway dilating and chest wall pumping muscles are involved. Our preliminary data provide evidence that leptin, a neurohumoral substance with anorexigenic properties, modulates respiratory drive via an area in the brain that is above the brain stem. Thus, we hypothesize that leptin activates neurons in the hypothalamus that project to a common respiratory-related network within the medulla oblongata to alter respiratory patterns and/or responses to hypercapnia. In Specific Aim 1, we will identify the neurochemical content of hypothalamic neurons that are activated by leptin and project to a respiratory rhythm-generating region in the medulla by combining neuroanatomical and physiological techniques. The goal of Specific Aim 2 is to determine the effects of stimulation of hypothalamic cells that are activated by leptin on inspiratory-related neuronal activity in the respiratory-related network and on phrenic and hypoglossal nerves that control the activity of upper airway dilating and chest wall pumping muscles. In Specific Aim 3, we will use neurochemical, molecular, pharmacologic, and physiologic techniques to test our hypothesis that leptin affects respiratory activity and alters ventilatory responses to changes in chemical drive via hypothalamic neurons that are activated by leptin and project to the respiratory rhythm-generating region in the medulla. This information may serve as a basis for designing new evidence-based therapeutic strategies that can reduce or alleviate severe cardiopulmonary consequences of respiratory disorders.

  Website: http://crisp.cit.nih.gov/crisp/Crisp_Query.Generate_Screen

- **Project Title: HYPOXIA INDUCIBLE VEGF PRODUCTION IN SLEEP APNEA**

  Principal Investigator & Institution: Levy, Andrew P.;; Technion-Israel Institute of Technology Technion City Haifa,

  Timing: Fiscal Year 2002; Project Start 30-SEP-2000; Project End 31-AUG-2004

  Summary: Angiogenesis is the physiological adaptive response of a tissue to hypoxia. The coronary collateral circulation of the heart represents such an adaptive response and is an important determinant in the extent of tissue damage following myocardial infarction. Autopsy studies have shown that only 50 percent of patients with coronary artery stenosis develop collaterals. A fundamental challenge in understanding the angiogenic response to ischemia in the clinical setting is to elucidate the basis for interindividual differences in the degree of collateral blood vessel formation. Recent evidence demonstrates the importance of differences between patients in the hypoxic regulation of the angiogenic growth factor, vascular endothelial growth factor (VEGF) in determining the extent of collateral blood vessel formation. Specifically, individuals who upregulate VEGF to a greater degree with hypoxia have more collateral blood vessels. The investigators intend to investigate the mechanism for this heterogeneity in the hypoxic regulation of VEGF. Accordingly, the specific aims of this project are: (1) Analysis of interindividual heterogeneity in hypoxia-inducible VEGF production in patients with **obstructive sleep apnea** syndrome (OSAS) in vivo and in vitro and its relationship to coronary collaterals; (2) Determination of the molecular mechanism for interindividual heterogeneity in VEGF production in response to hypoxia. These studies may lead to the development of new strategies to increase VEGF production in the setting of ischemic heart disease and thereby promote therapeutic angiogenesis. In addition, understanding the mechanism of interindividual heterogeneity in VEGF production in response to hypoxia would be of tremendous importance for understanding and predicting the natural history of a wide variety of diseases involving VEGF including tumor angiogenesis, diabetic retinopathy, rheumatoid arthritis, and inflammatory bowel disease.

  Website: http://crisp.cit.nih.gov/crisp/Crisp_Query.Generate_Screen

- **Project Title: HYPOXIA-INDUCED AKT SIGNALING MODULE IN NEURONAL CELLS.**

  Principal Investigator & Institution: Gozal, Evelyne; Pediatrics; University of Louisville Jouett Hall, Belknap Campus Louisville, Ky 40292

Timing: Fiscal Year 2003; Project Start 01-AUG-2003; Project End 31-JUL-2007

Summary: (provided by applicant): The purpose of this proposal is to elucidate hypoxia-induced Akt-related pathways induced in neuronal PC- 12 and RN46A neuronal cells by sustained hypoxia and by intermittent hypoxia, and to determine how these signaling pathways affect cell survival. We will test the hypothesis that hypoxia-induced interactions between different signaling molecules within the Akt signaling module, modulate tolerance or vulnerability to sustained and intermittent hypoxia in neuronal cells. We propose: (1) To identify, using proteomic approaches, members of the Akt signaling module in normoxic and hypoxic neuronal cells, and to identify differences in Akt-associated proteins during sustained and intermittent hypoxia; (2) To characterize protein-protein interactions within the Akt signaling modules; (3) To identify selective Akt - protein interactions within the signaling module that underlie neuronal survival to sustained and intermittent hypoxia; (4). To examine the effect of disruption of protein-protein interactions within the Akt signaling module on downstream genes involved in regulation of hypoxia-induced cellular apoptosis. We will use proteomic techniques, SDS-PAGE and MALDI-MS to identify the Akt-binding proteins co-immunoprecipitating with Akt in normoxic cells or cells exposed to sustained or intermittent hypoxia. Interactions of the components of the Akt signalosomes will be determined by TnT coupled transcription, translation, co-immunoprecipitation, and GST pull-down methods. Transformer kits will be used to make in frame and serial deletion mutants of Akt and its binding proteins in order to identify their Akt docking sites. Finally we will introduce into the cells TAT-fusion peptides corresponding to specific docking sites of targeted proteins binding to Akt signaling module, and disrupt their interaction with the Akt signaling complex to assess the effect of protein association/dissociation with the Akt signaling module, on cell survival to sustained and intermittent hypoxia. These studies will provide the groundwork for future intervention strategies aiming to prevent neuronal cell loss in diseases associated with intermittent and sustained hypoxia, such as **sleep apnea** and lung disease.

Website: http://crisp.cit.nih.gov/crisp/Crisp_Query.Generate_Screen

- **Project Title: IMPACT OF SLEEP DISORDERS ON HEALTH**

  Principal Investigator & Institution: Kryger, Meir H.;; University of Manitoba Winnipeg R3t 2N2, Canada Winnipeg, Mb

  Timing: Fiscal Year 2002; Project Start 01-APR-2000; Project End 31-MAR-2004

Summary: Sleep disorders are very common. The impact of these disorders on a person's long term health is unclear. The purpose of this project is to determine the cost to the health care system of patients with untreated sleep disorders and then to determine the change in cost with diagnosis and treatment. Hypotheses: Untreated sleep disorder patients (with **sleep apnea,** narcolepsy, and insomnia) are heavier consumers of health care services than age and sex matched controlled subjects and treatment will reduce these costs. Aims: The applicant will examine healthcare utilization data (and what patients were being treated for) of a large number of patients five years before diagnosis and five years after diagnosis and compare them to controls matched by age, gender, and postal code. The data will be obtained in a community with unrestricted access to medical care and where all the data is stored on a central database. To measure the use of medical services the applicant will analyze all doctors' claims and data from all hospitalization as well as use of prescription drugs. The applicant will establish whether treatment of these disorders reduces the consumption of healthcare services in these patients. The applicant expects to find fewer physicians visits, particularly for cardiovascular disease, neuro-psychiatric disease and general medical evaluations and for **sleep apnea,** fewer hospitalizations, particularly for cardiovascular disease and respiratory failure.

Website: http://crisp.cit.nih.gov/crisp/Crisp_Query.Generate_Screen

- **Project Title: INSULIN RESISTANCE IN PCOS--SEQUELAE AND TREATMENT**

  Principal Investigator & Institution: Legro, Richard S.; Associate Professor; Obstetrics-Gynecology; Pennsylvania State Univ Hershey Med Ctr 500 University Drive Hershey, Pa 170332390

  Timing: Fiscal Year 2002; Project Start 01-APR-2001; Project End 31-MAR-2006

  Summary: (Adapted from the applicant's description): The immediate goals of the PI are to expand the focus of his research from familial forms of polycystic ovary syndrome (PCOS), and genetic influences on the development of the syndrome into areas with even greater clinical impact. Specifically the goals of this application are to 1) identify other unrecognized morbidity that results from insulin resistance in PCOS and in the long term. 2) expand the clinical trials of improving insulin sensitivity as a primary treatment modality in PCOS. Another long-term goal is to develop within the medical center a cadre of investigators interested in PCOS patient-oriented research. The overall hypothesis of this proposal is that insulin resistance is the fundamental pathophysiologic defect in women with PCOS, that its effects can be protean and unrecognized, and that metabolic abnormalities worsen with age. Our preliminary studies suggest that insulin resistance is major contributor to both the etiology of PCOS and its association with **sleep apnea.** We propose further studies to clarify the role of insulin resistance in both PCOS and control female populations on sleep disorders. We theorize that there is enhanced steroidogenesis in endometrial glandular and stromal cells from women with PCOS and this is further stimulated by hyperinsulinemia. We intend to study these hypotheses in endometrial tissue form PCOS women and appropriate controls. Our preliminary experience suggests that insulin resistance over time will lead to a worsening of glucose tolerance and other metabolic markers in PCOS women with an improvement in reproductive abnormalities such as anovulation and hyperandrogenemia. We propose to identify clinical interventions in PCOS women that will improve insulin sensitivity and manifestations of the syndrome. Improving insulin action through diet and exercise, with and without weight loss, will result in lowered circulating insulin levels, lowered androgens and increased ovulatory frequency rate in PCOS women.

Website: http://crisp.cit.nih.gov/crisp/Crisp_Query.Generate_Screen

- **Project Title: INTERTRIGEMINAL REGION CONTROL OF APNEA**

  Principal Investigator & Institution: Radulovacki, Miodrag G.; Professor; Medicine; University of Illinois at Chicago 1737 West Polk Street Chicago, Il 60612

  Timing: Fiscal Year 2004; Project Start 01-JAN-2004; Project End 31-DEC-2007

  Summary: (provided by applicant): **Sleep apnea syndrome** affects at least 3% - 5% of the adult population in this country and available data suggest that significant morbidity and increased mortality result from this disorder. Despite 40 years of intensive investigation, the brainstem mechanisms responsible for, or permissive of, sleep-related apnea remain unknown. Our work to develop and characterize a rodent model of sleep-related breathing disorder makes it feasible to systematically examine the detailed brainstem mechanisms of apnea. A brainstem anatomical pathway recently has been demonstrated in which the intertrigeminal region (ITR) of the lateral pons is posited as a key regulatory site for apneic reflexes. The ITR is innervated by sensory subnuclei of the solitary tract that receive inputs from the ninth and tenth cranial nerves; each of which mediate airway-protective apneic reflexes. Moreover, the ITR sends direct projections to respiratory rhythm generating neurons in the medulla. Although the ITR thus may represent an important airway reflex integrating site, no physiological or pathophysiological role has yet been demonstrated for this region. We present novel preliminary evidence that the ITR dampens vagally-mediated reflex apnea, an effect that appears to be mediated by glutamatergic neurotransmission and may result from short term potentiation. Further, we show that focal lesions of the ITR lead to dramatically increased apnea expression during sleep. The overall goals of this proposal are 1) to identify the neural mechanisms by which the ITR modulates apneic reflexes, 2) to demonstrate the functional role of the ITR in **sleep apnea** genesis and 3) to establish the impact of sleep/wake state changes on ITR function. To achieve these goals, we will employ pressure microinjections to enhance and impair ITR functional activity and to test the strength of monoaminergic and cholinergic inputs on ITR function. The acute impact of these manipulations on respiratory pattern and apneic reflexes will be tested in anesthetized rats. Sustained effects following focal lesions will be tested by behavioral state and cardiorespiratory monitoring in sleeping rats. The proposed neurochemical manipulations of the ITR provide a systematic approach to define the importance of this region in modulating both reflexive and spontaneous sleep-related apnea and to identify the initial steps in the signaling pathway by which this region modulates apnea expression.

Website: http://crisp.cit.nih.gov/crisp/Crisp_Query.Generate_Screen

- **Project Title: IS INSOMNIA A MODIFIABLE RISK FACTOR FOR MDD?**

  Principal Investigator & Institution: Perlis, Michael L.; Psychiatry; University of Rochester Orpa - Rc Box 270140 Rochester, Ny 14627

  Timing: Fiscal Year 2004; Project Start 01-APR-2004; Project End 31-JAN-2007

  Summary: (provided by applicant): Recent studies have shown that insomnia may represent a vulnerability factor for Major Depression (MDD). These findings suggest that if remitted patients with recurrent MDD received treatment for their insomnia, this intervention might prevent or delay relapse/recurrence, or at least diminish the intensity of subsequent episodes. We propose to evaluate this hypothesis by undertaking a preliminary study on the effects of Behavioral treatment for insomnia on the clinical course of patients with remitted recurrent MDD. Specifically, we propose to randomly assign 45 patients with remitted recurrent Major Depression to one of two conditions behavioral treatment for insomnia (n=30) or to a contract control monitor only group (n=15) behavior therapy was selected because this treatment modality has demonstrated efficacy with respect to insomnia yet is not likely to have direct antidepressant effects. Sleep and depression symptoms will be monitored on a weekly basis prior to treatment initiation (3-4 weeks), during active treatment (8 weeks), and for a period of up to 33 months. Monitoring will require that subjects complete daily sleep diaries, weekly Beck Depression Inventories (BDI), and monthly clinical interviews. The BDI will be used to ascertain when subjects exhibit a worsening of their depressive symptoms and will serve as a prompt for a clinical evaluation to determine whether there has been a relapse/recurrence. Weekly diaries will be used to determine 1) the acute effects of the insomnia treatment, 2) the long term efficacy of the behavioral intervention, and 3) the extent to which sleep related complaints are prodromal to new onset episodes. Monthly interviews will be used to monitor and confirm clinical state. In addition, polysomnographic (PSG) data will be acquired prior to and following treatment. These data will be used to rule out occult sleep disorders (e.g., **sleep apnea** and PLMs), to objectively assess severity of insomnia symptoms prior to and following treatment, and to explore, in a preliminary way, the extent to which sleep architecture variables (e.g. reduced REM latency) independently predict treatment outcome, clinical course, and/or how these measures interact with self report sleep continuity measures. It is hypothesized that behavioral treatment for insomnia in patients with remitted MDD will be associated with less depressive symptomatology during remission, longer periods of remission, less severe new onset episodes and better responses to treatment for recurrent episodes Data for each of these hypotheses will be used to calculate effect sizes and to conduct power estimates. These analyses, if they provide good feasibility data, will be used as the foundation for a R01 level application. Ultimately, If one or more of these hypotheses are borne out in the larger follow up study, this will strongly suggest that 1) CBT for insomnia may be an important strategy for the management of recurrent MDD, and 2) insomnia is not only a symptom of MDD, but also a factor in the development of the disease.

Website: http://crisp.cit.nih.gov/crisp/Crisp_Query.Generate_Screen

- **Project Title: K+-CHANNELS REGULATING REM-RELATED CHOLINGERGIC NEURONS**

  Principal Investigator & Institution: Leonard, Christopher S.; Profesor; Physiology; New York Medical College Valhalla, Ny 10595

  Timing: Fiscal Year 2002; Project Start 30-SEP-1999; Project End 31-AUG-2004

  Summary: How and why we sleep are central unsolved questions in medicine. Nearly 40 million people in the United States are estimated to experience chronic or intermittent sleep disorders such as narcolepsy, **sleep apnea,** restless leg syndrome and insomnia. Traditional approaches have identified several neuronal populations whose interplay is important in generating sleep and wakefulness. How that interplay is established, how it is altered and its cellular and molecular consequences, remain poorly understood. The long-term objective of this proposal is to determine the molecular identity and function of ion channels and receptors expressed by sleep-related neurons in order to understand the molecular mechanisms controlling sleep generation. This application focuses on the identity and function of a family of K+ channels subunit genes in controlling activity of mesopontine cholinergic neurons which are believed to play a pivotal role in the generation of wakefulness and REM sleep. Our central hypothesis is that K+ channels formed by Kv3 subunits regulate action potential shape, intracellular Ca2+ levels, repetitive firing and the release of transmitter from mesopontine cholinergic neurons. To test this hypothesis we will use pharmacological methods with whole-cell patch clamp recordings in brain slices from wild-type and Kv3 knock-out mice. The results of these studies will 1) identify and verify the intrinsic electrophysiological properties of important REM-sleep related neurons in mouse; 2) determine the molecular identity and function of native K+ channels formed by Kv3 subunits; 3) elucidate new mechanisms controlling the activity and release of transmitter by REM sleep-related neurons; 4) identify novel functions of Kv3 channels which have previously been associated with the fast-spiking phenotype rather than broad-spiking phenotype of brainstem cholinergic neurons. These results will contribute to our understanding of the molecular basis of sleep regulation as well as advancing the mouse as a platform for future sleep research.

Website: http://crisp.cit.nih.gov/crisp/Crisp_Query.Generate_Screen

- **Project Title: LONGITUDINAL STUDY--SLEEP-DISORDERED BREATHING/PREGNANCY**

  Principal Investigator & Institution: Pien, Grace W.; Medicine; University of Pennsylvania 3451 Walnut Street Philadelphia, Pa 19104

  Timing: Fiscal Year 2002; Project Start 20-JAN-2002; Project End 31-DEC-2006

  Summary: (prepared by applicant): Candidate's Plans/Training: The patient-oriented research in sleep medicine and epidemiology. Training will include closely mentored completion of the research protocol, advanced epidemiological course work in patient-oriented research advanced training in sleep medicine and respiratory neurobiology. Environment: The University of Pennsylvania is a uniquely suited environment for this training award. The Center for Sleep and Respiratory Neurobiology will provide a mentored experience in patient-oriented research. The Center for Clinical Epidemiology and Biostatistics will provide advanced didactic training. Research: During pregnancy, physiologic changes including gestational weight gain take place that may place women at increased risk for the development of sleep-disordered breathing (SDB). Snoring, which is a common symptom of SDB, is a frequent complaint among pregnant women, experienced on a habitual b y as many as 23 percent of women by the end of the final trimester of pregnancy. The possibility regnant women snorers may manifest sleep-disordered breathing has remained largely unexplored. In general population, baseline obesity and weight gain are both associated with an increased risk for sleep-disordered breathing. It is our central hypothesis that pregnancy is a time of accelerated development of sleep disordered breathing in women, in which the degree of increase is likely to be larger in women with elevated baseline body mass index (BMI) or greater gestational weight gain. This protocol examines whether the number of sleep-disordered breathing events increases in women over the course of pregnancy and how baseline weight status and weight gain during pregnancy impact the degree of SDB. The specific aims of the study proposal are: 1) to test the hypothesis that the respiratory disturbance index (RDI), a measure of the number of abnormal respiratory events hourly during sleep, increases over the course of pregnancy; and to determine whether the degree of increase is greater in obese women; and 2) to identify specific clinical characteristics that influence the risk for clinically significant increases in the severity of SDB.

Website: http://crisp.cit.nih.gov/crisp/Crisp_Query.Generate_Screen

- **Project Title: MECHANISMS AND LOCALIZATION OF CO2 SENSITIVE CNS NEURONS**

  Principal Investigator & Institution: Richerson, George B.; Associate Professor; Neurology; Yale University 47 College Street, Suite 203 New Haven, Ct 065208047

  Timing: Fiscal Year 2002; Project Start 01-AUG-1995; Project End 31-JUL-2006

  Summary: (provided by applicant): The major source of feedback for control of breathing comes from central respiratory chemoreceptor that monitor blood CO2 levels. Dysfunction of these neurons occurs in many common diseases, including chronic obstructive pulmonary disease (COPD), **sleep apnea,** and possibly sudden infant death syndrome (SIDS). The first step in finding specific treatments for these diseases is to identify the neurons responsible for chemoreception, and define their mechanisms. Although the central chemoreceptors were localized to the ventrolateral medulla (VLM) 40 years ago, the specific neurons responsible have still not been clearly identified. We recently obtained evidence that serotonin-containing neurons within the VLM are central respiratory chemoreceptors, but the majority of neurons with identical properties are located in the medullary raphe. This is exciting, because chemosensitivity of serotonergic neurons could provide a biological basis for the interaction between sleep and breathing. The proposed work is aimed at further defining the cellular mechanisms of these neurons, and the role that they play in central chemoreception. We propose to use a combination of patch clamp recordings from neurons in tissue culture and brain slices, imaging of intracellular pH, immunohistochemistry, confocal microscopy, and computer modeling to address basic unanswered questions about chemosensitive raphe neurons. 1) Do medullary raphe neurons have properties that would make them uniquely specialized to sense changes in blood CO2? We will look at their anatomical relationship with blood vessels, the co-transmitters they contain, and their projections. 2) Are there differences between chemosensitive neurons in the medullary raphe and the VLM? 3) Does chemosensitivity of midbrain raphe neurons explain the arousal that occurs in response to hypercapnia during sleep? 4) What ion channels are responsible for chemosensitivity? 5) Does CO2 act through a change in intracellular pH alone? 6) Can the depression of breathing during sleep be explained in part by the effects of reticular activating system neurotransmitters on raphe neurons? Disturbances of breathing are common in human diseases, particularly during sleep. Understanding the basic mechanisms involved in modulation of neuronal activity by CO2, and the mechanisms by which breathing is affected by sleep, may help provide successful treatment for these diseases.

Website: http://crisp.cit.nih.gov/crisp/Crisp_Query.Generate_Screen

- **Project Title: MECHANISMS MEDIATING C/V DISEASE IN CHILDREN WITH OSA**

  Principal Investigator & Institution: Amin, Raouf S.;; Children's Hospital Med Ctr (Cincinnati) 3333 Burnet Ave Cincinnati, Oh 452293039

  Timing: Fiscal Year 2003; Project Start 01-APR-2003; Project End 31-MAR-2008

  Summary: (provided by applicant): **Obstructive sleep apnea** (OSA) is an important clinical disorder occurring in men, women, and children with a prevalence of 4%, 2% and 1-3%, respectively. OSA is under active study in adults and is definitely linked with increased cardiovascular morbidity, even in its mild to moderate clinical forms. In contrast, OSA has not been well studied in children and the potential deleterious consequences on cardiovascular function have received little or no attention. Our goal is to examine in children 1) The interaction between OSA and baroreflex dysfunction, 2) The relation of OSA severity and baroreflex dysfunction to abnormalities in blood pressure control during wakefulness and sleep, 3) The association of the diminished baroreflex gain and impaired blood pressure control with an index of end organ damage, the left ventricular mass index, and 4) Whether effective treatment of OSA results in significant improvement in baroreceptor function, blood pressure control and a decrease in left ventricular mass index. We will accomplish these aims by studying 8-12 year old children with OSA and a matched group of normal children in a cross-sectional design. We will study baroreceptor function, 24-hour ambulatory blood pressure and left ventricular mass index. Baroreceptor function will be measured by non-invasive techniques based on combined computer analysis of heart rate and blood pressure measured by portapres. 24-hour ambulatory blood pressure will be measured by a Spacelab monitor and left ventricular mass index will be measured by direct M-mode echocardiogram. In a longitudinal study we will study the effect of adequate treatment of OSA on baroreceptor function, daytime and nocturnal blood pressure and left ventricular mass index. We will follow a cohort of children with OSA and a matched group of normal controls for a period of 12 months after treatment of the disorder. Results are expected to show that children with OSA have decreased baroreceptor sensitivity, elevated nocturnal blood pressure and increased left ventricular mass index and that effective therapy for OSA, as determined by polysomnography, will improve or normalize baroreceptor sensitivity as well as nocturnal blood pressures and will lead to a decrease in left ventricular mass index.

Website: http://crisp.cit.nih.gov/crisp/Crisp_Query.Generate_Screen

- **Project Title: MECHANISMS OF DIFFERENTIAL SLEEPINESS IN SLEEP APNEA**

  Principal Investigator & Institution: Weaver, Terri E.;; University of Pennsylvania 3451 Walnut Street Philadelphia, Pa 19104

  Timing: Fiscal Year 2003; Project Start 15-SEP-2003; Project End 31-AUG-2008

  Summary: The purpose of this proposal is to explore potential operating mechanisms in the differential sleepiness observed in patients with equivalent degrees of **obstructive sleep apnea** (OSA). Within a given level of disease severity, i.e., number of respiratory disturbances during sleep, inter-individual differences, or differential vulnerability to sleepiness, have been noted in both subjectively measured and objectively measured daytime sleepiness. The reason for this phenomenon remains unclear. Critical to the management of patients with OSA is the understanding of mechanisms associated with the development of daytime sleepiness. We hypothesize that the variance in daytime sleepiness (EDS)will have a substantial trait component in addition to state-related factors among patients with equivalent levels of OSA severity. To systematically identify sources of EDS variance in sleepy and non-sleepy OSA patients, the specific aims of this study will determine: 1) state-specific variance related to sleep duration, obesity and fat distribution, specific comorbidities, and use of certain medications; 2) mis-estimation of severity of sleep disordered breathing from night-to-night variability in respiratory disturbances; 3) underlying trait associated with differential vulnerability to the sleepiness-producing effects of OSA. Using actigraphy and diaries to document sleep duration and both objective and subjective evaluations of sleepiness, Protocol A will classify 260 newly diagnosed OSA subjects as sleepy vs. non-sleepy and will document inter-individual differences in sleepiness among patients with similar disease severity caused by sleep history, obesity and fat distribution, specific comorbidities, and use of certain medications. Controlling for the variance identified in Protocol A, Protocol B will determine the degree to which inter-individual differences in sleepiness in 180 untreated OSA subjects with similar disease severity is a consequence of night-to-night variability in the occurrence of sleep disordered breathing documented by 7 consecutive nights of home sleep studies. Such night-to-night variability would reduce the reliability of single night determinations of apnea severity. Finally, in Protocol C we will determine if inter-individual differences in sleepiness remain after accounting for the variance explained by the clinical factors identified in Protocol A and the variance explained by mis-estimation of severity of sleep disordered breathing documented in Protocol B. In Protocol C, 60 patients (30 sleepy, 30 non-sleepy) will be matched on initial apnea severity and a set of a priori sleepiness factors will undergo 38 hrs of sleep deprivation in a laboratory to determine the existence of an underlying trait for daytime sleepiness.

Website: http://crisp.cit.nih.gov/crisp/Crisp_Query.Generate_Screen

- **Project Title: MENOPAUSE AND MIDLIFE AGING EFFECTS ON SLEEP DISORDERS**

  Principal Investigator & Institution: Young, Terry B.; Professor of Prventative Medicine; Population Health Sciences; University of Wisconsin Madison 750 University Ave Madison, Wi 53706

  Timing: Fiscal Year 2002; Project Start 15-JAN-1997; Project End 31-DEC-2006

Summary: (provided by applicant): The long-range goals of this ongoing longitudinal study of midlife aging in women are to accurately quantify the associations of menopause with the development and progression of **sleep apnea** and diminished sleep quality and to identify factors that influence the associations. Understanding the role of menopause in the development of **sleep apnea** and diminished sleep quality has important clinical and public health significance. **Sleep apnea** and diminished sleep quality are associated with significant cardiovascular morbidity, depression, and decrements in daytime performance. Because menopause will become a persistent state in nearly every woman during her lifetime, even a small effect on **sleep apnea** and insomnia, the major sleep disorders, would translate into significant morbidity. Furthermore, if associations are causal, understanding whether hormone replacement therapy or other factors significantly modify a menopause-sleep disorder link may lead to interventions that could reduce the occurrence and severity of sleep disorders in mid- and later life. The proposed study is designed to: 1) Test the hypothesis that changes over the continuum of pre to post menopause increase the incidence and progression of sleep disordered breathing, adjusted for baseline age, body composition, and other potential confounders, 2) investigate the effects of change in body composition during midlife on associations of menopause and **sleep apnea,** 3) quantify the risk of insomnia, hypersomnia and diminished sleep quality attributable to early, middle and late perimenopause and post menopause, 4) investigate protective effects of hormone replacement therapy on sleep problems, and 5) investigate genetic vulnerability to diminished sleep quality during menopause. To accomplish these aims, we propose additional research on our unique longitudinal cohort of midlife women, with 7-15 years of previously collected polysomnographic and other data with a) new data collected from overnight in-laboratory protocols with polysomnography conducted at 4-year intervals on 621 women enrolled in the Wisconsin Sleep Cohort Study, b) new data collected semi-annually by in-home polysomnography and other procedures and monthly diaries on menstrual characteristics and sleep problems on a subset of 280 women over their pre to peri to post menopausal years.

Website: http://crisp.cit.nih.gov/crisp/Crisp_Query.Generate_Screen

- **Project Title: MENTORED PATIENT-ORIENTED RESEARCH CAREER DEVELOPMENT AW**

  Principal Investigator & Institution: Gurubhagavatula, Indira Md; Medicine; University of Pennsylvania 3451 Walnut Street Philadelphia, Pa 19104

Timing: Fiscal Year 2002; Project Start 01-AUG-2000; Project End 31-JUL-2005

Summary: PROPOSAL (Adapted from the applicant's abstract): Characterized by intermittent airway closure during sleep, OSA is extremely prevalent, afflicting 2-4% of Americans. If left untreated, a large body of evidence convincingly shows that OSA can lead to daytime hypertension. In fact, 20-30% of patients with OSA will have hypertension, and 40% of patients with hypertension have occult OSA. The question then is how to identify patients who have OSA from among this high-risk population of individuals with hypertension. Polysomnography (PSG), the current diagnostic gold standard, is expensive and inconvenient. Several simple techniques to screen for OSA are available: questionnaires, craniofacial measurements, nocturnal oximetry and airflow monitoring devices. However, no one has compared their relative efficacies or costs in one unified population. The investigator proposes to compare these screening tools against full PSG's in a cohort of patients at high risk for OSA, i.e., outpatients with hypertension. Among the cases of OSA subsequently identified, the applicant next proposes to evaluate outcomes of treatment of OSA with continuous positive airway pressure (CPAP) in a randomized, placebo-controlled trial. The specific aims, therefore, are: 1) to compare the accuracy of several screening strategies for OSA in outpatients with hypertension; 2) to determine their relative economic costs; and 3) to determine the effect of CPAP therapy on blood pressure (BP) and sympathetic activity during sleep and awake states in OSA patients with hypertension. These projects are extraordinarily important. They have the potential to lead to dramatic changes in the approach to management of the patient with hypertension. Along with a complementary program of didactic training, they will constitute a strong foundation of experience for the applicant in her goal of becoming an independent clinical investigator.

Website: http://crisp.cit.nih.gov/crisp/Crisp_Query.Generate_Screen

- **Project Title: MICROCIRCULATORY EFFECTS OF INTERMITTENT HYPOXIA**

  Principal Investigator & Institution: Johnson, Paul C.; Professor and Head; Bioengineering; University of California San Diego La Jolla, Ca 920930934

  Timing: Fiscal Year 2003; Project Start 30-SEP-2000; Project End 31-AUG-2005

  Summary: The purpose of this study is to test certain hypotheses regarding the acute and chronic effects of intermittent hypoxia on microvascular and parenchymal cell function through in vivo microcirculatory studies. Using the cremaster muscle preparation of the anesthetized rat, Specific Aim 1 will test the hypothesis that reduction of oxygen concentration in the inspired air in the range of 7 percent to 10 percent for 30 s to 3 min duration causes microcirculatory hypoxia and changes in blood flow and vascular tone due to neural influences and local regulatory mechanisms. This aim will also test the hypothesis that chronic episodes of hypoxia alter normal control mechanisms that regulate vascular tone of arterioles in accordance with local oxygen levels; specifically prostaglandins, NO and metabolites of cytochrome P-450. Specific Aim 2 will test the hypothesis that reduction of oxygen in the inspired air causes oxygen levels in tissue surrounding the venous portion of the microvascular network to fall below critical levels, causing a shift in the redox state of mitochondria in the parenchymal cells. This aim will also test the hypothesis that intermittent hypoxia leads to tissue injury and increased expression of venular P-selectin, leukocyte adhesion and rolling oxidative stress, and parenchymal cell injury and death. Since some of the changes seen in sleep hypoxia are neural in origin, a subset of these studies will involve use of unanesthetized animals with an implanted window to study the microcirculation. By reproducing the hypoxic conditions in the microcirculation and tissue like present in **sleep apnea,** the investigators aim to identify key changes and provide a better rationale for treatment.

Website: http://crisp.cit.nih.gov/crisp/Crisp_Query.Generate_Screen

- **Project Title: NASAL OBSTRUCTION AND SLEEP APNEA TREATMENT OUTCOMES**

  Principal Investigator & Institution: Weaver, Edward M.; Otolaryngology/Head and Neck Surgery; University of Washington Grant & Contract Services Seattle, Wa 98105

  Timing: Fiscal Year 2003; Project Start 01-AUG-2003; Project End 31-JUL-2008

  Summary: (provided by applicant): **Obstructive sleep apnea** syndrome is characterized by symptomatic recurrent upper airway obstructions during sleep that may result in serious physiologic abnormalities, medical risks, and quality of life deficits. It occurs in 2 - 4% of adults and is a target disorder for Healthy People 2010. Providing continuous positive airway pressure (CPAP) represents first-line therapy. Surgical treatment may serve as an adjunct to CPAP or as a second line definitive therapy, but surgical effectiveness data are lacking. The principal investigator's long-term goal is to evaluate rigorously surgical treatment of the nasal, oral, hypopharyngeal, and laryngeal airways for **sleep apnea** as an independent investigator. For the period of this award, he proposes to develop sophisticated surgical outcomes research skills through a program of didactics, conferences, focused clinical activity in the Sleep Disorders Center, and hands-on research with the guidance of expert advisors. This research proposal focuses on the role of nasal obstruction, and its surgical correction, as a means of improving clinically important outcomes of CPAP therapy. The specific aims are to: 1. Determine whether nasal obstruction influences CPAP treatment outcomes above and beyond other behavioral and biomedical factors in a prospective inception cohort study. 2. Conduct a pilot trial to examine whether surgical treatment for nasal obstruction improves CPAP outcomes. This single-site pilot trial will provide the principal investigator with clinical trials experience as well as data on logistical, feasibility, and measurement issues for a definitive trial. Future independent investigations of other surgically correctible anatomic abnormalities associated with **sleep apnea** will follow the model of this proposed research plan.

Website: http://crisp.cit.nih.gov/crisp/Crisp_Query.Generate_Screen

- **Project Title: NEUROBEHAVIORAL CONSEQUENCES OF SLEEP APNEA IN CHILDREN**

  Principal Investigator & Institution: Gottlieb, Daniel J.; Associate Professor; Medicine; Boston University Medical Campus 715 Albany St, 560 Boston, Ma 02118

  Timing: Fiscal Year 2002; Project Start 20-SEP-1999; Project End 31-JUL-2004

  Summary: This abstract is not available.

  Website: http://crisp.cit.nih.gov/crisp/Crisp_Query.Generate_Screen

- **Project Title: NEUROMUSCULAR CONTROL OF THE PHARYNGEAL AIRWAY**

  Principal Investigator & Institution: Fregosi, Ralph F.; Associate Professor; Physiology; University of Arizona P O Box 3308 Tucson, Az 857223308

  Timing: Fiscal Year 2002; Project Start 10-APR-1998; Project End 31-MAR-2004

  Summary: (Adapted from the applicant's abstract): The long-term objective of this proposal is to test the hypothesis that the muscles that protrude and retract the tongue (genioglossus and hypoglossus/styloglossus muscles, respectively) are co-activated during inspiration, and that co-contraction contributes significantly to the maintenance of pharyngeal airway patency. The conceptual model is that co-contraction during inspiration stiffens the tongue as the antagonist muscles work against one another, thereby minimizing backward displacement of the tongue and subsequent occlusion of the pharynx. Significant new data showing respiratory-related co-activation of the protrudor and retractor muscles in animal models, as well as recent evidence showing improved inspiratory airflow with co-activation in human subjects with **obstructive sleep apnea,** provide strong support for this conceptual framework. Accordingly, the following Specific Aims are designed to rigorously test the co-activation hypothesis using an anesthetized rat model: Aim 1 is to demonstrate that the protrudor and retractor muscles of the tongue are co-activated during breathing and that they respond similarly to changes in respiratory related stimuli. Aim 2 is to show that co-activation of the extrinsic tongue muscles will improve pharyngeal airway mechanics more than the independent activation of either the protrudor or retractor muscles. Aim 3 is to demonstrate that the initial operating length of the tongue muscles will influence: a) the magnitude of respiratory related tongue movements, b) the ability of the tongue muscles to modulate pharyngeal airway flow mechanics, c) the fatigability of the tongue muscles. These experiments will lay the foundation for new and improved treatment strategies for persons with **obstructive sleep apnea** or with other conditions that are caused by malfunction of the tongue motor system.

Website: http://crisp.cit.nih.gov/crisp/Crisp_Query.Generate_Screen

- **Project Title: NEUROTRANSMITTER METABOLISM IN INTERMITTENT HYPOXIA**

  Principal Investigator & Institution: Kumar, Ganesh K.; Associate Professor; Case Western Reserve University 10900 Euclid Ave Cleveland, Oh 44106

  Timing: Fiscal Year 2002; Project Start 01-FEB-2002; Project End 31-DEC-2006

  Summary: (provided by applicant): The overall objective of the proposal is to broadly define post-translational mechanisms associated with changes in the activity of enzymes regulate the biosynthesis of neurotransmitters by chronic intermittent hypoxia (CIH). Mechanisms associated with CIH contribute to various physiological and pathophysiological conditions such as **sleep apnea** and leads to the development of hypertension. Neurotransmitters such as catecholamines, gamma-aminobutyric acid and amidated neuropeptides involve in the modulation of cardio-respiratory responses. The proposal tests the overall hypothesis that intermittent hypoxia alters neurotransmitter levels in the chemoafferent pathway by affecting the activity of enzymes associated with the synthesis of neurotransmitters via post-translational modifications. The hypothesis will be tested by focusing on tyrosine hydroxylase (TH), glutamate decarboxylase (GAD) and peptidylglycine alpha-amidating monooxygenase (PAM) the rate-limiting enzymes in the biosynthesis of catecholamines, GABA and amidated neuropeptides respectively. The experiments in specific aim 1 will compare the changes in the content of catecholamines (norepinephrine, dopamine and 5-hydroxytryptamine) and the activity of TH by CIH. Further, it will test the hypothesis that CIH induces phosphorylation of TH, thereby altering the enzyme activity. Potential alteration in enzymological properties of TH will be examined. Studies proposed under specific aim 2 focus on the mechanisms by which the activity of GAD is altered by CIH. Specifically, the aims of the proposed studies are to define changes in cofactor affinity and phosphorylation and dephosphorylation reactions of GAD. In specific aim 3, the effects of CIH on the redox chemistry of metal centers containing Cu2+ and the post-translational endoproteolytic modification of PAM will be investigated. Experiments will be performed in rats exposed to alternating cycles of hypoxia and normoxia for defined periods of time and rats exposed to similar duration of room air will serve as control. Tissues associated with the chemoafferent pathway such as brainstem, and carotid body will be investigated. It is anticipated that the results from studies proposed in this project may provide important new information and broaden our understanding of the effects of episodic hypoxia on enzymes associated with neurotransmitter metabolism in the chemoafferent pathway. The information from these studies will have the potential to identify new therapeutic targets for the intervention of sleep disorders associated with recurrent intermittent hypoxia.

Website: http://crisp.cit.nih.gov/crisp/Crisp_Query.Generate_Screen

- **Project Title: O2 SENSING BY MITOCHONDRIA DURING INTERMITTENT HYPOXIA**

  Principal Investigator & Institution: Schumacker, Paul T.; Professor; Medicine; University of Chicago 5801 S Ellis Ave Chicago, Il 60637

  Timing: Fiscal Year 2002; Project Start 30-SEP-2000; Project End 31-AUG-2004

  Summary: Obstructive **sleep apnea** (OSA) is a clinical syndrome characterized by repeated episodes of severe hypoxemia caused by intermittent closure of the upper airway during sleep. Complications of OSA include pulmonary hypertension caused by vascular remodeling in the lung. Repeated intermittent hypoxia is the most likely cause of this remodeling. The remodeling responses to hypoxia imply that a cellular O2 sensor exists that is capable of responding to rapid changes in [O2]. Studies from this laboratory indicate that mitochondria function as O2 sensors during hypoxia in diverse cells, releasing reactive oxygen species (ROS) to the cytoplasm that trigger intracellular signaling pathways leading to the activation of the transcription factors Nuclear Factor kappa B (NFkB) and Hypoxia-Inducible Factor (HIF- 1) in some cells, and that mediate adaptive metabolic responses in others. This application proposes that mitochondria also function as O2 sensors during intermittent hypoxia, by releasing ROS that lead to the activation of the transcription factors NFkB, HIF- I and AP- I that regulate genes involved in long-term vascular remodeling. Growth factors contribute to proliferation of cells in the vascular wall, and hypoxia amplifies their mitogenic response via an unknown mechanism. Mitochondrial ROS released during hypoxia could amplify the mitogenic response to growth factors by augmenting the oxidant signaling required for their proliferative response. Aim I will determine whether mitochondria function as O2 sensors by releasing ROS during intermittent hypoxia. Aim 2 will determine whether these ROS are necessary and sufficient for the activation of the transcription factors NFkB, HIF- I and AP- 1, and whether these factors mediate the subsequent transcriptional activation of target genes involved in vascular remodeling. Aim 3 will determine whether intermittent hypoxia amplifies the proliferative response to mitogens by stimulating mitochondrial ROS generation that augments growth factor-induced non-mitochondrial oxidant signaling. Collectively, these studies could identify a novel mechanism of O2 sensing in the lung, and provide a mechanistic explanation for the activation of gene transcritpion and cellular proliferation during intermittent hypoxia.

Website: http://crisp.cit.nih.gov/crisp/Crisp_Query.Generate_Screen

- **Project Title: O2-CHEMOSENSING BY REATIVE OXYGEN SPECIES/NADPH OXIDASE**

  Principal Investigator & Institution: Fidone, Salvatore J.; Professor of Physiology; Physiology; University of Utah Salt Lake City, Ut 84102

  Timing: Fiscal Year 2004; Project Start 01-JUL-1978; Project End 31-AUG-2008

  Summary: (provided by applicant): O2-sensing in the carotid body occurs in neuroectoderm-derived type I glomus cells where hypoxia elicits a complex chemotransduction cascade involving membrane depolarization, Ca 2+ entry and the release of excitatory neurotransmitters. Efforts to understand the exquisite O2-sensitivity of these cells focus primarily on the relationship between PO2 and the activity of K+-channels. A current hypothesis proposes that coupling between local PO2 and the open-closed state of K+-channels is mediated by a phagocytic-like multisubunit enzyme, NADPH oxidase, which produces reactive oxygen species (ROS) in proportion to the prevailing PO2. In O2-sensitive cells contained in lung neuroepithelial bodies (NEB), experiments have confirmed that ROS levels decrease in hypoxia, and that E M and K+-channel activity are indeed controlled by ROS produced by NADPH oxidase. However, recent studies in our laboratory suggest that ROS generated by a non-phagocytic form of NADPH oxidase, are important contributors to chemotransduction, but that their role in type I cells differs fundamentally from the mechanism utilized by NEB. We propose to test the hypothesis that in response to hypoxia, NADPH oxidase activity is increased in type I cells, and further, that increased ROS levels generated in response to low-O2 facilitate membrane re-polarization via the activation of a subset of K+-channels. In addition, we will examine the hypothesis that a non-phagocytic NADPH oxidase mediates adaptive morphological and physiological adjustments induced by exposure of the carotid body to chronic hypoxia (CH), a condition that occurs clinically in **sleep apnea** and chronic obstructive pulmonary disease (COPD). Studies will include: I. An examination of the sources and mechanisms of ROS production in type I cells, II. Evaluation of the involvement of NADPH oxidase and ROS in the carotid body response to acute hypoxia; III. The expression of NADPH oxidase subunits in the carotid body; and the effects of CH; and IV. The role of NADPH oxidase and ROS in carotid body adaptation to CH.

Website: http://crisp.cit.nih.gov/crisp/Crisp_Query.Generate_Screen

- **Project Title: OBSTRUCTIVE SLEEP APNEA IN CHILDREN**

  Principal Investigator & Institution: Glaze, Daniel G.; Associate Professor Pediatrics & Neurolo; Pediatrics; Baylor College of Medicine 1 Baylor Plaza Houston, Tx 77030

  Timing: Fiscal Year 2002; Project Start 20-SEP-1999; Project End 31-JUL-2004

  Summary: This abstract is not available.

  Website: http://crisp.cit.nih.gov/crisp/Crisp_Query.Generate_Screen

- **Project Title: OSA AND METABOLIC SYNDROME: ROLE OF OXIDATIVE STRESS**

  Principal Investigator & Institution: Sanders, Mark H.; Medicine; University of Pittsburgh at Pittsburgh 350 Thackeray Hall Pittsburgh, Pa 15260

Timing: Fiscal Year 2003; Project Start 30-SEP-2003; Project End 31-AUG-2007

Summary: (provided by applicant): The Metabolic Syndrome (Met. Syn.) has been defined as insulin resistance (I.R.), central obesity, systemic hypertension and dyslipidemia and is associated with increased cardio/cerebrovascular (CV) risk. I.R. may mediate much of this risk. Obstructive Sleep Apnea-Hypopnea (OSAH) is also associated with augmented CV risk and I.R. and plausibly, the CV risk of OSAH is mediated through I.R. Since OSAH is associated with both Oxidative Stress (O.S.) and pro-inflammatory processes, and O.S. is associated with I.Ro, it follows that O.S. and inflammation may link OSAH to I.R. and the Met. Syn. The Overall Goal of this research is to test the hypothesis that O.S and Inflammation link OSAH to I.R. as well as other CV risk-promoting conditions reflecting Met. Syn. We will specifically test if individual sleep consequences of OSAH, including Sleep Fragmentation and Intermittent Sleep Hypoxia, promote O.S. and Inflammation which in turn promote I.R. and other features of the Met. Syn. We propose: Specific Aim: la: To determine the effect of Sleep Fragmentation on O.S. and Inflammation and to explore the relationships between O.S. and Inflammation and I.R., dyslipidemia, sympathovagal tone and plasma cortisol, we will measure the following study variables: I.R., lipid profile, circulating & exhaled biomarkers of O.S., pro-inflammatory cytokines, plasma cortisol, & heart period variability before and after 2 consecutive nights with experimentally induced Sleep Fragmentation in normal subjects.Aim lb: To assess interaction between i) pre-existing Met. Syn., and ii) the overweight condition without Met. Syn., with regard to the effects of Sleep Fragmentation on the study variables, we will contrast the effect of experimentallyinduced sleep disruption in: non-OSAH/overweight individuals/(+)Met. Syn., non-OSAH/overweight individuals/(-)Met. Syn. and a control group of non-OSAH/normal weight/(-)Met. Syn.;Aim: 2: To evaluate the effect of Intermittent Sleep Hypoxia on O.S. and Inflammation and explore the relationships between O.S. and Inflammation and I.R., dyslipidemia, sympathovagal tone and plasma cortisol. OSAH patients on chronic positive airway pressure (PAP) therapy will have biomarkers of O.S., Inflammation and the other above study variables, measured under two conditions in random order: i) before and after 2 consecutive nights using PAP therapy but with experimentally induced Sleep Fragmentation (fragmentation+normoxia), ii) before and after 2 nights without PAP (fragmentation+hypoxia) to evaluate for an independent Intermittent Sleep Hypoxia effect.; Aim: 3: Using microarray data from peripheral monocytes, we will explore if specific gene expression profiles after the study conditions are associated with alterations consistent with Met. Syn.

Website: http://crisp.cit.nih.gov/crisp/Crisp_Query.Generate_Screen

- **Project Title: OSA IN OBESE TEENS AND PRETEENS: NEUROBEHAVIORAL EFFECTS**

  Principal Investigator & Institution: Beebe, Dean;; Children's Hospital Med Ctr (Cincinnati) 3333 Burnet Ave Cincinnati, Oh 452293039

  Timing: Fiscal Year 2004; Project Start 05-JAN-2004; Project End 31-DEC-2008

  Summary: (provided by applicant): The candidate, Dean W. Beebe, Ph.D., is an Assistant Professor of Pediatrics at Cincinnati Children's Hospital Medical Center. This K23 application will establish his independent research career in patient-oriented research into the nature, etiology and reversibility of the neurobehavioral effects of pediatric sleep disorders. This will be accomplished through a five-year training program and related research project. The training program has four specific objectives. First, the candidate will build a working knowledge of the biological processes that underlie normal and abnormal sleep in children and adolescents, with a particular focus on the mechanisms by which sleep pathology might cause neurobehavioral symptoms. This will provide an essential background in the physiology and pathophysiology of sleep, coupled with broad exposure to the diagnosis, measurement, and treatment of pediatric sleep disorders. Second, the candidate will enhance his training in longitudinal and epidemiological research design and analysis, with a particular focus on neurobehavioral outcome research. This will provide the skills needed to competently design and execute independent research in this area. Third, the candidate will improve his scientific writing and grant proposal skills. Finally, he will enhance his knowledge of the ethical conduct of clinical research. This training will take place under the guidance of faculty from a leading pediatric department and nearby medical school. The primary sponsor is an established researcher in the neurobehavioral effects of pediatric illness who has a history of successful career mentorship. Co-sponsors represent subspecialty divisions that are directly relevant to the research and career development plan. The proposed research plan focuses on an understudied population that is at high risk for **obstructive sleep apnea** (OSA): obese teens and preteens. This plan has been designed with two overarching goals: (1) to enhance scientific understanding of the presence, nature, and reversibility of neurobehavioral symptoms of OSA within this population, and (2) to expand the field's understanding of the effects of sleep pathology, broadly defined, on pediatric neurobehavioral functioning. Capitalizing on the unique combination of resources available to the candidate, this project will provide exceptional training in research linking the biological processes of sleep pathology with their neurobehavioral manifestations, while also generating much needed scientific data on a population that is rapidly growing and is at significant risk for both sleep disorders and poor neurobehavioral outcome.

Website: http://crisp.cit.nih.gov/crisp/Crisp_Query.Generate_Screen

- **Project Title: PAIN, OPIOIDS, AND SLEEP IN CANCER PATIENTS**

  Principal Investigator & Institution: Alley, Linda G.; Adult and Elder Health; Emory University 1784 North Decatur Road Atlanta, Ga 30322

  Timing: Fiscal Year 2002; Project Start 01-JUL-2002; Project End 31-MAR-2006

  Summary: (provided by applicant) Medical oncology patients experiencing pain frequently report nocturnal sleep disturbances and daytime sleepiness that adversely affect their functional health status (FHS) and quality of life (QOL). Furthermore, sleep disturbances may lead to increased subjective sensations of pain. Opioid analgesics are known to have intrinsic properties that negatively affect sleep quality. However, they can exert a positive effect on sleep by relieving pain. Therefore, pain and opioids can be viewed as two factors independently affecting nighttime sleep daytime wakefulness while also interacting with each other. The purposes of this descriptive comparative study are to examine pain and opioid use in relation to sleep and wakefulness and to examine associations between daytime and nocturnal sleep and FHS and QOL. The sample will include 80 medical oncology subjects who take opioid analgesics for cancer related pain and report a daily worst pain score or 6 on a scale of 10. All subjects who meet the entrance criteria will be screened by one night of laboratory-based polysomnography to eliminate those with severe periodic leg movement disorder or **sleep apnea syndrome.**. Those subjects meeting all criteria to continue in the study will undergo a laboratory based multiple sleep latency test the following day to index subjects' physiological sleepiness as well as complete brief pain and sleep surveys and QOL and FHS inventories with documented reliability and validity. Subjects will then be monitored for one 48 hour period in their usual home environments via ambulatory polysomnographic equipment and will make entries in a pain and sleep diary. The study will examine the extent to which pain intensity and opioid use are independently associated with day and night time sleep as well as the relationships between sleep and wakefulness and FHS and QOL. Given the centrality of opioids to cancer pain management, detailed analyses of the associations between pain and opioids and sleep and wakefulness in medical oncology patients are needed to develop optimal treatment regimens that maximize the benefits of pain relief while minimizing side effects of sleep disruption. Finally, the results of the study will assist in furthering the development of theory regarding sleep regulatory processes.

Website: http://crisp.cit.nih.gov/crisp/Crisp_Query.Generate_Screen

- **Project Title: PATHOGENESIS AND GENETICS OF OBSTRUCTIVE SLEEP APNEA**

  Principal Investigator & Institution: Schwab, Richard J.; Professor; Medicine; University of Pennsylvania 3451 Walnut Street Philadelphia, Pa 19104

  Timing: Fiscal Year 2002; Project Start 08-APR-2002; Project End 31-MAR-2007

  Summary: Although sleep disorders have been identified by the NIH as an area with tremendous scientific growth potential there are a paucity of patient oriented investigators studying sleep-related questions. The University of Pennsylvania is fortunate to have internationally recognized faculty and a strong infrastructure to support high quality patient-oriented research and training m sleep disorders. This infrastructure includes: Center for Sleep and Respiratory Neurobiology, Center for Clinical Epidemiology and Biostatistics, General Clinical Research Center, 3 Sleep Training Grants and the Pulmonary Imaging Group. Dr. Schwab is an integral part of each of these programs and is highly committed to a career in patient-oriented sleep research, proposing to study the genetics and biomechanical basis for **obstructive sleep apnea.** Dr. Schwab has made seminal observations about changes in the upper airway in patients with **sleep apnea** and he has successfully mentored several pulmonary fellows and junior faculty. Dr. Schwab through funding from this K24 can further develop into an academic leader and train others investigators that the sleep field desperately needs. Specifically this award would allow Dr. Schwab to develop further expertise in new radiologic techniques in upper airway imaging and computer-based volumetric analysis; further his expertise in genetic epidemiology and bioinformatics; allow increased time for mentoring young scientists and for developing new areas of collaboration with scientists. Dr. Schwab has developed a state-of-the-art upper airway imaging program focusing on understanding the pathogenesis and treatment of **obstructive sleep apnea.** Recently, Dr. Schwab has begun to apply his upper airway imaging expertise to study phenotypic risk factors for **sleep apnea.** He is the first to apply advanced quantitative MR Imaging techniques and novel volumetric computer image analysis techniques to study the genetic basis for **sleep apnea.** The scientific portion of this grant will utilize upper airway imaging to study both the pathogenesis and genetics of **sleep apnea.** My specific aims are: 1) to evaluate and compare upper airway soft tissue structural and biomechanical properties in apneics and normal weight-matched controls during wakefulness and sleep; 2) to quantify upper airway craniofacial structure, soft tissues and regional fat deposition using three dimensional magnetic resonance imaging in order to determine the intermediate traits associated with **obstructive sleep apnea** utilizing a case control design in normals and apneics; and 3) to determine the upper airway structural risk factors for **sleep apnea** that demonstrate family aggregation and are most likely to have a genetic component by comparing probands, siblings of probands, neighborhood controls and siblings of neighborhood controls. To address these specific aims, we have planned a logical series of studies that will provide insight in the pathogenesis of **obstructive sleep apnea** and the anatomic risk factors for this condition.

Website: http://crisp.cit.nih.gov/crisp/Crisp_Query.Generate_Screen

- **Project Title: PHARYNGEAL MECHANICS BY TAGGED MRI IN A ZUCKER RAT MODEL**

  Principal Investigator & Institution: Brennick, Michael J.; Ctr for Sleep and Respiratory Neurobiology; University of Pennsylvania 3451 Walnut Street Philadelphia, Pa 19104

  Timing: Fiscal Year 2003; Project Start 30-SEP-2003; Project End 31-AUG-2005

  Summary: (provided by applicant): The goal of the proposed research is to develop the technical, physiological and analytical techniques in advanced magnetic resonance imaging (MRI) to track tissue motion in the pharyngeal walls of anesthetized rats in order to establish a small animal model of pharyngeal airway mechanics. The model is relevant to the pathophysiology of **obstructive sleep apnea,** a prevalent respiratory disorder in humans characterized by the repetitive closure of the pharyngeal airway during sleep. Previous studies on the control of pharyngeal airway patency have been generally limited to measurements of airway size, shape, and collapsibility. Consequently, our understanding of the mechanical properties of the pharyngeal wall tissues that affect these airway changes is very limited. For example, although it is known that body mass index is the most important predictor of OSA, and that obesity is associated with an increase in airway collapsibility, we do not yet understand how obesity alters the mechanical properties of pharyngeal wall tissues to effect these changes. To address these gaps in our knowledge, the PI will adapt a novel magnetic resonance imaging (MRI) tissue tagging technique in anesthetized rats called spatial modulation of magnetization (SPAMM(r), developed at the University of Pennsylvania) to quantify pharyngeal wall tissue motion, i.e., tissue movement and tissue strain, and quantify how pharyngeal wall tissue motion produces changes in airway size and shape. We propose to develop novel technology that will enable us to examine pharyngeal wall tissue motion in anesthetized obese and non-obese Zucker rats, the obese genotype having a compromised pharyngeal airway similar to that in patients with OSA. Specific Aim 1 is to develop the techniques needed to use MRI with SPAMM to quantify pharyngeal wall tissue motion during spontaneous breathing in anesthetized, non-obese and obese Zucker rats under hyperoxic and hypoxic conditions. Specific Aim 2 is to develop the techniques needed to use MRI with SPAMM to quantify pharyngeal wall tissue motion in non-obese and obese Zucker rats during selective electrical stimulation of the hypoglossus nerve, and its branches that supply motor output to tongue protrudor (medial branch) and retractor (lateral branch) muscles. The global hypothesis for Aims 1 and 2 is that obesity compromises pharyngeal airway patency by reducing cross-sectional area and putting the pharyngeal muscles at a mechanical disadvantage. Our development of innovative methods to track tissue motion in the pharyngeal walls will reveal new insights into pharyngeal mechanics that increase our understanding of the role of obesity in the pathophysiology of OSA.

Website: http://crisp.cit.nih.gov/crisp/Crisp_Query.Generate_Screen

- **Project Title: PHYSIOLOGIC PHENOTYPES FOR OBSTRUCTIVE SLEEP APNEA**

  Principal Investigator & Institution: Schneider, Hartmut; Medicine; Johns Hopkins University 3400 N Charles St Baltimore, Md 21218

  Timing: Fiscal Year 2004; Project Start 05-JAN-2004; Project End 31-DEC-2008

  Summary: (provided by applicant): **Obstructive sleep apnea** is characterized by recurrent episodes of upper airway obstruction, leading to reductions in ventilation and disruption of sleep. As the severity of upper airway obstruction increases, ventilation decreases progressively, resulting in a spectrum of clinical disorders characterized by snoring and periodic obstructive hypopneas and apneas. Although obesity, and in particular central obesity, and male gender predispose to **obstructive sleep apnea,** the physiologic basis for these associations remains largely unknown. The current proposal will define the relationship between these risk factors and discrete intermediate physiologic traits during sleep that predispose to upper airway obstruction and hypoventilation. Our proposal is predicated on the concept that specific physiologic characteristics of upper airway function (critical pressure) and ventilatory control (maximum inspiratory airflow and inspiratory duty cycle) determine the level of ventilation during sleep. Preliminary Data indicate that obesity predisposes to alterations in critical pressure, whereas male gender is associated with disturbances in the neural control of ventilation. Our major hypothesis is that obesity and male gender predispose to specific mechanical alterations and neural responses that determine susceptibility to **obstructive sleep apnea.** To test this hypothesis, methods have been developed to rapidly assess baseline upper airway and ventilatory characteristics, and compensatory neural responses to upper airway obstruction during sleep. A major strength of our approach is that these physiologic phenotypes will be assessed in normal individuals who are free of confounding from **sleep apnea** and co-morbid conditions. In Specific Aim 1, we will determine the effect of obesity on intermediate physiologic traits that confer susceptibility to **sleep apnea** in normal subjects, and examine the effect of fat distribution on these phenotypes. In Specific Aim 2, we will elucidate the effect of gender on these physiologic traits, and the modulation of these characteristics by body fat distribution. Our experimental findings will lay the groundwork for further studies elucidating underlying physiologic mechanisms and phenotypic correlates of disease susceptibility in **obstructive sleep apnea.**

Website: http://crisp.cit.nih.gov/crisp/Crisp_Query.Generate_Screen

- **Project Title: POSTNATAL BRAIN SUSCEPTIBILITY TO INTERMITTENT HYPOXIA**

  Principal Investigator & Institution: Gozal, David; Professor and Vice-Chair for Research; Pediatrics; University of Louisville Jouett Hall, Belknap Campus Louisville, Ky 40292

  Timing: Fiscal Year 2002; Project Start 01-APR-2002; Project End 31-MAR-2007

  Summary: (provided by applicant): **Obstructive sleep apnea** syndrome (OSA) is a frequent condition affecting up to 2 percent of the pediatric population at ages that are characteristically associated with dynamic brain development and acquisition of important neurocognitive functions. OSA is characterized by repeated episodes of hypoxia during sleep, and when untreated it is associated with significant neurocognitive morbidities such as excessive restlessness and irritability, diminished intellectual performance, attention span, learning and vigilance. However, the relative contributions of chronic intermittent hypoxia (CIH) to OSA-associated neurocognitive dysfunction in children remain unclear. In adult rats, a CIII profile that mimics the intermittent hypoxia observed in patients with OSA during sleep leads to substantial reductions in spatial learning and retention as well as diminished ability to induce long-term potentiation in the CA1 region of the hippocampus. These neurobehavioral and physiological alterations correlate with anatomical changes developing in cortico-hippocampal regions., and we have found that such anatomical changes are particularly prominent in developing rat pups at post-natal ages that coincide with the peak prevalence of USA in children, suggesting that this period of brain maturation is uniquely vulnerable to CIH. We therefore hypothesized that the detrimental effects of CIH on memory and learning performances during this highly vulnerable developmental period are long-lasting, and will be manifest even during adulthood, long after the CIH exposure has ceased. Furthermore, these neurocognitive deficits will be associated and correlated with parallel electrophysiological alterations in the characteristics of long-term potentiation (LTP) of the CAl region of the hippocampus, as well as with disruption of normal ionotropic glutamate receptor expression and binding characteristics within the cortex and hippocampus. We propose to: (1) examine the short-term and long-term consequences of CIH on behavioral patterning and on water maze task acquisition and retention. (2) To assess the short-term and long-lasting effects of CIH on LTP characteristics of the CA1 region of the hippocampus.; (3) To establish changes in NMDA glutamate receptor expression and binding characteristics in neocortical and hippocampal regions associated with CIH, and following long-term recovery; (4) To determine whether exposure to CIH during a critically-vulnerable period of development will elicit time-dependent glial and neuronal stem cell proliferation within cortical and hippocampal regions. These studies will characterize concomitant structural and phenotypic changes induced by CIH in a developmental rodent model of OSA, and provide initial insights into the role of CIH in short-term and long-term neurobehavioral morbidity of USA in children.

Website: http://crisp.cit.nih.gov/crisp/Crisp_Query.Generate_Screen

- **Project Title: PREDICTORS OF ADVERSE METABOLIC EFFECTS OF SLEEP LOSS**

  Principal Investigator & Institution: Spiegel, Karine;; Free University of Brussels 50 Ave Franklin Roosevelt Brussels,

  Timing: Fiscal Year 2003; Project Start 30-SEP-2003; Project End 31-JUL-2007

  Summary: (provided by applicant): Chronic sleep loss, obesity and sleep-disordered breathing (SDB) are increasingly common in industrialized countries. Sleep curtailment in healthy young lean adults results in the development of components of the metabolic syndrome, including reduced glucose tolerance and/or insulin resistance, elevated evening cortisol levels, increased cardiac sympatho-vagal balance, and a risk of weight gain resulting from reduced leptin levels and increased hunger and appetite. The studies proposed in the present application build on novel findings from our group that indicate that obese individuals may be more at risk for further weight gain than lean individuals in conditions of sleep loss, and that individuals levels of slow wave activity (SWA), a stable trait-dependent marker of deep sleep, may predict subjective vulnerability to sleep loss, and are also likely to predict the severity of adverse metabolic and cardiovascular consequences of sleep loss. We therefore propose to characterize sleep architecture, autonomic nervous system (ANS) activity, and biomarkers of the metabolic syndrome in three groups of middle aged (35-50 years old) subjects studied while they follow their usual sleep habits as well as during 4 days of sleep restriction and sleep extension, presented in randomized order in a cross-over design. The three groups of subjects will be healthy lean men and women, gender-matched individuals who are obese, and gender-matched individuals who are obese and also suffer from SDB. The specific aims are: 1. To test the hypothesis that baseline levels of SWA are lower in obese adults than in lean controls, and are even lower in obese subjects with SDB, and examine correlations between levels of SWA and sleep duration, ANS activity and biomarkers of the metabolic syndrome. 2. To test the hypothesis that sleep restriction, as compared to sleep extension, has adverse effects on biomarkers of the metabolic syndrome in lean adults, obese adults, and obese adults with SDB. 3. To test the hypothesis that the adverse impact of partial sleep loss on components of the metabolic syndrome is more important for obese adults than in lean adults, and more severe in obese adults with SDB than in those without SDB. This project capitalizes on our experience with human studies of "sleep debt" and on our extensive expertise in assessment of ANS activity to evaluate the role of the ANS as a mediator of the adverse health effects of chronic sleep loss.

Website: http://crisp.cit.nih.gov/crisp/Crisp_Query.Generate_Screen

- **Project Title: PREVALENCE AND CORRELATES OF CHILDHOOD SLEEP APNEA**

  Principal Investigator & Institution: Quan, Stuart F.; Professor of Medicine; None; University of Arizona P O Box 3308 Tucson, Az 857223308

  Timing: Fiscal Year 2002; Project Start 15-AUG-1999; Project End 31-DEC-2003

  Summary: This abstract is not available.

  Website: http://crisp.cit.nih.gov/crisp/Crisp_Query.Generate_Screen

- **Project Title: PREVALENCE OF SLEEP DISORDERED BREATHING IN CHILDREN**

  Principal Investigator & Institution: Bixler, Edward O.; Professor; Psychiatry; Pennsylvania State Univ Hershey Med Ctr 500 University Drive Hershey, Pa 170332390

  Timing: Fiscal Year 2002; Project Start 01-AUG-2001; Project End 31-JUL-2006

  Summary: (provided by applicant): The objectives of this proposal are to: 1) establish the prevalence of different types of sleep disordered breathing (SDB) in a large general random sample of children; 2) identify important risk factors of SDB; (3) establish the family history of various risk factors associated with children with SDB; (4) assess the impact of SDB on clinical, psychometric and behavioral/academic outcomes; and 5) identify characteristics which will assist in identifying those children at risk for SDB for possible early intervention. Several studies evaluating select populations have suggested that various severe consequences are associated with SDB in children. These consequences include: cardiovascular complications such as pulmonary hypertension, cor pulmonale, and arrhythmia; behavioral abnormalities such as excessive daytime sleepiness, poor school performance, hyperactivity, aggressive behavior, and social withdrawal; and growth disturbances which at times are reversed by successful treatment. To date, there have been only four studies evaluating the prevalence of **sleep apnea** using objective sleep evaluation methods in general random samples of children. Three studies evaluated a limited age range of 6 mos to 6 yrs, while the fourth assessed a range of 2-18 years. These studies employed relatively small samples in their sleep laboratory phase (N=lO, 11, 132, and 126, respectively). Thus, they could not adequately assess clinical significance. None of these studies evaluated: general development (eg height, weight, age adjusted BMI); the effects of SDB on physical health (eg blood pressure); academic achievement; or electrophysiologic defined sleep stages as possible outcome measures. Only one study reported a possible association with daytime sleepiness and behavior. Thus, the prevalence and clinical impact of SDB in school age children is unknown. In order to establish the prevalence and clinical significance of SDB in children aged 6 - 12 years with reasonable precision, we propose to employ a protocol similar to that used to establish the prevalence and clinical significance in two previously NIH supported protocols in adults. The proposed study will employ a two-phase protocol: 1) questionnaire completed by the parents of every child enrolled in local elementary school which will assess general sleep, behavior and learning problems; 2) a random sample (n= 1,000) selected from the first sample based on risk for SDB and evaluated in the sleep laboratory to determine the presence of SDB. The second phase will receive a thorough pediatric ENT and pulmonary evaluation and school records and behavior will be assessed. The parents of this group will be interviewed for the family history of risk factors associated with SDB in children. This strategy will yield adequate power to establish the prevalence and clinical significance of SDB in children.

Website: http://crisp.cit.nih.gov/crisp/Crisp_Query.Generate_Screen

- **Project Title: PROGESTERONE AND SLEEP IN OLDER WOMEN**

  Principal Investigator & Institution: Moe, Karen E.; Psychiatry and Behavioral Scis; University of Washington Grant & Contract Services Seattle, Wa 98105

  Timing: Fiscal Year 2002; Project Start 01-FEB-2002; Project End 31-DEC-2004

  Summary: Sleep complaints increase significantly with age in women. Many older women experience difficulty falling asleep, more night-time awakenings, and less restful sleep. Sleep studies verify that disturbed sleep patterns are observed even in healthy older women. Sleep disturbances are associated with increased daytime drowsiness, increased accident risk, increased use of health care, and reduced quality of life. Older women receive a disproportionate number of sedative-hypnotic medications, which can exacerbate **sleep apnea** and have daytime carryover effects such as sedation, falls and subsequent fractures, and cognitive impairment. A better understanding of the sleep changes experienced by older women is sorely needed. One contributing factor may be menopause-related changes in sex steroids such as estrogen and progesterone. Research attention has focused on estrogen. However, progesterone may also participate in the control of sleep. Clinical reports indicate that women often feel drowsy after they take oral progesterone - an effect which is undesirable during the day, but may be positive at night. To date there are no published studies of progesterone's effect on the objectively-measured sleep and daytime drowsiness of older women. The proposed study will take a systematic, multi-dimensional approach to determining the effect of progesterone on the sleep and drowsiness of older women. Objective techniques (polysomnography, Multiple Sleep Latency Test) will be used to measure sleep and daytime drowsiness following evening or morning administration of 300 mg micronized progesterone, in 40 postmenopausal women who are at least 5 years past menopause and who are not experiencing hot flashes. Attention, memory, subjective sleepiness, and blood levels of progesterone and its metabolite (allopregnanolone) will also be measured. This study is part of a long-term research plan to assess (1) how the very low postmenopausal levels of estrogen and progesterone contribute to sleep difficulties of older women, and (2) how hormone replacement therapy affects the sleep of women. An ongoing placebo-controlled study is investigating the effects of estrogen on the sleep of older women. The proposed study will complement the estrogen study. It will enhance our limited understanding of the relationship between sex steroids and sleep, and the factors that contribute to sleep problems in older women.

Website: http://crisp.cit.nih.gov/crisp/Crisp_Query.Generate_Screen

- **Project Title: PROTEOMIC ANALYSIS OF HIPPOCAMPAL HYPOXIC VULNERABILITY**

  Principal Investigator & Institution: Klein, Jon B.; Professor; Medicine; University of Louisville Jouett Hall, Belknap Campus Louisville, Ky 40292

  Timing: Fiscal Year 2002; Project Start 30-SEP-2000; Project End 31-AUG-2004

  Summary: Obstructive **sleep apnea syndrome** (OSAS) is a frequent condition affecting up to 5 percent of the population, and is characterized by repeated episodes of hypoxia and recurrent EEG/behavioral arousal, particularly during REM sleep. When untreated, OSAS is associated with significant neurocognitive morbidities such as excessive daytime sleepiness and diminished intellectual performance, attention span, learning and vigilance. Although some experimental evidence suggest that chronic continuous hypoxia (CCH) may elicit neural dysfunction, the relative contributions of episodic hypoxia to OSAS-associated neurocognitive dysfunction remain unclear. In a rat model, regional differences in susceptibility of the hippocampal formation to chronic intermittent hypoxia (CIH) emerged. The CA1 region of the hippocampus displayed major increases in apoptosis and anatomical disruption while the CA3 hippocampal region was unaffected. Similarly, c-Fos protein was markedly enhanced in CA1 but not in CA3. Recent developments in 2-dimensional electrophoresis, mass spectroscopy, and bioinformatics permit the large scale analysis of proteins, termed proteomics. To test the hypothesis that a restricted number of identifiable proteins accounts for the differential susceptibility of the CA1 and CA3 regions of the hippocampus to CIH, the project proposes to examine the following specific aims: (1) To characterize the protein expression patterns of CA1 and CA3 regions of the hippocampus in the adult rat, by establishing a proteomic database of these 2 regions; (2) To determine differences in temporal changes of protein expression between the CA1 and CA3 regions of the hippocampus in adult rats exposed to CIH by comparing the changes in the proteomic databases within each region; (3) To determine differences in temporal changes of protein expression between the CA1 and CA3 regions of the hippocampus in adult rats exposed to CCH by comparing proteomic datasets established during CCH. In addition, differential proteomic analysis will be conducted between CCH and CIH. These studies will characterize changes in protein expression and post-translational modifications that may have important implications for cell survival and/or adaption to intermittent and sustained hypoxia.

Website: http://crisp.cit.nih.gov/crisp/Crisp_Query.Generate_Screen

- **Project Title: PULMONARY HYPERTENSION FOLLOWING INTERMITTENT HYPOXIA**

  Principal Investigator & Institution: Fagan, Karen A.; Medicine; University of Colorado Hlth Sciences Ctr P.O. Box 6508, Grants and Contracts Aurora, Co 800450508

  Timing: Fiscal Year 2003; Project Start 01-AUG-2003; Project End 31-JUL-2007

  Summary: (provided by applicant): Pulmonary hypertension (PHTN) is common in diseases characterized by chronic hypoxia (CH) (i.e. COPD, IPF) and occurs in 15-40% of patients with **sleep apnea.** Intermittent hypoxia (IH) mimicking the hypoxia-reoxygenation cycles of **sleep apnea** causes systemic hypertension and altered regulation of systemic vascular tone. However, the effect of intermittent hypoxia on the pulmonary circulation is unknown. Recently, patients with sleep apnea-induced PHTN were found to have exaggerated hypoxic pulmonary vasoconstriction. Unlike in chronic hypoxia, hypoxia in **sleep apnea** is not continuous, thus the mechanisms causing sleep apnea-induced PHTN are likely different from chronic hypoxia-induced PHTN. We therefore hypothesize that intermittent hypoxia leads to pulmonary hypertension by differential expression of genes important in regulating pulmonary vascular tone. Specifically, we hypothesize that oxidant stress in IH increases NOS and decreases SOD leading to PHTN through increased formation of peroxynitrite thus decreasing NO available for cellular effects such as attenuating vasoconstriction and mediating vasodilation. We further hypothesize that IH activates redox sensitive transcription factors leading to differential lung gone expression compared to CH. We will present data showing IH-induced PHTN in both rats and mice. We also will present data showing differential expression of NOS (nitric oxide synthase) and SOD (superoxide dismutase) in the lung following IH compared to CH, which may contribute to IH-induced PHTN through increased oxidant stress and decreased NO activity. This proposal will address the questions: 1) does repetitive hypoxia-reoxygenation causes pulmonary hypertension, 2) that despite increased NOS, NO appears to be insufficient to prevent IH-induced PHTN, 3) decreased SOD may contribute to IH-induced PHTN by increasing oxidant stress and formation of peroxynitrite, and 4) does IH leads to differential gene expression through activation of specific signaling pathways compared to CH. We will correlate physiologic measures of PHTN and pulmonary vascular tone with expression and activity of NOS and SOD, measurements of oxidant stress and NO, and activation of specific signaling pathways leading to altered gone expression in IH. This proposal, for the first time, will identify the consequences of IH in the pulmonary circulation. Understanding mechanisms contributing to the development of PHTN in IH may lead improved cardiovascular morbidity and mortality in this common disease.

Website: http://crisp.cit.nih.gov/crisp/Crisp_Query.Generate_Screen

- **Project Title: REGULATION OF GENE EXPRESSION IN INTERMITTENT HYPOXIA**

  Principal Investigator & Institution: Czyzyk-Krzeska, Maria F.; Associate Professor; Molecular and Cellular Physio; University of Cincinnati 2624 Clifton Ave Cincinnati, Oh 45221

  Timing: Fiscal Year 2002; Project Start 30-SEP-2000; Project End 31-AUG-2004

  Summary: Obstructive **sleep apnea** (OSA) is a relatively common disorder that is characterized by repetitive episodes of upper-airway obstruction that occur during sleep and cause repetitive episodes of oxygen desaturation of arterial blood (hypoxia). Chronically, OSA syndrome can result in a number of serous cardiovascular problems including systemic arterial hypertension. There is evidence that the OSA-induced hypertension is neurogenic, that it emanates from the oxygen chemoreceptor cells in the carotid body, and involves the catecholaminergic cells within the peripheral sympathetic nervous system and adrenal medulla. This application proposes that intermittent hypoxia stimulates gene expression in these tissues, and that this may be involved in the pathogenesis of hypertension associated with OSA. This is supported by the previous finding that brief periods (<1hr) of sustained hypoxia stimulates expression of several genes in the oxygen-sensitive type 1 cells of the carotid body, including tyrosine hydroxylase (TH), the rate-limiting enzyme in catecholamine synthesis. Enhanced catecholamine biosynthesis in the sympathetic nervous system is a potential mechanism for hypertension. The present research will test the hypothesis that very brief episodes (20 sec) of re-occurring hypoxia are sufficient to increase gene expression in the carotid body, superior cervical ganglion, and the adrenal gland. It is hypothesized that intermittent hypoxia regulates gene expression in these tissues and results in the OSA-induced hypertension. Specific Aim 1 will focus on the characterizing the effects of intermittent hypoxia on a known hypoxia-regulated gene that has been implicated in hypertension, namely TH and some of its known transcriptional regulators, including c-fos, junB, and CREB. This aim will also test the hypothesis that gene expression induced by intermittent hypoxia in the superior cervical ganglion and adrenal gland requires synaptic input that originates in the carotid body. It is further hypothesized that coordinate regulation of many genes and proteins mediates the cellular response to such a complex stimulus as intermittent hypoxia. This possibility will be explored in Specific Aim 2, which will focus on identifying the gene and protein expression pattern in the carotid body, superior cervical ganglion and adrenal gland using unique cDNA libraries and high-throughout genomics (cDNA microarray) and proteomics (2-D protein gels and mass spectrometer) analysis. The findings from this study may provide new insight concerning the role of intermittent hypoxia on regulation of gene expression and possible targets for mediating the pathogenesis of OSA-induced hypertension.

Website: http://crisp.cit.nih.gov/crisp/Crisp_Query.Generate_Screen

- **Project Title: RURAL DWELLING OLDER ADULTS: CPAP ADHERENCE SUPPORT**

  Principal Investigator & Institution: Smith, Carol E.; Professor; None; University of Kansas Medical Center Msn 1039 Kansas City, Ks 66160

  Timing: Fiscal Year 2002; Project Start 01-APR-2000; Project End 31-MAR-2005

  Summary: Obstructive **Sleep Apnea** (OSA) is the most prevalent and costly sleep disorder in essentially healthy older adults. OSA is assoicated with cardiovascular and neurocognitive sequaela and with public safety losses due to traffic fatalities and other accidents that cost 43 to 56 billion dollars annually (National Commission Sleep Report, number 1, 1993). OSA is controlled with nightly Continuous Positive Airway Pressure (CPAP) ventilation, the treatment of choice (National Commission on Sleep Report number 2, 1994). The primary aim of this randomized clinical trial is to determine the long-term adherence, health, quality of life outcomes, and cost-benefit of a comprehensive intervention on CPAP ventilation in 168 rural dwelling older adults with OSA. Adherence is measured by microprocessor pressure-sensor timer/recorder as patient hours of nightly CPAP use. The Secondary Aim is to assess relationships among CPAP adherence, quality of life, family caregiving, use of a decision aid for driving safety and accidents. The intervention was derived from Triandis and Smith models and each intervention step has been tested in older adults. The intervention steps gradually increase in intensity from self-directed and focused counseling to in home 2-way telehealth monitoring that allows a nurse to direct CPAP care and assess for physical and emotional barriers to adherence and internet interaction. Intervention steps in this proposed study are administered per criteria only if the patient is not adhering to the prescribed CPAP treatment. The steps use music and focused imagery for CPAP habit initiation and sensitization to physiologic and affective benefits from CPAP and mobilizing the family to overcome barriers to CPAP use. Through the internet, subjects connect to peer and professional counselors, engage in interactive adherence support activities, obtain accurate information when seeking unproven cures and use decision aids for driving. An established Univ. of Ks. multidisciplinary team will conduct the study with a subcontract with the Univ. of Wisc. The long-term goal of this proposed study is to validate a CPAP adherence support system that will ultimately improve patient and family caregiver quality of life and public safety, as well as reduce patient and family caregivers' morbidity and the 100 billion dollars spent annually on non-adherence.

Website: http://crisp.cit.nih.gov/crisp/Crisp_Query.Generate_Screen

- **Project Title: SDB, METABOLIC SYNDROME, AND VASCULAR FUNCTION**

  Principal Investigator & Institution: Nieto, F Javier.; Helfaer Professor of Public Health; Population Health Sciences; University of Wisconsin Madison 750 University Ave Madison, Wi 53706

  Timing: Fiscal Year 2003; Project Start 30-SEP-2003; Project End 31-JUL-2007

  Summary: (provided by applicant): Insulin resistance and the metabolic syndrome share risk factors and pathogenetic mechanisms with vascular endothelial dysfunction and atherosclerosis. Sleep disorder breathing (SDB) might be associated with this pathogenetic milieu in complex and intricate ways, both as a consequence (via obesity) and as a cause (via hypoxemia, oxidative stress, and sympathetic overload). The primary objective of this proposal is to study the longitudinal association between SDB and the incidence of the metabolic syndrome and vascular dysfunction in a nested case-cohort sample of participants in the Wisconsin Sleep Cohort (WSC) Study, a community-based sample of middle-age individuals who have undergone repeated full polysomnography studies over the last 15 years, up to four in each participants, four years apart. Additional existing data on these individuals include extensive data on sleep habits, repeat blood pressure measurements (including both sitting and ambulatory blood pressure), anthropometric data, measures of fasting serum glucose, insulin, leptin, ghrelin, inflammatory markers, ApoE-E4, and non-invasive markers of subclinical atherosclerosis (ankle-arm index). A total of 600 participants who have had at least 2 visit in the WSC will be recruited into the study, including a) about 150 cases of incident metabolic syndrome, and b) a random sample of about 450-470 members of the cohort. These participants will undergo non-invasive measures of vascular function in different vascular beds, including: (1) brachial artery reactivity; (2) cerebral artery responsiveness to hypercapnia; and (3) retinal arteriolar/venular ratio. In addition, we will assess possible mediating mechanisms by measuring markers of hypoxic stress (VEGF), oxidative stress (urinary isoprostane), and markers of sympathetic and hypothalamic-pituitary-adrenal axis function (heart rate variability, urinary norepinephrine, urinary cortisol). The proposed study will test, with adequate statistical power, the hypothesis that recent or past SDB (assessed by AHI, hypoxemia index) predict incident metabolic syndrome and is related to the degree of insulin resistance (HOMA-IR), and vascular or endothelial dysfunction while controlling for potential confounders or explanatory variables, including the existing and newly acquired covariate information.

Website: http://crisp.cit.nih.gov/crisp/Crisp_Query.Generate_Screen

- **Project Title: SLEEP ACADEMIC AWARD--RECOGNITION OF SLEEP DISORDERS**

  Principal Investigator & Institution: Strohl, Kingman P.; Professor of Medicine and Anatomy; Medicine; Case Western Reserve University 10900 Euclid Ave Cleveland, Oh 44106

  Timing: Fiscal Year 2002; Project Start 01-SEP-1998; Project End 31-AUG-2004

  Summary: The goals of this SLEEP ACADEMIC AWARD are to implement and assess a knowledge system for sleep and sleep disorders. The proposal links educational specialists, training programs, and sleep research at Case Western Reserve University with medical undergraduate and post-graduate education in Northeast Ohio. The Specific Aims are: 1. Implement and evaluate a medical curriculum on the causes and consequences of sleepiness, both a common experience and a symptom common to many sleep disorders. The P.I. will improve knowledge construction and assess exposure to and recognition of sleepiness and sleep disorders in the internal medicine clerkship, before and after interventions aimed at increasing knowledge synthesis and problem solving. Outcome assessments are identified at several intermediate and final end-points. Two stations in a structured clinical examination for all third year medical students will evaluate knowledge use of sleep and sleepiness, and tabulation of patient logs will identify exposure to and recognition of fatigue and **sleep apnea,** in comparison to other common disorders. Interventions include a case-management tutorial and computerized patient management modules. Additional assessments include a sleep quiz and attitude questionnaire about sleep problems. Data will be analyzed using the analysis of variance and covariance models with results pooled across clerkships for the class (n= 140). Change over time will be examined. Special student groups will be targeted to address research and minority health needs. 2. Implement an instruction tool ("Sleep Disorders Structured Clinical Instruction Module") in Internal Medicine/Family Medicine house staff training. 3. Expand knowledge of sleep disorders in Cleveland area primary care physicians by active experimentation. We will enhance current practice by assessment of patients for sleep habits and developing with Northeast Ohio physicians strategies for recognition of sleepiness and sleep disorders. 4. Examine the impact of sleep habits on academic performance in an Ohio public school system as well as in professional education. This program will assess the impact of snoring and chronic sleepiness on results of common tests for promotion and competency before and after interventions designed to promote sleep health. For each aim, there are plans to implement new or recast existing educational and evaluative tools, and assess attitude and/or behavior. We will disseminate of educational assessments, patient-oriented material, and clinical pathways through local and national consultants in both the public and private sector, as well as through interaction with other awardees.

Website: http://crisp.cit.nih.gov/crisp/Crisp_Query.Generate_Screen

- **Project Title: SLEEP APNEA & HYPERTENSION--ROLE OF SYMP NERVOUS SYSTEM**

  Principal Investigator & Institution: Dimsdale, Joel E.; Professor; Psychiatry; University of California San Diego La Jolla, Ca 920930934

  Timing: Fiscal Year 2002; Project Start 01-AUG-1991; Project End 31-JUL-2004

  Summary: (adapted from investigator's abstract): This competing renewal examines the effect of chemoreceptor (CHEMO) and sympathetic nervous system (SNS) physiology in four groups of individuals: apneics and non-apneics, with and without hypertension. A total of 80 individuals will be studied in terms of their CHEMO and SNS function, sleep physiology, and quality of life. They will then be randomized to receive either nocturnal oxygen supplementation or nocturnal room-air supplementation and they will be restudied after 24 hours and after one week. Studies will include measurement of plasma and urinary catecholamines, beta adrenergic receptors on lymphocytes, plasma endothelin-1. CHEMO activity will be characterized while breathing room-air, while stimulating CHEMO with a brief period of hypoxia, and while blocking CHEMO with a brief period of hyperoxia. Using tritiated norepinephrine, norepinephrine release rate will be calculated during each of these CHEMO manipulations. Using impedance cardiography, cardiac hemodynamics will be characterized at rest and in response to behavioral stressors. The study will measure heart rate and tidal volume responses to infused isoproterenol. Baroreflexes will be characterized after stimuli that transiently increase and decrease blood pressure. Blood pressure will be characterized with ambulatory blood pressure monitoring. Sleep will be characterized with polysomnography. The effect of nocturnal oxygen treatment will be studied in terms of patient satisfaction, compliance, and quality of life.

Website: http://crisp.cit.nih.gov/crisp/Crisp_Query.Generate_Screen

- **Project Title: SLEEP APNEA IN LOOK AHEAD PARTICIPANTS**

  Principal Investigator & Institution: Foster, Gary D.; Associate Professor of Psychiatry; Psychiatry; University of Pennsylvania 3451 Walnut Street Philadelphia, Pa 19104

  Timing: Fiscal Year 2002; Project Start 30-SEP-2001; Project End 31-JUL-2006

  Summary: (provided by applicant): Weight loss is a frequently recommended treatment for obese patients with **obstructive sleep apnea** (OSA). The empirical support for this recommendation is lacking. Based on descriptive studies, weight loss appears to improve but not abolish sleep disordered breathing. Moreover, the degree of improvement in OSA is quite variable and not directly proportional to weight loss. The lack of randomized trials, the study of predominantly male samples, and the absence of follow-up evaluations leave physicians and patients unsure about the utility of weight loss treatment in obese OSA patients. The research proposed in this application will assess the effects of weight loss on sleep disordered breathing in 120 obese, Type 2 diabetics with OSA (RDI greater than or equal to 15) who are randomly assigned to either weight loss (n=60) or usual care (n=60) treatments within the context of the Look AHEAD study. Home polysomnography studies will be performed before treatment and at 1 and 2 years. Among the 60 weight loss subjects, we will assess the relative importance of changes in neck and abdominal fat in explaining the variability of changes in sleep disordered breathing after weight loss. Finally, we will examine the relationship between changes in sleep-disordered breathing and changes in blood pressure after weight loss in the 60 weight loss participants. Specifically, this research will: 1) determine the efficacy of a weight loss program in reducing sleep disordered breathing in obese Type 2 diabetics; 2) identify sources of variability in sleep disordered breathing associated with weight loss; and 3) examine the role of sleep disordered breathing in mediating changes in blood pressure associated with weight loss. The results of this study will provide an empirical basis for making recommendations about the effectiveness of weight loss in Type 2 diabetics with OSA.

Website: http://crisp.cit.nih.gov/crisp/Crisp_Query.Generate_Screen

- **Project Title: SLEEP DISORDERED BREATHING AND VASOMOTOR REGULATION**

  Principal Investigator & Institution: Morgan, Barbara J.; Assistant Professor; Kinesiology; University of Wisconsin Madison 750 University Ave Madison, Wi 53706

  Timing: Fiscal Year 2004; Project Start 01-APR-2004; Project End 31-MAR-2008

  Summary: (provided by applicant): Sleep-disordered breathing has emerged as a risk factor for many forms of cardiovascular disease; however, the underlying mechanisms are incompletely understood. Our goal is to determine whether sleep-disordered breathing alters structure and function of resistance vessels in the cerebral and skeletal muscle circulations. We will investigate the time course and reversibility of these vascular alterations and examine the causative roles played by oxidant stress and sympathetic neural activation. Humans subjects with **obstructive sleep apnea** and rats exposed to chronic intermittent hypoxia (CIH) will be studied to address 4 specific aims. In Aim 1, we will perform in vitro studies of isolated, perfused middle cerebral and gracilis arteries of the rat to determine the time course and potential for reversibility of CIH-induced impairments in vascular structure and function. In addition, we will assess the roles of sleep fragmentation and cyclic dexoygenation/reoxygenation in causing CIH-induced alterations in vascular function. In Aim 2, we will use similar in vitro methods to determine whether oxidant stress contributes importantly to CIH-induced vascular dysfunction. In Aim 3, we use chemical and surgical sympathectomy and angiotensin II receptor blockade to assess the role of the sympathetic nervous system causing CIH-induced vascular dysfunction. In Aim 4, we will explore the functional consequences of

CIH-induced vascular dysfunction in humans by assessing vasodilatory responses to acute episodes of hypoxia and hypercapnia before and after treatment of **obstructive sleep apnea.** The results of these experiments will further define the pathogenetic link between sleep-disordered breathing and cardiovascular disease and may lead to the development of a more rational approach to therapy for this common clinical condition.

Website: http://crisp.cit.nih.gov/crisp/Crisp_Query.Generate_Screen

- **Project Title: SLEEP DISORDERED BREATHING, APOE AND LIPID METABOLISM**

  Principal Investigator & Institution: Mignot, Emmanuel J.; Director; Psychiatry and Behavioral Sci; Stanford University Stanford, Ca 94305

  Timing: Fiscal Year 2002; Project Start 21-SEP-2002; Project End 31-JUL-2006

  Summary: (provided by applicant): Recent findings suggest interrelationships between **obstructive sleep apnea,** lipid metabolism, and neurodegeneration. Apolipoprotein E epsilon4 (APOE e4), a genetic marker linked to increased cardiovascular disease (CVD) risk and Alzheimer's disease (AD), is associated with a two fold increased risk of sleep disordered breathing (SDB), and an increase in severity of apnea symptoms. Preliminary data suggest that this association is stronger between the ages of 50 and 65. Other experiments suggest dysregulated leptin levels in **obstructive sleep apnea** (OSA). Taken together, these findings suggest common pathophysiological mechanisms involving dysregulated lipid metabolism in OSA. An understanding of these mechanisms is essential for the prevention and treatment of SDB. In this project, we will: 1) extend our finding that APOE e4 increases the risk of **sleep apnea** in the general population using case/control and family designs; 2) examine if polymorphisms in other genes regulating lipid levels are associated with **sleep apnea;** 3) study the relationship between lipid regulatory gene polymorphisms, lipid profile (LDL- cholesterol, HDL-cholesterol, triglycerides), plasma leptin (and other lipid regulatory hormones), and **sleep apnea** levels. These studies will be critical to extend our understanding of the association between **sleep apnea** and the metabolic syndrome. This application will focus on one arm of this complex equation, the relationship between lipid metabolism and SDB. With lipid metabolism being critical to cardiovascular risk, this application will also trigger further studies focusing on cardiovascular impact with adequate control of SDB.

  Website: http://crisp.cit.nih.gov/crisp/Crisp_Query.Generate_Screen

- **Project Title: SLEEP HEART HEALTH STUDY**

  Principal Investigator & Institution: O'connor, George T.; Associate Professor; Medicine; Boston University Medical Campus 715 Albany St, 560 Boston, Ma 02118

  Timing: Fiscal Year 2002; Project Start 30-SEP-1994; Project End 31-AUG-2004

  Summary: The Sleep Heart Health Study (SHHS) was started in 1994 as a multicenter cohort study of the cardiovascular consequences of sleep-disordered breathing (SDB). The study's principal aims are to assess SDB as a risk factor for adverse cardiovascular outcomes, including incident coronary heart disease events, stroke, and hypertension, and accelerated increase in blood pressure with age. The SHHS protocol added an assessment of SDB to ongoing cohort studies of cardiovascular and other diseases, including the Framingham Offspring and Omni cohorts, the Hagerstown and Minneapolis/St. Paul sites of the Atherosclerosis Risk in Communities (ARIC) Study, the Hagerstown, Sacramento, and Pittsburgh sites of the Cardiovascular Health Study (CHS), the Strong Heart Study (SHS) sites South Dakota, Oklahoma, and Arizona, and cohort studies of respiratory disease in Tucson and of hypertension in New York. During its first four years (1994-1998), the SHHS was successfully started with full and high quality polysomnography (PSG) data obtained in the home from 6,440 participants, exceeding the recruitment target. The SHHS cohort, includes 3,039 men and 3,401 women 40 years of age or more, of whom 8.2 percent are African American, 9.6 percent are Native American, 1.3 percent are Asian, and 4.2 percent are Hispanic. In addition to PSG, data collection covered snoring and sleepiness and quality of life (QOL). Outcome assessment protocols are in place for all cohorts and the second SHHS examination is now in progress. Initial cross-sectional findings show that SDB is common and associated with hypertension and self-reported cardiovascular disease (CVD). This application requests five years additional support to continue the SHHS. Further follow-up is needed to have sufficient power to test the primary SHHS hypotheses. Additionally in Years 7-9, PSG will be repeated to further characterize SDB in the participants and to describe the natural history of SDB. During the first five years, the SHHS has shown that large-scale research on sleep, SDB, and disease risk can be conducted in the community. Follow-up of the SHHS cohort will provide the data needed to characterize the cardiovascular consequences of SDB, along with its natural history.

  Website: http://crisp.cit.nih.gov/crisp/Crisp_Query.Generate_Screen

- **Project Title: SLEEP HEART HEALTH STUDY**

  Principal Investigator & Institution: Resnick, Helaine E.; Director; Missouri Breaks Research, Inc. Timber Lake, Sd 57656

  Timing: Fiscal Year 2002; Project Start 30-SEP-1999; Project End 31-AUG-2004

  Summary: This abstract is not available.

  Website: http://crisp.cit.nih.gov/crisp/Crisp_Query.Generate_Screen

- **Project Title: SLEEP REGULATION AND TUMOR NECROSIS FACTOR**

  Principal Investigator & Institution: Krueger, James M.; Professor; Vet & Comp Anat/Pharm/Physiol; Washington State University 423 Neill Hall Pullman, Wa 99164

  Timing: Fiscal Year 2002; Project Start 01-AUG-1993; Project End 31-JUL-2005

  Summary: (provided by applicant): Sleep is of central importance to neurobiology because to understand how the brain works, we will have to decipher the mechanisms and functions of sleep. The function(s) of sleep remain unknown and the humoral and neural mechanisms of sleep are incompletely understood. Most people intuitively recognize that sleep increases after sleep loss or during the course of an infection. There is much evidence that those sleep responses, as well as physiological sleep, are regulated, in part, by humoral mechanisms. We hypothesize that tumor necrosis factor alpha (TNF-alpha) is one of the key substances in sleep regulation. This hypothesis is based on studies showing: 1) TNF-alpha induces non-rapid eye movement sleep (NREMS); 2) inhibition of TNF-alpha inhibits spontaneous sleep and sleep responses induced by sleep loss or bacterial products; 3) TNF mRNA and TNF brain levels correlate with sleep propensity; 4) in humans, circulating TNF levels correlate with electroencephalogram slow-wave activity and increase after sleep loss or during several pathologies with associated fatigue, e.g., **sleep apnea,** rheumatoid arthritis, pre-eclampsia, multiple sclerosis. The proposed experiments seek to understand in mechanistic detail how TNF-alpha is involved in sleep regulation. We will determine whether blocking TNF-alpha or TNF-alpha production centrally attenuates systemic TNF-alpha-induced sleep responses; preliminary data show that vagotomy attenuates systemic TNF-alpha-induced NREMS (Specific Aim #1). We will investigate TNF-alpha regulation of NREMS within specific TNF-active sites in brain (Specific Aim #2). Preliminary data indicate that microinjection of TNF-alpha into the preoptic area enhances NREMS, whereas microinjection of an inhibitor of TNF-alpha reduces NREMS.

Pharmacologic blockage of prostaglandins, adenosine, and interleukin-1, and sleep manipulation using sleep deprivation and acute mild increases in ambient temperature to enhance sleep, will be combined with microinjections of TNF-alpha or TNF-alpha inhibitors. We will also use gene arrays to determine the time course of sleep-sensitive changes in brain for TNF and TNF superfamily member mRNAs. Anticipated results will provide molecular-mechanistic advances to understand sleep regulation as well as aid our general understanding of cytokine regulation in the brain. We anticipate that results will be directly relevant to therapeutics, e.g., a TNF soluble receptor has already been shown to reduce fatigue associated with rheumatoid arthritis.

Website: http://crisp.cit.nih.gov/crisp/Crisp_Query.Generate_Screen

- **Project Title: SLEEP, METABOLIC, AND CARDIOVASCULAR DYSFUNCTION IN PCOS**

  Principal Investigator & Institution: Ehrmann, David A.; Associate Professor; Medicine; University of Chicago 5801 S Ellis Ave Chicago, Il 60637

  Timing: Fiscal Year 2003; Project Start 30-SEP-2003; Project End 31-JUL-2007

  Summary: (provided by applicant): Polycystic ovary syndrome (PCOS) affects 5-10% of women and may be viewed as the combination of hyperandrogenism with the classical features of the metabolic syndrome in young women. PCOS presents a unique opportunity to dissect the relationship between metabolic and cardiovascular risk and sleep disordered breathing (SDB) in a population where intrinsic effects of aging have not yet developed. Because a relationship between **obstructive sleep apnea,** insulin resistance and elevated testosterone levels has also been observed in men and in women without PCOS, insights gained from studies in PCOS will have broad implications. the Specific Aims of the present application are: Specific Aim 1: to test the hypothesis that sleep disturbances are caused by hyperandrogenemia and hyperinsulinemia that characterize PCOS. Following a detailed baseline evaluation of sleep, hormonal, metabolic and cardiovascular parameters, women with PCOS will be randomized to an 8-week treatment phase with pioglitazone or depot leuprolide plus estrogerdprogestin replacement or placebo. Pioglitazone will reduce insulin levels, and consequently androgen levels, in PCOS. We will compare the effects of androgen reduction alone (depot leuprolide plus estrogerdprogestin) to those of insulin plus androgen reduction achieved with pioglitazone. Primary comparisons will be the change in sleep parameters from baseline between: placebo & pioglitazone; placebo &

leuprolide/estrogen/progestin; pioglitazone & leuprolide/estrogen/progestin. Specific Aim 2: to test the hypothesis that sleep disturbances cause the hormonal, metabolic and cardiovascular alterations seen in women with PCOS. PCOS women with SDB and matched control women with SDB will be evaluated at baseline and following 8 weeks of CPAP treatment. The primary comparison will be between baseline and post-treatment parameters in PCOS women. The secondary comparison will be the post-treatment change from baseline between PCOS and control women to test the hypothesis that for the same degree in improvement in SDB, the magnitude of change in metabolic and cardiovascular measures will be greater in PCOS than in controls. Specific Aim 3: to test the hypothesis that in normal young women, experimental manipulation of sleep that recapitulates the sleep disturbances characteristic of women with PCOS will result in metabolic, hormonal, and cardiovascular alterations that are typical of the metabolic syndrome. A group of healthy young women will be studied twice using a randomized cross-over design. In one study, REM sleep will be fragmented by experimentally induced microarousals for 3 consecutive nights and non- REM sleep will be left undisturbed. In the other, slow wave activity will be suppressed without awakening the subject and REM sleep will be left undisturbed. Each study will be preceded by 2 nights of basetine sleep.

Website: http://crisp.cit.nih.gov/crisp/Crisp_Query.Generate_Screen

- **Project Title: SLEEP-DISORDERED BREATHING & THE METABOLIC SYNDROME**

  Principal Investigator & Institution: Saad, Mohammed F.; Professor; Medicine; University of California Los Angeles 10920 Wilshire Blvd., Suite 1200 Los Angeles, Ca 90024

  Timing: Fiscal Year 2003; Project Start 30-SEP-2003; Project End 31-JUL-2007

  Summary: (provided by applicant): Sleep-disordered breathing (SDB) and the metabolic syndrome commonly co-exist. It is possible that the increased sympathetic activity and neuroendocrine changes associated with SDB contribute to development or worsening of insulin resistance and/or other components of the metabolic syndrome. Alternatively, adiposity and increased visceral obesity could link the metabolic syndrome and SBD. Furthermore, both the metabolic syndrome and SDB aggregate in families, and these two conditions could share some genetic determinants. This proposal will test the hypotheses that in African Americans: 1) SDB and the metabolic syndrome share common determinants; and 2) genetic factors contribute to the association between

SDB and the metabolic syndrome. To achieve this goal, we will examine inter-relationships between the metabolic syndrome and SDB in a large well-defined cohort of African American families participating in the Insulin Resistance Atherosclerosis Family Study (IRAS Family Study), an ongoing study funded by NHLBI. In the IRAS Family Study, the UCLA center recruited 34 large extended African American families comprising 523 subjects and providing 479 sib-pairs and 1257 avuncular pairs. Insulin sensitivity and other components of the metabolic syndrome were measured in all subjects and a genome-wide scan has been performed. SDB will be assessed with polysomnography in 400 subjects which will provide more than 350 sib-pairs and 1,000 avuncular pairs. We will also repeat measuring components of the metabolic syndrome in these subjects so that they will be concurrent with measures of SDB. The specific aims are to: 1) Determine the association between SDB and the metabolic syndrome and its components in African American families participating in the IRAS Family Study; 2) Determine the heritability of SDB and the effects of shared genes, shared environments, or both on the association between SDB and the metabolic syndrome in African Americans; and 3) Determine candidate regions of the human genome which could contribute to SDB and the association between SDB and the metabolic syndrome in African Americans using a systemic linkage mapping approach utilizing the available genome scan. Success of this work will lead to better understanding of the interaction and the pathogenesis of the two conditions and could lead to better preventive and therapeutic modalities.

Website: http://crisp.cit.nih.gov/crisp/Crisp_Query.Generate_Screen

- **Project Title: THE METABOLIC SYNDROME IN PEDIATRIC OBSTRUCTIVE APNEA**

  Principal Investigator & Institution: Waters, Karen A.;; Children's Hospital at Westmead Locked Bag 4001 New South Wales,

  Timing: Fiscal Year 2002; Project Start 01-SEP-2002; Project End 31-JUL-2006

  Summary: (provided by applicant): This project will evaluate the association between **obstructive sleep apnea** (OSA) in childhood, and the presence of the "metabolic syndrome". Our aims are: 1. To confirm the association between OSA in children and the presence of known risk factors for future cardiovascular disease. 2. To confirm that the physiological disruptions caused by OSA can induce the same metabolic abnormalities in an animal model, and 3. To confirm that treatment of OSA can reverse the abnormalities underlying the metabolic syndrome. The metabolic syndrome is a combination of hypertension, insulin resistance, and dyslipidemia. The first abnormality to appear in children is insulin resistance. The presence of insulin resistance in children has been associated with development of all three abnormalities in adulthood, and thus with increased risk for later cardiovascular disease. Studying OSA in children provides a unique opportunity to study the mechanisms underlying the association between OSA, the metabolic syndrome, and cardiovascular disease. The majority of children with OSA are NOT obese, so it is possible to determine the relative contribution of factors including obesity, chronic sympathetic activation, and chronic inflammation, if a sufficiently large group is studied. Children who present to a sleep unit already have some combination of symptoms suggestive of OSA. Therefore, a parallel study will seek to understand the earliest associations between OSA and the metabolic syndrome. To do this, piglets will be exposed to repetitive hypercapnic hypoxia, and equivalent studies of metabolic abnormalities will be undertaken. This component of the study will examine the specific sequence of disturbances underlying the metabolic syndrome, with the goal of determining preventative strategies that could be translated into the clinical setting. Finally, children who have OSA will undergo treatment, followed by re-evaluation. If treatment of OSA can reverse the metabolic disturbances present in association with OSA, this will support the need for early and aggressive intervention in childhood OSA.

Website: http://crisp.cit.nih.gov/crisp/Crisp_Query.Generate_Screen

- **Project Title: THE ROLE OF CYTOKINES IN SLEEPINESS AND SLEEP APNEA**

  Principal Investigator & Institution: Vgontzas, Alexandros N.; Professor; Psychiatry; Pennsylvania State Univ Hershey Med Ctr 500 University Drive Hershey, Pa 170332390

  Timing: Fiscal Year 2002; Project Start 01-AUG-2000; Project End 31-JUL-2004

  Summary: (applicant's abstract): Excessive daytime sleepiness (EDS) is a major public health concern, in part because individuals suffering from EDS often are not productive at work, are more susceptible to accidents, and generally are unable to function normally during the day. EDS is one of the major manifestations of individuals suffering from **obstructive sleep apnea** (OSA) and is frequently reported by obese individuals without **sleep apnea.** The mechanisms underlying EDS observed in both types of these individuals are not clear. We have recently demonstrated that the pro-inflammatory and fatigue-inducing cytokines, tumor necrosis factor-alpha (TNFalpha) and interleukin-6 (IL-6), assayed in single plasma samples, are elevated in subjects with disorders of EDS. In addition, in preliminary studies, we demonstrated that these two cytokines are elevated in obese, compared to lean subjects, and that both sleep disturbance and obesity contribute to the cytokine elevation. More recently, we showed that daytime plasma levels of IL-6 are elevated in experimentally-induced EDS by the use of sleep deprivation and that a good night's sleep is associated with decreased daytime levels in healthy young subjects. There is a large literature implicating several pro-inflammatory cytokines in the regulation of sleep in animals; however, cytokine research on sleep in humans has been very limited. The fundamental hypothesis to be tested by the proposed studies is that the pro-inflammatory cytokines, TNFalpha and IL-6, are associated with and may contribute to EDS. We will test this hypothesis by determining the circadian secretory patterns of TNFalpha and IL-6 in plasma obtained from subjects that exhibit EDS associated with OSA or obesity. Also, we will determine whether nighttime nasal CPAP reduces daytime plasma TNFalpha and IL-6 concentrations in sleep apneics. In addition, we will experimentally induce EDS in healthy young subjects by the use of total sleep deprivation or one week of sleep restriction, which mimics real life-situations, to determine the relationship between the pattern of daytime plasma TNFalpha and IL-6 concentrations and daytime sleepiness as measured objectively using MSLT. Finally, we will assess the effects of daytime napping, in healthy subjects, on post-nap sleepiness and TNFalpha and IL-6 secretion. In these studies, we will use a series of experimental techniques including nighttime polysomnography, MSLT, computerized EEG, actigraphy, 24-hour blood sampling, 24-hour recording of core body temperature, and assays for TNFalpha and IL-6. These studies collectively will provide additional evidence for a role of TNFalpha and IL-6 in EDS and lay the foundation for the development of potential therapeutic interventions.

Website: http://crisp.cit.nih.gov/crisp/Crisp_Query.Generate_Screen

- **Project Title: THE SLEEP HEART HEALTH STUDY**

  Principal Investigator & Institution: Shahar, Eyal; Associate Professor; Epidemiology; University of Minnesota Twin Cities 200 Oak Street Se Minneapolis, Mn 554552070

  Timing: Fiscal Year 2002; Project Start 30-SEP-1994; Project End 31-AUG-2004

  Summary: This abstract is not available.

  Website: http://crisp.cit.nih.gov/crisp/Crisp_Query.Generate_Screen

- **Project Title: TRANSFERRING BEHAV RESEARCH INTO NURSING HOME PRACTICE**

  Principal Investigator & Institution: Ouslander, Joseph G.; Professor; Medicine; Emory University 1784 North Decatur Road Atlanta, Ga 30322

  Timing: Fiscal Year 2002; Project Start 01-SEP-1999; Project End 31-AUG-2004

  Summary: This abstract is not available.

  Website: http://crisp.cit.nih.gov/crisp/Crisp_Query.Generate_Screen

- **Project Title: VALIDATION OF IN-HOME SLEEP APNEA RISK EVALUATION SYSTEM**

  Principal Investigator & Institution: Levendowski, Daniel J.;; Advanced Brain Monitoring, Inc. 2850 Pio Pico Dr, Ste a Carlsbad, Ca 920081554

  Timing: Fiscal Year 2002; Project Start 01-FEB-2001; Project End 31-JAN-2004

  Summary: Phase II completes development of the Apnea Risk Evaluation System (ARES), an integrated method, including: a) a physiological data acquisition device, easily self-applied to the forehead and comfortably worn throughout the night to collect data to screen for SA (Sp02, pulse, snoring and head position), b) software to identify respiratory events and distinguish movement artifacts, c) a questionnaire with Profile Analysis to assess SA risk factors, and d) expert system logic to quantify level of risk for SA. ARES will be compared directly to overnight polysomnography (PSG) on 400 patients referred to a sleep clinic, 50 patients diagnosed with hypertension, diabetes and depression with symptoms similar to SA and 10 healthy subjects. ARES Questionnaires from 100 healthy subjects will be acquired to cross-validate the Profile Analysis with PSG to verify subjects classified Profile Analysis "at-risk" for SA. Since AIRES is designed to be easily self-applied and worn at home, 20 healthy subjects and 50 SA patients will complete the questionnaire and wear the ARES Device at home, following instructions for self application. In home data will be compared to in lab PSG and ARES. Clarity of instructions, ease of application and comfort of the device when worn at home will also be evaluated. PROPOSED COMMERCIAL APPLICATION: **Sleep Apnea** is a serious, prevalent, under-diagnosed, but treatable disorder, creating a significant market demand for accurate, inexpensive and easy-to-administer assessment methods. The ARES willbe marketed to Managed care providers, HMOs and other medical professionals, including those involved with Occupational and Industrial Medicine and epidemiology. The ARES will also be marketed directly-to-consumers as an in-home risk assessment for SA.

Website: http://crisp.cit.nih.gov/crisp/Crisp_Query.Generate_Screen

- **Project Title: VASCULAR CONSEQUENCES OF SYMPATHETIC NEURAL ACTIVATION IN OBESITY**

  Principal Investigator & Institution: Haynes, William G.; Associate Professor; University of Iowa Iowa City, Ia 52242

  Timing: Fiscal Year 2003; Project Start 21-JAN-2003; Project End 31-DEC-2007

  Summary: The mechanisms underlying the association between obesity and hypertension are unclear, but increased sympathetic neural drive to skeletal muscle circulation and kidney has been implicated. This insight has been derived from direct intraneural recordings of sympathetic nerve activity and regional norepinephrine turnover. It has been assumed that the increases in sympathetic nerve activity (SNA) directly translate into elevated sympathetic vasoconstrictor tone, but these assumptions have not been rigorously tested. We have recently obtained preliminary data using maximal alpha-adrenergic receptor blockade of the forearm vasculature that demonstrates no increase in sympathetic vascular tone in normotensive obese humans despite increased muscle SNA. This suggests that there is dissociation between sympathetic neural outflow and sympathetically mediated vasoconstrictor tone. Interestingly, we also have preliminary data indicating that in obese hypertensive humans, increased muscle SNA is associated with increased sympathetic vasoconstrictor tone. This suggests that a predisposition to hypertension interacts with obesity to permit the increased SNA to be expressed as increased sympathetic vascular tone. This project will test the hypothesis that the vasoconstrictor effects of SNA are attenuated in obesity but preserved in obese humans with a predisposition to hypertension, with these specific aims: 1) What are the effects of hypertension, **obstructive sleep apnea** and visceral adiposity on the resistance vessel expression of elevated SNA? 2) Is endothelial nitric oxide generation responsible for attenuated effects of SNA on vascular tone in obese compared to lean normotensive humans, and is the modulating influence of nitric oxide attenuated in obese hypertensive humans? 3) What are the effects of different dietary components on SNA and sympathetically mediated vasoconstrictor tone in obese normotensive and hypertensive subjects? Sympathetic nerve traffic to skin and skeletal muscle will be assessed by microneurography. Sympathetic vasoconstrictor tone will be assessed by the vasodilator response of skin (laser Doppler flux) and skeletal muscle (oxygenation measured by near infra-red oximetry) to intra-arterial infusion of an alpha-adrenergic antagonist. These studies should provide new insights into the cardiovascular effects of obesity and the factors that predispose to obesity-related hypertension.

Website: http://crisp.cit.nih.gov/crisp/Crisp_Query.Generate_Screen

- **Project Title: WORKING MEMORY IN OBSTRUCTIVE SLEEP APNEA-AN FMRI STUDY**

  Principal Investigator & Institution: Thomas, Robert J.;; Beth Israel Deaconess Medical Center St 1005 Boston, Ma 02215

  Timing: Fiscal Year 2002; Project Start 30-SEP-2002; Project End 31-JUL-2007

  Summary: (provided by applicant): **Obstructive sleep apnea** (OSA) is associated with abnormalities of higher order executive cognitive functions. The precise neuroanatomical localization of these deficits is unknown. The physiological correlates of executive cognitive dysfunction are poorly defined, and recovery following therapy may be incomplete. This project proposes the novel use of a neuroimaging technology, functional magnetic resonance imaging (fMRI), and precise neurobehavioral protocols, to localize the neuroanatomical site of dysfunction. Additional protocols will isolate specific physiological correlates of these neurocognitive abnormalities such as sleep fragmentation, sleep deprivation, and nocturnal oxygen desaturation and will relate them to altered regional cortical function. We will examine the cause of incomplete recovery of executive function while on therapy with nasal positive airway pressure. Working memory is a brain system that provides temporary storage and manipulation of information necessary to execute complex cognitive tasks, and it contributes to several executive functions. The n-back paradigm is an extensively used probe of working memory in MU studies, and is normally associated with activation of dorsolateral prefrontal cortex (DLPFC), anterior cingulate and posterior parietal cortex. We have adapted this task at the 2- back level of difficulty for use in OSA patients. Our preliminary data suggest a reversible (with treatment) reduction of working memory capacity in OSA patients that may be secondary to selective dysfunction in the DLPFC, relative to other nodes in the executive control network. Based on this data we hypothesize that: 1) Patients with OSA have reduced activation of the DLPFC, relative to posterior parietal cortex during tests of working memory. 2) Sleep deprivation or fragmentation but not nocturnal hypoxia disrupts working memory in normal subjects. 3). Post-treatment residual abnormalities are caused by persisting sleep fragmentation, not prior hypoxic exposure. The P.I. has training in general medicine, neurology, sleep disorders and functional neuroimaging. The proposed projects will be performed under the direct guidance of experts in sleep disorders, cognitive neuroscience, and fMRI within the Harvard system. The relevant research environment is particularly rich at the participating institutions-basic and applied neurobiology of sleep, clinical sleep disorders, behavioral neurology, and fMRI. The career development plan will include training in MRI physics, applied MRI, statistics and research methodology, ethics, planning of clinical research, and cognitive neuroscience. The immediate career goal is to acquire the necessary skills for applied clinical fMRI and determine the functional neurocircuitry of the localization, etiology and recovery of reduced working memory capacity in patients with OSA using the 2-back task paradigm. The longterm career goal is to develop a model of the function of sleep by demonstrating the functional consequences of sleep disruption in conditions such as depression, age-related memory dysfunction, and attention deficit hyperactivity disorder.

Website: http://crisp.cit.nih.gov/crisp/Crisp_Query.Generate_Screen

- **Project Title: WRIST- WORN AMBULATORY OXIMETER**

  Principal Investigator & Institution: Krausman, David T.; Vice Prsident & Ceo; Individual Monitoring Sys, Inc. (Im Sys) 1055 Taylor Ave, Ste 300 Baltimore, Md 21286

  Timing: Fiscal Year 2002; Project Start 30-SEP-1999; Project End 31-AUG-2004

  Summary: The problems in sleep disorder medicine caused by the cost, access and variety of sleep laboratory testing have led to increasing use of home testing with oximeters for screening and triage of patients with suspected **sleep apnea.** Current oximeters are designed for hospital use and not for sleep medicine. They are complex and difficult to use for unattended recordings. They process the signal to reduce movement artifacts thereby reducing accuracy for apneas. This project will develop a new fully ambulatory oximeter (OxiTrac) designed for unattended recording in the home for two or more consecutive nights. OxiTrac will be worn like a wristwatch with a short cable connecting to a finger probe. Activity monitoring will be fully integrated into the unit for direct artifact detection reducing errors introduced by the amount of signal processing in current oximeters. Heart rate, SaO2, and activity will be stored in the unit and later downloaded to a computer for display and automatic analyses. In phase I the OxiTrac prototype was developed and successfully used, establishing feasibility. In phase II the unit will be improved, automatic artifact detection and data analyses developed and clinical evaluation completed. PROPOSED COMMERCIAL APPLICATIONS: The prevalence of the **sleep apnea syndrome** (SAS) is estimated at between 4 to 8% of the population. The high consequences of this disease and the cost of polysomnography make simplified recording techniques for screening and diagnosing imperative. Pulse oximetry has become a primary measure of choice in the evaluation of SAS and other sleep-related breathing disorders. The OxiTrac unit if established as a standard, would be suitable for use by the specialist, family doctor, nurse and most clinical staff and sold to virtually all sleep disorder centers, researchers, physicians, home testing agencies and similar clinical environments.

Website: http://crisp.cit.nih.gov/crisp/Crisp_Query.Generate_Screen

E-Journals: PubMed Central[17]

PubMed Central (PMC) is a digital archive of life sciences journal literature developed and managed by the National Center for Biotechnology Information (NCBI) at the U.S. National Library of Medicine (NLM).[18] Access to this growing archive of e-journals is free and unrestricted.[19] To search, go to **http://www.ncbi.nlm.nih.gov/entrez/query.fcgi?db=Pmc**, and type "sleep apnea" (or synonyms) into the search box. This search gives you access to full-text articles. The following is a sample of items found for sleep apnea in the PubMed Central database:

- **Obstructive sleep apnea and vascular disease.** by Lanfranchi P, Somers VA.; 2001; http://www.pubmedcentral.gov/articlerender.fcgi?tool=pmcentrez&artid=64798
- **Parasomnias and sleep disordered breathing in Caucasian and Hispanic children -- the Tucson children's assessment of sleep apnea study.** by Goodwin JL, Kaemingk KL, Fregosi RF, Rosen GM, Morgan WJ, Smith T, Quan SF.; 2004; http://www.pubmedcentral.gov/articlerender.fcgi?tool=pmcentrez&artid=419382

---

[17] Adapted from the National Library of Medicine: **http://www.pubmedcentral.nih.gov/about/intro.html**.

[18] With PubMed Central, NCBI is taking the lead in preservation and maintenance of open access to electronic literature, just as NLM has done for decades with printed biomedical literature. PubMed Central aims to become a world-class library of the digital age.

[19] The value of PubMed Central, in addition to its role as an archive, lies the availability of data from diverse sources stored in a common format in a single repository. Many journals already have online publishing operations, and there is a growing tendency to publish material online only, to the exclusion of print.

The National Library of Medicine: PubMed

One of the quickest and most comprehensive ways to find academic studies in both English and other languages is to use PubMed, maintained by the National Library of Medicine. The advantage of PubMed over previously mentioned sources is that it covers a greater number of domestic and foreign references. It is also free to the public.[20] If the publisher has a Web site that offers full text of its journals, PubMed will provide links to that site, as well as to sites offering other related data. User registration, a subscription fee, or some other type of fee may be required to access the full text of articles in some journals.

To generate your own bibliography of studies dealing with sleep apnea, simply go to the PubMed Web site at **www.ncbi.nlm.nih.gov/pubmed**. Type "sleep apnea" (or synonyms) into the search box, and click "Go." The following is the type of output you can expect from PubMed for "sleep apnea" (hyperlinks lead to article summaries):

- **A comparison of radiofrequency treatment schemes for obstructive sleep apnea syndrome.**
  Author(s): Steward DL, Weaver EM, Woodson BT.
  Source: Otolaryngology and Head and Neck Surgery. 2004 May; 130(5): 579-85.
  http://www.ncbi.nlm.nih.gov/entrez/query.fcgi?cmd=Retrieve&db=pubmed&dopt=Abstract&list_uids=15138424

- **A large pleomorphic adenoma of soft palate causing sleep apnea syndrome--a case report.**
  Author(s): Murthy SV, Murthy NC, Belagavi CS, Munishwara GB.
  Source: Indian J Pathol Microbiol. 2003 July; 46(3): 466-7.
  http://www.ncbi.nlm.nih.gov/entrez/query.fcgi?cmd=Retrieve&db=pubmed&dopt=Abstract&list_uids=15025309

[20] PubMed was developed by the National Center for Biotechnology Information (NCBI) at the National Library of Medicine (NLM) at the National Institutes of Health (NIH). The PubMed database was developed in conjunction with publishers of biomedical literature as a search tool for accessing literature citations and linking to full-text journal articles at Web sites of participating publishers. Publishers that participate in PubMed supply NLM with their citations electronically prior to or at the time of publication.

- **A mandibular protruding device in obstructive sleep apnea and snoring.**
  Author(s): Fransson A.
  Source: Swed Dent J Suppl. 2003; (163): 1-49. Review.
  http://www.ncbi.nlm.nih.gov/entrez/query.fcgi?cmd=Retrieve&db=pubmed&dopt=Abstract&list_uids=14713187

- **A modified monobloc for treatment of young children with obstructive sleep apnea.**
  Author(s): Cozza P, Ballanti F, Prete L.
  Source: J Clin Orthod. 2004 April; 38(4): 241-7. No Abstract Available.
  http://www.ncbi.nlm.nih.gov/entrez/query.fcgi?cmd=Retrieve&db=pubmed&dopt=Abstract&list_uids=15115898

- **A practical method for describing patterns of tongue-base narrowing (modification of Fujita) in awake adult patients with obstructive sleep apnea.**
  Author(s): Moore KE, Phillips C.
  Source: Journal of Oral and Maxillofacial Surgery : Official Journal of the American Association of Oral and Maxillofacial Surgeons. 2002 March; 60(3): 252-60; Discussion 260-1. Erratum In: J Oral Maxillofac Surg 2002 May; 60(5): 610.
  http://www.ncbi.nlm.nih.gov/entrez/query.fcgi?cmd=Retrieve&db=pubmed&dopt=Abstract&list_uids=11887133

- **A prospective 8 week trial of nasal interfaces vs. a novel oral interface (Oracle) for treatment of obstructive sleep apnea hypopnea syndrome.**
  Author(s): Khanna R, Kline LR.
  Source: Sleep Medicine. 2003 July; 4(4): 333-8.
  http://www.ncbi.nlm.nih.gov/entrez/query.fcgi?cmd=Retrieve&db=pubmed&dopt=Abstract&list_uids=14592306

- **A randomized trial of auto-titrating CPAP and fixed CPAP in the treatment of obstructive sleep apnea-hypopnea.**
  Author(s): Hussain SF, Love L, Burt H, Fleetham JA.
  Source: Respiratory Medicine. 2004 April; 98(4): 330-3.
  http://www.ncbi.nlm.nih.gov/entrez/query.fcgi?cmd=Retrieve&db=pubmed&dopt=Abstract&list_uids=15072173

- **A randomized, controlled crossover trial of two oral appliances for sleep apnea treatment.**
  Author(s): Bloch KE, Iseli A, Zhang JN, Xie X, Kaplan V, Stoeckli PW, Russi EW.
  Source: American Journal of Respiratory and Critical Care Medicine. 2000 July; 162(1): 246-51.
  http://www.ncbi.nlm.nih.gov/entrez/query.fcgi?cmd=Retrieve&db=pubmed&dopt=Abstract&list_uids=10903249

- **A randomized, double-blind clinical trial comparing continuous positive airway pressure with a novel bilevel pressure system for treatment of obstructive sleep apnea syndrome.**
  Author(s): Gay PC, Herold DL, Olson EJ.
  Source: Sleep. 2003 November 1; 26(7): 864-9.
  http://www.ncbi.nlm.nih.gov/entrez/query.fcgi?cmd=Retrieve&db=pubmed&dopt=Abstract&list_uids=14655921
- **A sleep apnea syndrome detection system.**
  Author(s): Ishida R, Yonczawa Y, Maki H, Ogawa H, Hahn AW, Caldwell WM.
  Source: Biomed Sci Instrum. 2004; 40: 458-62.
  http://www.ncbi.nlm.nih.gov/entrez/query.fcgi?cmd=Retrieve&db=pubmed&dopt=Abstract&list_uids=15134001

- **Access to diagnosis and treatment of patients with suspected sleep apnea.**
  Author(s): Flemons WW, Douglas NJ, Kuna ST, Rodenstein DO, Wheatley J.
  Source: American Journal of Respiratory and Critical Care Medicine. 2004 March 15; 169(6): 668-72.
  http://www.ncbi.nlm.nih.gov/entrez/query.fcgi?cmd=Retrieve&db=pubmed&dopt=Abstract&list_uids=15003950

- **Accuracy of an unattended home CPAP titration in the treatment of obstructive sleep apnea.**
  Author(s): Series F.
  Source: American Journal of Respiratory and Critical Care Medicine. 2000 July; 162(1): 94-7.
  http://www.ncbi.nlm.nih.gov/entrez/query.fcgi?cmd=Retrieve&db=pubmed&dopt=Abstract&list_uids=10903226

- **Acoustic pharyngometry patterns of snoring and obstructive sleep apnea patients.**
  Author(s): Kamal I.
  Source: Otolaryngology and Head and Neck Surgery. 2004 January; 130(1): 58-66.
  http://www.ncbi.nlm.nih.gov/entrez/query.fcgi?cmd=Retrieve&db=pubmed&dopt=Abstract&list_uids=14726911

- **Adenotonsillectomy improves neurocognitive function in children with obstructive sleep apnea syndrome.**
  Author(s): Friedman BC, Hendeles-Amitai A, Kozminsky E, Leiberman A, Friger M, Tarasiuk A, Tal A.
  Source: Sleep. 2003 December 15; 26(8): 999-1005.
  http://www.ncbi.nlm.nih.gov/entrez/query.fcgi?cmd=Retrieve&db=pubmed&dopt=Abstract&list_uids=14746381

- **Adenotonsillectomy in children with obstructive sleep apnea syndrome reduces health care utilization.**
  Author(s): Tarasiuk A, Simon T, Tal A, Reuveni H.
  Source: Pediatrics. 2004 February; 113(2): 351-6.
  http://www.ncbi.nlm.nih.gov/entrez/query.fcgi?cmd=Retrieve&db=pubmed&dopt=Abstract&list_uids=14754948

- **Airway inflammation in patients affected by obstructive sleep apnea syndrome.**
  Author(s): Salerno FG, Carpagnano E, Guido P, Bonsignore MR, Roberti A, Aliani M, Vignola AM, Spanevello A.
  Source: Respiratory Medicine. 2004 January; 98(1): 25-8.
  http://www.ncbi.nlm.nih.gov/entrez/query.fcgi?cmd=Retrieve&db=pubmed&dopt=Abstract&list_uids=14959810

- **Aldosterone excretion among subjects with resistant hypertension and symptoms of sleep apnea.**
  Author(s): Calhoun DA, Nishizaka MK, Zaman MA, Harding SM.
  Source: Chest. 2004 January; 125(1): 112-7.
  http://www.ncbi.nlm.nih.gov/entrez/query.fcgi?cmd=Retrieve&db=pubmed&dopt=Abstract&list_uids=14718429

- **Annual review of patients with sleep apnea/hypopnea syndrome--a pragmatic randomised trial of nurse home visit versus consultant clinic review.**
  Author(s): Palmer S, Selvaraj S, Dunn C, Osman LM, Cairns J, Franklin D, Hulks G, Godden DJ.
  Source: Sleep Medicine. 2004 January; 5(1): 61-5.
  http://www.ncbi.nlm.nih.gov/entrez/query.fcgi?cmd=Retrieve&db=pubmed&dopt=Abstract&list_uids=14725828

- **Antioxidant capacity in obstructive sleep apnea patients.**
  Author(s): Sleep Med. 2003 Jul;4(4):361-6
  Source: Sleep Medicine. 2003 May; 4(3): 225-8.
  http://www.ncbi.nlm.nih.gov/entrez/query.fcgi?cmd=Retrieve&db=pubmed&dopt=Abstract&list_uids=14592314

- **Assessment of closed-loop ventilatory stability in obstructive sleep apnea.**
  Author(s): Asyali MH, Berry RB, Khoo MC.
  Source: Ieee Transactions on Bio-Medical Engineering. 2002 March; 49(3): 206-16.
  http://www.ncbi.nlm.nih.gov/entrez/query.fcgi?cmd=Retrieve&db=pubmed&dopt=Abstract&list_uids=11878312

- **Bariatric surgery for treatment of sleep apnea syndrome in 15 morbidly obese patients: long-term results.**
  Author(s): Scheuller M, Weider D.
  Source: Otolaryngology and Head and Neck Surgery. 2001 October; 125(4): 299-302.
  http://www.ncbi.nlm.nih.gov/entrez/query.fcgi?cmd=Retrieve&db=pubmed&dopt=Abstract&list_uids=11593162

- **Behavioral and pharmacologic therapy of obstructive sleep apnea.**
  Author(s): Magalang UJ, Mador MJ.
  Source: Clinics in Chest Medicine. 2003 June; 24(2): 343-53. Review.
  http://www.ncbi.nlm.nih.gov/entrez/query.fcgi?cmd=Retrieve&db=pubmed&dopt=Abstract&list_uids=12800788

- **Benefit of atrial pacing in sleep apnea syndrome.**
  Author(s): Garrigue S, Bordier P, Jais P, Shah DC, Hocini M, Raherison C, Tunon De Lara M, Haissaguerre M, Clementy J.
  Source: The New England Journal of Medicine. 2002 February 7; 346(6): 404-12. Erratum In: N Engl J Med 2002 March 14; 346(11): 872.
  http://www.ncbi.nlm.nih.gov/entrez/query.fcgi?cmd=Retrieve&db=pubmed&dopt=Abstract&list_uids=11832528

- **Beyond systemic hypertension: understanding cardiac dysfunction in obstructive sleep apnea.**
  Author(s): Hudgel DW.
  Source: Respiration; International Review of Thoracic Diseases. 2000; 67(4): 360-1.
  http://www.ncbi.nlm.nih.gov/entrez/query.fcgi?cmd=Retrieve&db=pubmed&dopt=Abstract&list_uids=11001709

- **Bilateral leg edema, obesity, pulmonary hypertension, and obstructive sleep apnea.**
  Author(s): Blankfield RP, Hudgel DW, Tapolyai AA, Zyzanski SJ.
  Source: Archives of Internal Medicine. 2000 August 14-28; 160(15): 2357-62. Erratum In: Arch Intern Med 2000 September 25; 160(17): 2650.
  http://www.ncbi.nlm.nih.gov/entrez/query.fcgi?cmd=Retrieve&db=pubmed&dopt=Abstract&list_uids=10927734

- **Bilateral leg edema, pulmonary hypertension, and obstructive sleep apnea: a cross-sectional study.**
  Author(s): Blankfield RP, Zyzanski SJ.
  Source: The Journal of Family Practice. 2002 June; 51(6): 561-4.
  http://www.ncbi.nlm.nih.gov/entrez/query.fcgi?cmd=Retrieve&db=pubmed&dopt=Abstract&list_uids=12100781

- **Binswanger's disease: its association with hypertension and obstructive sleep apnea.**
  Author(s): Matthews KD, Richter RW.
  Source: J Okla State Med Assoc. 2003 June; 96(6): 265-8; Quiz 269-70.
  http://www.ncbi.nlm.nih.gov/entrez/query.fcgi?cmd=Retrieve&db=pubmed&dopt=Abstract&list_uids=12858817

- **Blood levels of vascular endothelial growth factor in obstructive sleep apnea-hypopnea syndrome.**
  Author(s): Gunsilius E, Petzer AL, Gastl GA.
  Source: Blood. 2002 January 1; 99(1): 393-4.
  http://www.ncbi.nlm.nih.gov/entrez/query.fcgi?cmd=Retrieve&db=pubmed&dopt=Abstract&list_uids=11783437

- **Blood pressure elevation associated with sleep-related breathing disorder in a community sample of white and Hispanic children: the Tucson Children's Assessment of Sleep Apnea study.**
  Author(s): Enright PL, Goodwin JL, Sherrill DL, Quan JR, Quan SF; Tucson Children's Assessment of Sleep Apnea study.
  Source: Archives of Pediatrics & Adolescent Medicine. 2003 September; 157(9): 901-4.
  http://www.ncbi.nlm.nih.gov/entrez/query.fcgi?cmd=Retrieve&db=pubmed&dopt=Abstract&list_uids=12963596

- **Blood pressure variability in obstructive sleep apnea: role of sympathetic nervous activity and effect of continuous positive airway pressure.**
  Author(s): Bao X, Nelesen RA, Loredo JS, Dimsdale JE, Ziegler MG.
  Source: Blood Pressure Monitoring. 2002 December; 7(6): 301-7.
  http://www.ncbi.nlm.nih.gov/entrez/query.fcgi?cmd=Retrieve&db=pubmed&dopt=Abstract&list_uids=12488649

- **Blood pressure, cardiac structure and severity of obstructive sleep apnea in a sleep clinic population.**
  Author(s): Kraiczi H, Peker Y, Caidahl K, Samuelsson A, Hedner J.
  Source: Journal of Hypertension. 2001 November; 19(11): 2071-8.
  http://www.ncbi.nlm.nih.gov/entrez/query.fcgi?cmd=Retrieve&db=pubmed&dopt=Abstract&list_uids=11677374

- **Blood viscosity and platelet function in patients with obstructive sleep apnea syndrome treated with nasal continuous positive airway pressure.**
  Author(s): Reinhart WH, Oswald J, Walter R, Kuhn M.
  Source: Clinical Hemorheology and Microcirculation. 2002; 27(3-4): 201-7.
  http://www.ncbi.nlm.nih.gov/entrez/query.fcgi?cmd=Retrieve&db=pubmed&dopt=Abstract&list_uids=12454377

- **Body fat distribution, serum leptin, and cardiovascular risk factors in men with obstructive sleep apnea.**
  Author(s): Schafer H, Pauleit D, Sudhop T, Gouni-Berthold I, Ewig S, Berthold HK.
  Source: Chest. 2002 September; 122(3): 829-39.
  http://www.ncbi.nlm.nih.gov/entrez/query.fcgi?cmd=Retrieve&db=pubmed&dopt=Abstract&list_uids=12226021

- **Body position and obstructive sleep apnea in children.**
  Author(s): Fernandes do Prado LB, Li X, Thompson R, Marcus CL.
  Source: Sleep. 2002 February 1; 25(1): 66-71.
  http://www.ncbi.nlm.nih.gov/entrez/query.fcgi?cmd=Retrieve&db=pubmed&dopt=Abstract&list_uids=11833863

- **Body position and obstructive sleep apnea syndrome.**
  Author(s): Cuhadaroglu C, Keles N, Erdamar B, Aydemir N, Yucel E, Oguz F, Deger K.
  Source: Pediatric Pulmonology. 2003 October; 36(4): 335-8.
  http://www.ncbi.nlm.nih.gov/entrez/query.fcgi?cmd=Retrieve&db=pubmed&dopt=Abstract&list_uids=12950048

- **Brahms' lullaby revisited. Did the composer have obstructive sleep apnea?**
  Author(s): Margolis ML.
  Source: Chest. 2000 July; 118(1): 210-3.
  http://www.ncbi.nlm.nih.gov/entrez/query.fcgi?cmd=Retrieve&db=pubmed&dopt=Abstract&list_uids=10893381

- **Brain morphology associated with obstructive sleep apnea.**
  Author(s): Macey PM, Henderson LA, Macey KE, Alger JR, Frysinger RC, Woo MA, Harper RK, Yan-Go FL, Harper RM.
  Source: American Journal of Respiratory and Critical Care Medicine. 2002 November 15; 166(10): 1382-7.
  http://www.ncbi.nlm.nih.gov/entrez/query.fcgi?cmd=Retrieve&db=pubmed&dopt=Abstract&list_uids=12421746

- **Breathhold cine MRI of left ventricular function in patients with obstructive sleep apnea: work-in-progress.**
  Author(s): Mintorovitch J, Duerinckx AJ, Goldman MD, Meissner HH.
  Source: Magnetic Resonance Imaging. 2000 January; 18(1): 81-7.
  http://www.ncbi.nlm.nih.gov/entrez/query.fcgi?cmd=Retrieve&db=pubmed&dopt=Abstract&list_uids=10642105

- **Breath-to-breath variability correlates with apnea-hypopnea index in obstructive sleep apnea.**
  Author(s): Kowallik P, Jacobi I, Jirmann A, Meesmann M, Schmidt M, Wirtz H.
  Source: Chest. 2001 February; 119(2): 451-9.
  http://www.ncbi.nlm.nih.gov/entrez/query.fcgi?cmd=Retrieve&db=pubmed&dopt=Abstract&list_uids=11171722

- **By the way, doctor. Three years ago, my husband went to a sleep clinic for his snoring. He was diagnosed with moderate sleep apnea and given a continuous positive airway pressure (CPAP) device. He has been sleeping like a baby ever since--and so have I. Here's my question: when he reapplied for life insurance, his rating went from super-preferred to borderline insurable. Is there that much risk, even though he faithfully wears his mask every night? I would warn anyone who has a snoring problem to get life insurance before going to the sleep clinic!**
  Author(s): Lee TH.
  Source: Harvard Health Letter / from Harvard Medical School. 2003 September; 28(11): 8.
  http://www.ncbi.nlm.nih.gov/entrez/query.fcgi?cmd=Retrieve&db=pubmed&dopt=Abstract&list_uids=14505972

- **Cardiovascular disease and obstructive sleep apnea: implications for physicians.**
  Author(s): Foresman BH, Gwirtz PA, McMahon JP.
  Source: J Am Osteopath Assoc. 2000 June; 100(6): 360-9. Review.
  http://www.ncbi.nlm.nih.gov/entrez/query.fcgi?cmd=Retrieve&db=pubmed&dopt=Abstract&list_uids=10902407

- **Cardiovascular disease associated with obstructive sleep apnea.**
  Author(s): Fletcher EC.
  Source: Monaldi Arch Chest Dis. 2003 July-September; 59(3): 254-61. No Abstract Available.
  http://www.ncbi.nlm.nih.gov/entrez/query.fcgi?cmd=Retrieve&db=pubmed&dopt=Abstract&list_uids=15065329

- **Catecholaminergic neurons in the brain-stem and sleep apnea in SIDS victims.**
  Author(s): Sawaguchi T, Ozawa Y, Patricia F, Kadhim H, Groswasser J, Sottiaux M, Takashima S, Nishida H, Kahn A.
  Source: Early Human Development. 2003 December; 75 Suppl: S41-50.
  http://www.ncbi.nlm.nih.gov/entrez/query.fcgi?cmd=Retrieve&db=pubmed&dopt=Abstract&list_uids=14693390

- **Central sleep apnea and chronic heart failure.**
  Author(s): Andreas S.
  Source: Sleep. 2000 June 15; 23 Suppl 4: S220-3. Review.
  http://www.ncbi.nlm.nih.gov/entrez/query.fcgi?cmd=Retrieve&db=pubmed&dopt=Abstract&list_uids=10893107

- **Change in periodic limb movement index during treatment of obstructive sleep apnea with continuous positive airway pressure.**
  Author(s): Baran AS, Richert AC, Douglass AB, May W, Ansarin K.
  Source: Sleep. 2003 Sep15; 26(6): 717-20.
  http://www.ncbi.nlm.nih.gov/entrez/query.fcgi?cmd=Retrieve&db=pubmed&dopt=Abstract&list_uids=14572125

- **Changes in brain morphology associated with obstructive sleep apnea.**
  Author(s): Morrell MJ, McRobbie DW, Quest RA, Cummin AR, Ghiassi R, Corfield DR.
  Source: Sleep Medicine. 2003 September; 4(5): 451-4.
  http://www.ncbi.nlm.nih.gov/entrez/query.fcgi?cmd=Retrieve&db=pubmed&dopt=Abstract&list_uids=14592287

- **Changes in quality of life and respiratory disturbance after extended uvulopalatal flap surgery in patients with obstructive sleep apnea.**
  Author(s): Li HY, Chen NH, Shu YH, Wang PC.
  Source: Archives of Otolaryngology--Head & Neck Surgery. 2004 February; 130(2): 195-200.
  http://www.ncbi.nlm.nih.gov/entrez/query.fcgi?cmd=Retrieve&db=pubmed&dopt=Abstract&list_uids=14967750

- **Clinical predictors in obstructive sleep apnea patients with computer-assisted quantitative videoendoscopic upper airway analysis.**
  Author(s): Hsu PP, Tan BY, Chan YH, Tay HN, Lu PK, Blair RL.
  Source: The Laryngoscope. 2004 May; 114(5): 791-9.
  http://www.ncbi.nlm.nih.gov/entrez/query.fcgi?cmd=Retrieve&db=pubmed&dopt=Abstract&list_uids=15126732

- **Clinicopathological correlation between brainstem gliosis using GFAP as a marker and sleep apnea in the sudden infant death syndrome.**
  Author(s): Sawaguchi T, Patricia F, Kadhim H, Groswasser J, Sottiaux M, Nishida H, Kahn A.
  Source: Early Human Development. 2003 December; 75 Suppl: S3-11.
  http://www.ncbi.nlm.nih.gov/entrez/query.fcgi?cmd=Retrieve&db=pubmed&dopt=Abstract&list_uids=14693386

- **Combined uvulopalatopharyngoplasty and radiofrequency tongue base reduction for treatment of obstructive sleep apnea/hypopnea syndrome.**
  Author(s): Friedman M, Ibrahim H, Lee G, Joseph NJ.
  Source: Otolaryngology and Head and Neck Surgery. 2003 December; 129(6): 611-21.
  http://www.ncbi.nlm.nih.gov/entrez/query.fcgi?cmd=Retrieve&db=pubmed&dopt=Abstract&list_uids=14663425

- **Comparison of obstructive sleep apnea syndrome in children with cleft palate following Furlow palatoplasty or pharyngeal flap for velopharyngeal insufficiency.**
  Author(s): Liao YF, Noordhoff MS, Huang CS, Chen PK, Chen NH, Yun C, Chuang ML.
  Source: The Cleft Palate-Craniofacial Journal : Official Publication of the American Cleft Palate-Craniofacial Association. 2004 March; 41(2): 152-6.
  http://www.ncbi.nlm.nih.gov/entrez/query.fcgi?cmd=Retrieve&db=pubmed&dopt=Abstract&list_uids=14989690

- **Comparison of the NovaSom QSG, a new sleep apnea home-diagnostic system, and polysomnography.**
  Author(s): Reichert JA, Bloch DA, Cundiff E, Votteri BA.
  Source: Sleep Medicine. 2003 May; 4(3): 213-8.
  http://www.ncbi.nlm.nih.gov/entrez/query.fcgi?cmd=Retrieve&db=pubmed&dopt=Abstract&list_uids=14592324

- **Compliance, education, monitoring in the treatment of obstructive sleep apnea by nasal continuous positive airway pressure.**
  Author(s): Delguste P, Rodenstein DO.
  Source: Sleep. 2000 June 15; 23 Suppl 4: S158-60. Review. No Abstract Available.
  http://www.ncbi.nlm.nih.gov/entrez/query.fcgi?cmd=Retrieve&db=pubmed&dopt=Abstract&list_uids=10893093

- **Comprehensive reconstructive surgery for obstructive sleep apnea.**
  Author(s): Colin WB.
  Source: J Ky Med Assoc. 2004 April; 102(4): 154-62.
  http://www.ncbi.nlm.nih.gov/entrez/query.fcgi?cmd=Retrieve&db=pubmed&dopt=Abstract&list_uids=15125302

- **Computed tomographic evaluation of the role of craniofacial and upper airway morphology in obstructive sleep apnea in Chinese.**
  Author(s): Lam B, Ooi CG, Peh WC, Lauder I, Tsang KW, Lam WK, Ip MS.
  Source: Respiratory Medicine. 2004 April; 98(4): 301-7.
  http://www.ncbi.nlm.nih.gov/entrez/query.fcgi?cmd=Retrieve&db=pubmed&dopt=Abstract&list_uids=15072170

- **Con: Sleep apnea does not cause cardiovascular disease.**
  Author(s): Stradling J.
  Source: American Journal of Respiratory and Critical Care Medicine. 2004 January 15; 169(2): 148-9; Discussion 150.
  http://www.ncbi.nlm.nih.gov/entrez/query.fcgi?cmd=Retrieve&db=pubmed&dopt=Abstract&list_uids=14718234

- **Controlled trial of continuous positive airway pressure in obstructive sleep apnea and heart failure.**
  Author(s): Mansfield DR, Gollogly NC, Kaye DM, Richardson M, Bergin P, Naughton MT.
  Source: American Journal of Respiratory and Critical Care Medicine. 2004 February 1; 169(3): 361-6. Epub 2003 November 03.
  http://www.ncbi.nlm.nih.gov/entrez/query.fcgi?cmd=Retrieve&db=pubmed&dopt=Abstract&list_uids=14597482

- **Correlation between the Ki-67 antigen in the brainstem and physiological data on sleep apnea in SIDS victims.**
  Author(s): Sawaguchi T, Patricia F, Kadhim H, Groswasser J, Sottiaux M, Nishida H, Kahn A.
  Source: Early Human Development. 2003 December; 75 Suppl: S119-27.
  http://www.ncbi.nlm.nih.gov/entrez/query.fcgi?cmd=Retrieve&db=pubmed&dopt=Abstract&list_uids=14693398

- **CSF hypocretin measures in patients with obstructive sleep apnea.**
Author(s): Kanbayashi T, Inoue Y, Kawanishi K, Takasaki H, Aizawa R, Takahashi K, Ogawa Y, Abe M, Hishikawa Y, Shimizu T.
Source: Journal of Sleep Research. 2003 December; 12(4): 339-41.
http://www.ncbi.nlm.nih.gov/entrez/query.fcgi?cmd=Retrieve&db=pubmed&dopt=Abstract&list_uids=14633246

- **Current treatment practices in obstructive sleep apnea and snoring.**
Author(s): Gupta VK, Reiter ER.
Source: American Journal of Otolaryngology. 2004 January-February; 25(1): 18-25.
http://www.ncbi.nlm.nih.gov/entrez/query.fcgi?cmd=Retrieve&db=pubmed&dopt=Abstract&list_uids=15011202

- **Decision rules for diagnosis of sleep apnea.**
Author(s): Lewis KE.
Source: American Journal of Respiratory and Critical Care Medicine. 2004 March 15; 169(6): 771; Author Reply 771.
http://www.ncbi.nlm.nih.gov/entrez/query.fcgi?cmd=Retrieve&db=pubmed&dopt=Abstract&list_uids=15003952

- **Decreased pituitary-gonadal secretion in men with obstructive sleep apnea.**
Author(s): Luboshitzky R, Aviv A, Hefetz A, Herer P, Shen-Orr Z, Lavie L, Lavie P.
Source: The Journal of Clinical Endocrinology and Metabolism. 2002 July; 87(7): 3394-8.
http://www.ncbi.nlm.nih.gov/entrez/query.fcgi?cmd=Retrieve&db=pubmed&dopt=Abstract&list_uids=12107256

- **Dental and skeletal changes after 4 years of obstructive sleep apnea treatment with a mandibular advancement device: a prospective, randomized study.**
Author(s): Ringqvist M, Walker-Engstrom ML, Tegelberg A, Ringqvist I.
Source: American Journal of Orthodontics and Dentofacial Orthopedics : Official Publication of the American Association of Orthodontists, Its Constituent Societies, and the American Board of Orthodontics. 2003 July; 124(1): 53-60.
http://www.ncbi.nlm.nih.gov/entrez/query.fcgi?cmd=Retrieve&db=pubmed&dopt=Abstract&list_uids=12867898

- **Dental devices; classification for intraoral devices for snoring and/or obstructive sleep apnea. Final rule.**
  Author(s): Food and Drug Administration, HHS.
  Source: Federal Register. 2002 November 12; 67(218): 68510-2.
  http://www.ncbi.nlm.nih.gov/entrez/query.fcgi?cmd=Retrieve&db=pubmed&dopt=Abstract&list_uids=12428642

- **Determining the site of airway obstruction in obstructive sleep apnea with airway pressure measurements during sleep.**
  Author(s): Demin H, Jingying Y, Jun W, Qingwen Y, Yuhua L, Jiangyong W.
  Source: The Laryngoscope. 2002 November; 112(11): 2081-5.
  http://www.ncbi.nlm.nih.gov/entrez/query.fcgi?cmd=Retrieve&db=pubmed&dopt=Abstract&list_uids=12439185

- **Development of the obstructive sleep apnea knowledge and attitudes (OSAKA) questionnaire.**
  Author(s): Schotland HM, Jeffe DB.
  Source: Sleep Medicine. 2003 September; 4(5): 443-50.
  http://www.ncbi.nlm.nih.gov/entrez/query.fcgi?cmd=Retrieve&db=pubmed&dopt=Abstract&list_uids=14592286

- **Diagnosis and treatment of obstructive sleep apnea in a stroke rehabilitation unit: a feasibility study.**
  Author(s): Disler P, Hansford A, Skelton J, Wright P, Kerr J, O'Reilly J, Hepworth J, Middleton S, Sullivan C.
  Source: American Journal of Physical Medicine & Rehabilitation / Association of Academic Physiatrists. 2002 August; 81(8): 622-5.
  http://www.ncbi.nlm.nih.gov/entrez/query.fcgi?cmd=Retrieve&db=pubmed&dopt=Abstract&list_uids=12172072

- **Diagnosis of sleep apnea.**
  Author(s): Stevenson JE.
  Source: Wmj. 2003; 102(1): 25-7, 46. Review.
  http://www.ncbi.nlm.nih.gov/entrez/query.fcgi?cmd=Retrieve&db=pubmed&dopt=Abstract&list_uids=12679967

- **Diastolic blood pressure is the first to rise in association with early subclinical obstructive sleep apnea: lessons from periodic examination screening.**
  Author(s): Sharabi Y, Scope A, Chorney N, Grotto I, Dagan Y.
  Source: American Journal of Hypertension : Journal of the American Society of Hypertension. 2003 March; 16(3): 236-9.
  http://www.ncbi.nlm.nih.gov/entrez/query.fcgi?cmd=Retrieve&db=pubmed&dopt=Abstract&list_uids=12620704

- **Difficult endotracheal intubation in patients with sleep apnea syndrome.**
  Author(s): Siyam MA, Benhamou D.
  Source: Anesthesia and Analgesia. 2002 October; 95(4): 1098-102, Table of Contents.
  http://www.ncbi.nlm.nih.gov/entrez/query.fcgi?cmd=Retrieve&db=pubmed&dopt=Abstract&list_uids=12351303

- **Difficult-to-control asthma and obstructive sleep apnea.**
  Author(s): Yigla M, Tov N, Solomonov A, Rubin AH, Harlev D.
  Source: The Journal of Asthma : Official Journal of the Association for the Care of Asthma. 2003 December; 40(8): 865-71.
  http://www.ncbi.nlm.nih.gov/entrez/query.fcgi?cmd=Retrieve&db=pubmed&dopt=Abstract&list_uids=14736085

- **Discriminative power of phrenic twitch-induced dynamic response for diagnosis of sleep apnea during wakefulness.**
  Author(s): Verin E, Similowski T, Teixeira A, Series F.
  Source: Journal of Applied Physiology (Bethesda, Md. : 1985). 2003 January; 94(1): 31-7. Epub 2002 September 06.
  http://www.ncbi.nlm.nih.gov/entrez/query.fcgi?cmd=Retrieve&db=pubmed&dopt=Abstract&list_uids=12391097

- **Distraction osteogenesis in correction of micrognathia accompanying obstructive sleep apnea syndrome.**
  Author(s): Wang X, Wang XX, Liang C, Yi B, Lin Y, Li ZL.
  Source: Plastic and Reconstructive Surgery. 2003 November; 112(6): 1549-57; Discussion 1558-9.
  http://www.ncbi.nlm.nih.gov/entrez/query.fcgi?cmd=Retrieve&db=pubmed&dopt=Abstract&list_uids=14578784

- **Diurnal hypercapnia in patients with obstructive sleep apnea syndrome.**
  Author(s): Golpe R, Jimenez A, Carpizo R.
  Source: Chest. 2002 September; 122(3): 1100-1; Author Reply 1101.
  http://www.ncbi.nlm.nih.gov/entrez/query.fcgi?cmd=Retrieve&db=pubmed&dopt=Abstract&list_uids=12226064

- **Does cognitive dysfunction conform to a distinctive pattern in obstructive sleep apnea syndrome?**
  Author(s): Antonelli Incalzi R, Marra C, Salvigni BL, Petrone A, Gemma A, Selvaggio D, Mormile F.
  Source: Journal of Sleep Research. 2004 March; 13(1): 79-86.
  http://www.ncbi.nlm.nih.gov/entrez/query.fcgi?cmd=Retrieve&db=pubmed&dopt=Abstract&list_uids=14996039

- **Does sleep deprivation worsen mild obstructive sleep apnea?**
  Author(s): Desai AV, Marks G, Grunstein R.
  Source: Sleep. 2003 December 15; 26(8): 1038-41.
  http://www.ncbi.nlm.nih.gov/entrez/query.fcgi?cmd=Retrieve&db=pubmed&dopt=Abstract&list_uids=14746387

- **Does sleep deprivation worsen mild obstructive sleep apnea?**
  Author(s): McEvoy RD.
  Source: Sleep. 2003 December 15; 26(8): 937-8. No Abstract Available.
  http://www.ncbi.nlm.nih.gov/entrez/query.fcgi?cmd=Retrieve&db=pubmed&dopt=Abstract&list_uids=14746370

- **Doppler measurement of blood flow velocities in extraocular orbital vessels in patients with obstructive sleep apnea syndrome.**
  Author(s): Erdem CZ, Altin R, Erdem LO, Kargi S, Kart L, Cinar F, Ayoglu F.
  Source: Journal of Clinical Ultrasound : Jcu. 2003 June; 31(5): 250-7.
  http://www.ncbi.nlm.nih.gov/entrez/query.fcgi?cmd=Retrieve&db=pubmed&dopt=Abstract&list_uids=12767020

- **Dynamics of heart rate and sleep stages in normals and patients with sleep apnea.**
  Author(s): Penzel T, Kantelhardt JW, Lo CC, Voigt K, Vogelmeier C.
  Source: Neuropsychopharmacology : Official Publication of the American College of Neuropsychopharmacology. 2003 July; 28 Suppl 1: S48-53. Review.
  http://www.ncbi.nlm.nih.gov/entrez/query.fcgi?cmd=Retrieve&db=pubmed&dopt=Abstract&list_uids=12827144

- **Dysphagia, obstructive sleep apnea, and difficult fiberoptic intubation secondary to diffuse idiopathic skeletal hyperostosis.**
  Author(s): Naik B, Lobato EB, Sulek CA.
  Source: Anesthesiology. 2004 May; 100(5): 1311-2.
  http://www.ncbi.nlm.nih.gov/entrez/query.fcgi?cmd=Retrieve&db=pubmed&dopt=Abstract&list_uids=15114233

- **Early predictors of CPAP use for the treatment of obstructive sleep apnea.**
  Author(s): Lewis KE, Seale L, Bartle IE, Watkins AJ, Ebden P.
  Source: Sleep. 2004 February 1; 27(1): 134-8.
  http://www.ncbi.nlm.nih.gov/entrez/query.fcgi?cmd=Retrieve&db=pubmed&dopt=Abstract&list_uids=14998250

- **ECG analysis for sleep apnea detection.**
  Author(s): Zywietz CW, Von Einem V, Widiger B, Joseph G.
  Source: Methods of Information in Medicine. 2004; 43(1): 56-9.
  http://www.ncbi.nlm.nih.gov/entrez/query.fcgi?cmd=Retrieve&db=pubmed&dopt=Abstract&list_uids=15026838

- **Effect of continuous positive airway pressure treatment on elderly Chinese patients with obstructive sleep apnea in the prethrombotic state.**
  Author(s): Zhang X, Yin K, Wang H, Su M, Yang Y.
  Source: Chinese Medical Journal. 2003 September; 116(9): 1426-8.
  http://www.ncbi.nlm.nih.gov/entrez/query.fcgi?cmd=Retrieve&db=pubmed&dopt=Abstract&list_uids=14527381

- **Effect of nasal valve dilation on effective CPAP level in obstructive sleep apnea.**
  Author(s): Schonhofer B, Kerl J, Suchi S, Kohler D, Franklin KA.
  Source: Respiratory Medicine. 2003 September; 97(9): 1001-5.
  http://www.ncbi.nlm.nih.gov/entrez/query.fcgi?cmd=Retrieve&db=pubmed&dopt=Abstract&list_uids=14509553

- **Effect of oral appliance therapy on upper airway collapsibility in obstructive sleep apnea.**
  Author(s): Ng AT, Gotsopoulos H, Qian J, Cistulli PA.
  Source: American Journal of Respiratory and Critical Care Medicine. 2003 July 15; 168(2): 238-41. Epub 2003 April 30.
  http://www.ncbi.nlm.nih.gov/entrez/query.fcgi?cmd=Retrieve&db=pubmed&dopt=Abstract&list_uids=12724125

- **Effects of a mandibular protruding device on the sleep of patients with obstructive sleep apnea and snoring problems: a 2-year follow-up.**
  Author(s): Fransson AM, Tegelberg A, Leissner L, Wenneberg B, Isacsson G.
  Source: Sleep & Breathing = Schlaf & Atmung. 2003 September; 7(3): 131-41.
  http://www.ncbi.nlm.nih.gov/entrez/query.fcgi?cmd=Retrieve&db=pubmed&dopt=Abstract&list_uids=14569524

- **Effects of an anteriorly titrated mandibular position on awake airway and obstructive sleep apnea severity.**
  Author(s): Tsuiki S, Lowe AA, Almeida FR, Fleetham JA.
  Source: American Journal of Orthodontics and Dentofacial Orthopedics : Official Publication of the American Association of Orthodontists, Its Constituent Societies, and the American Board of Orthodontics. 2004 May; 125(5): 548-55.
  http://www.ncbi.nlm.nih.gov/entrez/query.fcgi?cmd=Retrieve&db=pubmed&dopt=Abstract&list_uids=15127023

- **Effects of gender on upper airway collapsibility and severity of obstructive sleep apnea.**
  Author(s): Mohsenin V.
  Source: Sleep Medicine. 2003 November; 4(6): 523-9.
  http://www.ncbi.nlm.nih.gov/entrez/query.fcgi?cmd=Retrieve&db=pubmed&dopt=Abstract&list_uids=14607346

- **Effects of hypoxia on the brain: neuroimaging and neuropsychological findings following carbon monoxide poisoning and obstructive sleep apnea.**
  Author(s): Gale SD, Hopkins RO.
  Source: Journal of the International Neuropsychological Society : Jins. 2004 January; 10(1): 60-71.
  http://www.ncbi.nlm.nih.gov/entrez/query.fcgi?cmd=Retrieve&db=pubmed&dopt=Abstract&list_uids=14751008

- **Effects of obstructive sleep apnea syndrome on serum aminotransferase levels in obese patients.**
  Author(s): Chin K, Nakamura T, Takahashi K, Sumi K, Ogawa Y, Masuzaki H, Muro S, Hattori N, Matsumoto H, Niimi A, Chiba T, Nakao K, Mishima M, Ohi M, Nakamura T.
  Source: The American Journal of Medicine. 2003 April 1; 114(5): 370-6.
  http://www.ncbi.nlm.nih.gov/entrez/query.fcgi?cmd=Retrieve&db=pubmed&dopt=Abstract&list_uids=12714126

- **Effects of oxygen administration on the circulating vascular endothelial growth factor (VEGF) levels in patients with obstructive sleep apnea syndrome.**
  Author(s): Teramoto S, Kume H, Yamamoto H, Ishii T, Miyashita A, Matsuse T, Akishita M, Toba K, Ouchi Y.
  Source: Intern Med. 2003 August; 42(8): 681-5.
  http://www.ncbi.nlm.nih.gov/entrez/query.fcgi?cmd=Retrieve&db=pubmed&dopt=Abstract&list_uids=12924491

- **Elongated uvula with a pleomorphic adenoma: a rare cause of obstructive sleep apnea syndrome.**
  Author(s): Motomura H, Harada T, Muraoka M, Taniguchi T.
  Source: Annals of Plastic Surgery. 2000 July; 45(1): 61-3.
  http://www.ncbi.nlm.nih.gov/entrez/query.fcgi?cmd=Retrieve&db=pubmed&dopt=Abstract&list_uids=10917100

- **Endoscopic examination of obstructive sleep apnea syndrome patients during drug-induced sleep.**
  Author(s): Iwanaga K, Hasegawa K, Shibata N, Kawakatsu K, Akita Y, Suzuki K, Yagisawa M, Nishimura T.
  Source: Acta Otolaryngol Suppl. 2003; (550): 36-40.
  http://www.ncbi.nlm.nih.gov/entrez/query.fcgi?cmd=Retrieve&db=pubmed&dopt=Abstract&list_uids=12737340

- **Endothelial function in obstructive sleep apnea and response to treatment.**
  Author(s): Ip MS, Tse HF, Lam B, Tsang KW, Lam WK.
  Source: American Journal of Respiratory and Critical Care Medicine. 2004 February 1; 169(3): 348-53. Epub 2003 October 09.
  http://www.ncbi.nlm.nih.gov/entrez/query.fcgi?cmd=Retrieve&db=pubmed&dopt=Abstract&list_uids=14551167

- **Enuresis in children with sleep apnea.**
  Author(s): Brooks LJ, Topol HI.
  Source: The Journal of Pediatrics. 2003 May; 142(5): 515-8.
  http://www.ncbi.nlm.nih.gov/entrez/query.fcgi?cmd=Retrieve&db=pubmed&dopt=Abstract&list_uids=12756383

- **Esophageal foreign bodies causing obstructive sleep apnea in a patient with Sturge-Weber syndrome.**
  Author(s): Watson NF, Kapur V.
  Source: Chest. 2003 July; 124(1): 400-3.
  http://www.ncbi.nlm.nih.gov/entrez/query.fcgi?cmd=Retrieve&db=pubmed&dopt=Abstract&list_uids=12853553

- **Evaluation of diagnostic device for obstructive sleep apnea.**
  Author(s): Cunnington D.
  Source: Chest. 2003 October; 124(4): 1623.
  http://www.ncbi.nlm.nih.gov/entrez/query.fcgi?cmd=Retrieve&db=pubmed&dopt=Abstract&list_uids=14555606

- **Evaluation of the accuracy of SNAP technology sleep sonography in detecting obstructive sleep apnea in adults compared to standard polysomnography.**
  Author(s): Liesching TN, Carlisle C, Marte A, Bonitati A, Millman RP.
  Source: Chest. 2004 March; 125(3): 886-91.
  http://www.ncbi.nlm.nih.gov/entrez/query.fcgi?cmd=Retrieve&db=pubmed&dopt=Abstract&list_uids=15006946

- **Evidence for lipid peroxidation in obstructive sleep apnea.**
  Author(s): Lavie L, Vishnevsky A, Lavie P.
  Source: Sleep. 2004 February 1; 27(1): 123-8.
  http://www.ncbi.nlm.nih.gov/entrez/query.fcgi?cmd=Retrieve&db=pubmed&dopt=Abstract&list_uids=14998248

- **Executive summary on the systematic review and practice parameters for portable monitoring in the investigation of suspected sleep apnea in adults.**
  Author(s): ATS/ACCP/AASM Taskforce Steering Committee.
  Source: American Journal of Respiratory and Critical Care Medicine. 2004 May 15; 169(10): 1160-3. Review.
  http://www.ncbi.nlm.nih.gov/entrez/query.fcgi?cmd=Retrieve&db=pubmed&dopt=Abstract&list_uids=15132960

- **Facial patterns of obstructive sleep apnea patients using Ricketts' method.**
  Author(s): Kikuchi M, Higurashi N, Miyazaki S, Itasaka Y.
  Source: Psychiatry and Clinical Neurosciences. 2000 June; 54(3): 336-7.
  http://www.ncbi.nlm.nih.gov/entrez/query.fcgi?cmd=Retrieve&db=pubmed&dopt=Abstract&list_uids=11186102

- **Factors associated with sleep apnea in men with spinal cord injury: a population-based case-control study.**
  Author(s): Burns SP, Kapur V, Yin KS, Buhrer R.
  Source: Spinal Cord : the Official Journal of the International Medical Society of Paraplegia. 2001 January; 39(1): 15-22.
  http://www.ncbi.nlm.nih.gov/entrez/query.fcgi?cmd=Retrieve&db=pubmed&dopt=Abstract&list_uids=11224009

- **Factors related to the efficacy of an adjustable oral appliance for the treatment of obstructive sleep apnea.**
  Author(s): Liu Y, Lowe AA.
  Source: Chin J Dent Res. 2000 November; 3(3): 15-23.
  http://www.ncbi.nlm.nih.gov/entrez/query.fcgi?cmd=Retrieve&db=pubmed&dopt=Abstract&list_uids=11314530

- **Falling asleep while driving and automobile accidents among patients with obstructive sleep apnea-hypopnea syndrome.**
  Author(s): Shiomi T, Arita AT, Sasanabe R, Banno K, Yamakawa H, Hasegawa R, Ozeki K, Okada M, Ito A.
  Source: Psychiatry and Clinical Neurosciences. 2002 June; 56(3): 333-4.
  http://www.ncbi.nlm.nih.gov/entrez/query.fcgi?cmd=Retrieve&db=pubmed&dopt=Abstract&list_uids=12047620

- **Familial link seen in obstructive sleep apnea.**
  Author(s): Lamberg L.
  Source: Jama : the Journal of the American Medical Association. 2003 December 10; 290(22): 2925-6.
  http://www.ncbi.nlm.nih.gov/entrez/query.fcgi?cmd=Retrieve&db=pubmed&dopt=Abstract&list_uids=14665642

- **Familial predisposition and cosegregation analysis of adult obstructive sleep apnea and the sudden infant death syndrome.**
  Author(s): Gislason T, Johannsson JH, Haraldsson A, Olafsdottir BR, Jonsdottir H, Kong A, Frigge ML, Jonsdottir GM, Hakonarson H, Gulcher J, Stefansson K.
  Source: American Journal of Respiratory and Critical Care Medicine. 2002 September 15; 166(6): 833-8.
  http://www.ncbi.nlm.nih.gov/entrez/query.fcgi?cmd=Retrieve&db=pubmed&dopt=Abstract&list_uids=12231493

- **Fatigue associated with obstructive sleep apnea in a patient with sarcoidosis.**
  Author(s): Drent M, Verbraecken J, van der Grinten C, Wouters E.
  Source: Respiration; International Review of Thoracic Diseases. 2000; 67(3): 337-40.
  http://www.ncbi.nlm.nih.gov/entrez/query.fcgi?cmd=Retrieve&db=pubmed&dopt=Abstract&list_uids=10867608

- **Fatigue in obstructive sleep apnea: driven by depressive symptoms instead of apnea severity?**
  Author(s): Bardwell WA, Moore P, Ancoli-Israel S, Dimsdale JE.
  Source: The American Journal of Psychiatry. 2003 February; 160(2): 350-5.
  http://www.ncbi.nlm.nih.gov/entrez/query.fcgi?cmd=Retrieve&db=pubmed&dopt=Abstract&list_uids=12562583

- **Feasibility of using unattended polysomnography in children for research--report of the Tucson Children's Assessment of Sleep Apnea study (TuCASA).**
  Author(s): Goodwin JL, Enright PL, Kaemingk KL, Rosen GM, Morgan WJ, Fregosi RF, Quan SF.
  Source: Sleep. 2001 December 15; 24(8): 937-44.
  http://www.ncbi.nlm.nih.gov/entrez/query.fcgi?cmd=Retrieve&db=pubmed&dopt=Abstract&list_uids=11766164

- **Feasibility study of Flextube reflectometry for localisation of upper airway obstruction in obstructive sleep apnea.**
  Author(s): Hessel NS, Laman M, van Ammers VC, van Duijn H, de Vries N.
  Source: Rhinology. 2003 June; 41(2): 87-90.
  http://www.ncbi.nlm.nih.gov/entrez/query.fcgi?cmd=Retrieve&db=pubmed&dopt=Abstract&list_uids=12868373

- **Fiberoptic nasopharyngolaryngoscopy for airway monitoring after obstructive sleep apnea surgery.**
  Author(s): Li KK, Riley RW, Powell NB, Zonato A.
  Source: Journal of Oral and Maxillofacial Surgery : Official Journal of the American Association of Oral and Maxillofacial Surgeons. 2000 December; 58(12): 1342-5; Discussion 1345-6.
  http://www.ncbi.nlm.nih.gov/entrez/query.fcgi?cmd=Retrieve&db=pubmed&dopt=Abstract&list_uids=11117680

- **Fibrinogen levels and obstructive sleep apnea in ischemic stroke.**
  Author(s): Wessendorf TE, Thilmann AF, Wang YM, Schreiber A, Konietzko N, Teschler H.
  Source: American Journal of Respiratory and Critical Care Medicine. 2000 December; 162(6): 2039-42.
  http://www.ncbi.nlm.nih.gov/entrez/query.fcgi?cmd=Retrieve&db=pubmed&dopt=Abstract&list_uids=11112110

- **Fibrinogen, stroke, and obstructive sleep apnea: an evolving paradigm of cardiovascular risk.**
  Author(s): Shamsuzzaman AS, Somers VK.
  Source: American Journal of Respiratory and Critical Care Medicine. 2000 December; 162(6): 2018-20. Review.
  http://www.ncbi.nlm.nih.gov/entrez/query.fcgi?cmd=Retrieve&db=pubmed&dopt=Abstract&list_uids=11112100

- **First place--resident clinical science award 1999. Quality of life for children with obstructive sleep apnea.**
  Author(s): Franco RA Jr, Rosenfeld RM, Rao M.
  Source: Otolaryngology and Head and Neck Surgery. 2000 July; 123(1 Pt 1): 9-16.
  http://www.ncbi.nlm.nih.gov/entrez/query.fcgi?cmd=Retrieve&db=pubmed&dopt=Abstract&list_uids=10889473

- **Fluticasone for obstructive sleep apnea.**
  Author(s): Wheeler AJ, van Someren V.
  Source: The Journal of Pediatrics. 2002 April; 140(4): 489; Author Reply 489-90.
  http://www.ncbi.nlm.nih.gov/entrez/query.fcgi?cmd=Retrieve&db=pubmed&dopt=Abstract&list_uids=12006973

- **fMRI responses to cold pressor challenges in control and obstructive sleep apnea subjects.**
  Author(s): Harper RM, Macey PM, Henderson LA, Woo MA, Macey KE, Frysinger RC, Alger JR, Nguyen KP, Yan-Go FL.
  Source: Journal of Applied Physiology (Bethesda, Md. : 1985). 2003 April; 94(4): 1583-95. Epub 2003 January 03.
  http://www.ncbi.nlm.nih.gov/entrez/query.fcgi?cmd=Retrieve&db=pubmed&dopt=Abstract&list_uids=12514164

- **Follow-up and outcomes of nasal CPAP therapy in patients with sleep apnea syndrome.**
  Author(s): McNicholas WT.
  Source: Monaldi Arch Chest Dis. 2001 December; 56(6): 535-9. Review.
  http://www.ncbi.nlm.nih.gov/entrez/query.fcgi?cmd=Retrieve&db=pubmed&dopt=Abstract&list_uids=11980286

- **Frequency of snoring and symptoms of sleep apnea among Pakistani medical students.**
  Author(s): Pasha SN, Khan UA.
  Source: J Ayub Med Coll Abbottabad. 2003 January-March; 15(1): 23-5.
  http://www.ncbi.nlm.nih.gov/entrez/query.fcgi?cmd=Retrieve&db=pubmed&dopt=Abstract&list_uids=12870311

- **From snoring to sleep apnea in a Singapore population.**
  Author(s): Puvanendran K, Goh KL.
  Source: Sleep Res Online. 1999; 2(1): 11-4.
  http://www.ncbi.nlm.nih.gov/entrez/query.fcgi?cmd=Retrieve&db=pubmed&dopt=Abstract&list_uids=11382877

- **Functional magnetic resonance imaging responses to expiratory loading in obstructive sleep apnea.**
  Author(s): Macey PM, Macey KE, Henderson LA, Alger JR, Frysinger RC, Woo MA, Yan-Go F, Harper RM.
  Source: Respiratory Physiology & Neurobiology. 2003 November 14; 138(2-3): 275-90.
  http://www.ncbi.nlm.nih.gov/entrez/query.fcgi?cmd=Retrieve&db=pubmed&dopt=Abstract&list_uids=14609516

- **Gastric bypass is an effective treatment for obstructive sleep apnea in patients with clinically significant obesity.**
  Author(s): Rasheid S, Banasiak M, Gallagher SF, Lipska A, Kaba S, Ventimiglia D, Anderson WM, Murr MM.
  Source: Obesity Surgery : the Official Journal of the American Society for Bariatric Surgery and of the Obesity Surgery Society of Australia and New Zealand. 2003 February; 13(1): 58-61.
  http://www.ncbi.nlm.nih.gov/entrez/query.fcgi?cmd=Retrieve&db=pubmed&dopt=Abstract&list_uids=12630614

- **Gastroesophageal reflux and obstructive sleep apnea.**
  Author(s): Senior BA, Khan M, Schwimmer C, Rosenthal L, Benninger M.
  Source: The Laryngoscope. 2001 December; 111(12): 2144-6.
  http://www.ncbi.nlm.nih.gov/entrez/query.fcgi?cmd=Retrieve&db=pubmed&dopt=Abstract&list_uids=11802013

- **Gastroesophageal reflux common in patients with sleep apnea rather than snorers without sleep apnea.**
  Author(s): Teramoto S, Yamamoto H, Ouchi Y.
  Source: Chest. 2003 August; 124(2): 767; Author Reply 767-8.
  http://www.ncbi.nlm.nih.gov/entrez/query.fcgi?cmd=Retrieve&db=pubmed&dopt=Abstract&list_uids=12907575

- **Gender and obstructive sleep apnea syndrome, part 1: Clinical features.**
  Author(s): Kapsimalis F, Kryger MH.
  Source: Sleep. 2002 June 15; 25(4): 412-9.
  http://www.ncbi.nlm.nih.gov/entrez/query.fcgi?cmd=Retrieve&db=pubmed&dopt=Abstract&list_uids=12071542

- **Gender and obstructive sleep apnea syndrome, part 2: mechanisms.**
  Author(s): Kapsimalis F, Kryger MH.
  Source: Sleep. 2002 August 1; 25(5): 499-506. Review.
  http://www.ncbi.nlm.nih.gov/entrez/query.fcgi?cmd=Retrieve&db=pubmed&dopt=Abstract&list_uids=12150315

- **Gender differences in sleep apnea: epidemiology, clinical presentation and pathogenic mechanisms.**
  Author(s): Jordan AS, McEvoy RD.
  Source: Sleep Medicine Reviews. 2003 October; 7(5): 377-89. Review.
  http://www.ncbi.nlm.nih.gov/entrez/query.fcgi?cmd=Retrieve&db=pubmed&dopt=Abstract&list_uids=14573374

- **Gender differences in sleep apnea: the role of neck circumference.**
  Author(s): Dancey DR, Hanly PJ, Soong C, Lee B, Shepard J Jr, Hoffstein V.
  Source: Chest. 2003 May; 123(5): 1544-50.
  http://www.ncbi.nlm.nih.gov/entrez/query.fcgi?cmd=Retrieve&db=pubmed&dopt=Abstract&list_uids=12740272

- **Gender differences in symptoms related to sleep apnea in a general population and in relation to referral to sleep clinic.**
  Author(s): Larsson LG, Lindberg A, Franklin KA, Lundback B.
  Source: Chest. 2003 July; 124(1): 204-11.
  http://www.ncbi.nlm.nih.gov/entrez/query.fcgi?cmd=Retrieve&db=pubmed&dopt=Abstract&list_uids=12853524

- **Gender differences in the polysomnographic features of obstructive sleep apnea.**
  Author(s): O'Connor C, Thornley KS, Hanly PJ.
  Source: American Journal of Respiratory and Critical Care Medicine. 2000 May; 161(5): 1465-72.
  http://www.ncbi.nlm.nih.gov/entrez/query.fcgi?cmd=Retrieve&db=pubmed&dopt=Abstract&list_uids=10806140

- **Gender, age and menopause effects on the prevalence and the characteristics of obstructive sleep apnea in obesity.**
  Author(s): Resta O, Caratozzolo G, Pannacciulli N, Stefano A, Giliberti T, Carpagnano GE, De Pergola G.
  Source: European Journal of Clinical Investigation. 2003 December; 33(12): 1084-9.
  http://www.ncbi.nlm.nih.gov/entrez/query.fcgi?cmd=Retrieve&db=pubmed&dopt=Abstract&list_uids=14636291

- **General physicians' perspective of sleep apnea from a developing country.**
  Author(s): Hussain SF, Zahid S, Haqqee R, Khan JA.
  Source: Southeast Asian J Trop Med Public Health. 2003 June; 34(2): 420-3.
  http://www.ncbi.nlm.nih.gov/entrez/query.fcgi?cmd=Retrieve&db=pubmed&dopt=Abstract&list_uids=12971574

- **Genioglossal activation in patients with obstructive sleep apnea versus control subjects. Mechanisms of muscle control.**
  Author(s): Fogel RB, Malhotra A, Pillar G, Edwards JK, Beauregard J, Shea SA, White DP.
  Source: American Journal of Respiratory and Critical Care Medicine. 2001 December 1; 164(11): 2025-30.
  http://www.ncbi.nlm.nih.gov/entrez/query.fcgi?cmd=Retrieve&db=pubmed&dopt=Abstract&list_uids=11739130

- **Genioglossal advancement--a simple surgical procedure for sleep apnea. Case report and literature review.**
  Author(s): Nagler RM, Laufer D.
  Source: European Surgical Research. Europaische Chirurgische Forschung. Recherches Chirurgicales Europeennes. 2002 September-October; 34(5): 373-7.
  http://www.ncbi.nlm.nih.gov/entrez/query.fcgi?cmd=Retrieve&db=pubmed&dopt=Abstract&list_uids=12364822

- **Genioglossus activity in children with obstructive sleep apnea during wakefulness and sleep onset.**
  Author(s): Katz ES, White DP.
  Source: American Journal of Respiratory and Critical Care Medicine. 2003 September 15; 168(6): 664-70. Epub 2003 July 11.
  http://www.ncbi.nlm.nih.gov/entrez/query.fcgi?cmd=Retrieve&db=pubmed&dopt=Abstract&list_uids=12857721

- **Genomic approaches to understanding obstructive sleep apnea.**
  Author(s): Palmer LJ, Redline S.
  Source: Respiratory Physiology & Neurobiology. 2003 May 30; 135(2-3): 187-205. Review.
  http://www.ncbi.nlm.nih.gov/entrez/query.fcgi?cmd=Retrieve&db=pubmed&dopt=Abstract&list_uids=12809619

- **Glaucoma in patients with sleep apnea.**
  Author(s): Pearson J.
  Source: Ophthalmology. 2000 May; 107(5): 816-7.
  http://www.ncbi.nlm.nih.gov/entrez/query.fcgi?cmd=Retrieve&db=pubmed&dopt=Abstract&list_uids=10811063

- **Glossoptosis (posterior displacement of the tongue) during sleep: a frequent cause of sleep apnea in pediatric patients referred for dynamic sleep fluoroscopy.**
  Author(s): Donnelly LF, Strife JL, Myer CM 3rd.
  Source: Ajr. American Journal of Roentgenology. 2000 December; 175(6): 1557-60. Erratum In: Ajr Am J Roentgenol 2001 February; 176(2): 548.
  http://www.ncbi.nlm.nih.gov/entrez/query.fcgi?cmd=Retrieve&db=pubmed&dopt=Abstract&list_uids=11090374

- **Growth and biochemical markers of growth in children with snoring and obstructive sleep apnea.**
  Author(s): Nieminen P, Lopponen T, Tolonen U, Lanning P, Knip M, Lopponen H.
  Source: Pediatrics. 2002 April; 109(4): E55.
  http://www.ncbi.nlm.nih.gov/entrez/query.fcgi?cmd=Retrieve&db=pubmed&dopt=Abstract&list_uids=11927728

- **Haptoglobin polymorphism is a risk factor for cardiovascular disease in patients with obstructive sleep apnea syndrome.**
  Author(s): Lavie L, Lotan R, Hochberg I, Herer P, Lavie P, Levy AP.
  Source: Sleep. 2003 August 1; 26(5): 592-5.
  http://www.ncbi.nlm.nih.gov/entrez/query.fcgi?cmd=Retrieve&db=pubmed&dopt=Abstract&list_uids=12938813

- **Health care services utilization in children with obstructive sleep apnea syndrome.**
Author(s): Reuveni H, Simon T, Tal A, Elhayany A, Tarasiuk A.
Source: Pediatrics. 2002 July; 110(1 Pt 1): 68-72.
http://www.ncbi.nlm.nih.gov/entrez/query.fcgi?cmd=Retrieve&db=pubmed&dopt=Abstract&list_uids=12093948

- **Heart block in patients after bariatric surgery accompanying sleep apnea.**
Author(s): Block M, Jacobson LB, Rabkin RA.
Source: Obesity Surgery : the Official Journal of the American Society for Bariatric Surgery and of the Obesity Surgery Society of Australia and New Zealand. 2001 October; 11(5): 627-30.
http://www.ncbi.nlm.nih.gov/entrez/query.fcgi?cmd=Retrieve&db=pubmed&dopt=Abstract&list_uids=11594108

- **Heart failure and sleep apnea: emphasis on practical therapeutic options.**
Author(s): Javaheri S.
Source: Clinics in Chest Medicine. 2003 June; 24(2): 207-22. Review.
http://www.ncbi.nlm.nih.gov/entrez/query.fcgi?cmd=Retrieve&db=pubmed&dopt=Abstract&list_uids=12800779

- **Heart rate variability during sleep stages in normals and in patients with sleep apnea.**
Author(s): Penzel T, Bunde A, Grote L, Kantelhardt JW, Peter JH, Voigt K.
Source: Stud Health Technol Inform. 2000; 77: 1256-60.
http://www.ncbi.nlm.nih.gov/entrez/query.fcgi?cmd=Retrieve&db=pubmed&dopt=Abstract&list_uids=11187524

- **Heart rate variability in obstructive sleep apnea: a prospective study and frequency domain analysis.**
Author(s): Gula LJ, Krahn AD, Skanes A, Ferguson KA, George C, Yee R, Klein GJ.
Source: Annals of Noninvasive Electrocardiology : the Official Journal of the International Society for Holter and Noninvasive Electrocardiology, Inc. 2003 April; 8(2): 144-9.
http://www.ncbi.nlm.nih.gov/entrez/query.fcgi?cmd=Retrieve&db=pubmed&dopt=Abstract&list_uids=12848796

- **Heated humidification during nasal continuous positive airway pressure for obstructive sleep apnea syndrome: objective evaluation of efficacy with nasal peak inspiratory flow measurements.**
  Author(s): Winck JC, Delgado JL, Almeida JM, Marques JA.
  Source: American Journal of Rhinology. 2002 May-June; 16(3): 175-7.
  http://www.ncbi.nlm.nih.gov/entrez/query.fcgi?cmd=Retrieve&db=pubmed&dopt=Abstract&list_uids=12141777

- **Hemostatic alterations in patients with obstructive sleep apnea and the implications for cardiovascular disease.**
  Author(s): von Kanel R, Dimsdale JE.
  Source: Chest. 2003 November; 124(5): 1956-67. Review.
  http://www.ncbi.nlm.nih.gov/entrez/query.fcgi?cmd=Retrieve&db=pubmed&dopt=Abstract&list_uids=14605073

- **High leg motor activity in sleep apnea hypopnea patients: efficacy of clonazepam combined with nasal CPAP on polysomnographic variables.**
  Author(s): Noseda A, Nouvelle M, Lanquart JR, Kempenaers Ch, De Maertelaer V, Linkowski R, Kerkhofs M.
  Source: Respiratory Medicine. 2002 September; 96(9): 693-9.
  http://www.ncbi.nlm.nih.gov/entrez/query.fcgi?cmd=Retrieve&db=pubmed&dopt=Abstract&list_uids=12243315

- **Higher prevalence of smoking in patients diagnosed as having obstructive sleep apnea.**
  Author(s): Kashyap R, Hock LM, Bowman TJ.
  Source: Sleep & Breathing = Schlaf & Atmung. 2001 December; 5(4): 167-72.
  http://www.ncbi.nlm.nih.gov/entrez/query.fcgi?cmd=Retrieve&db=pubmed&dopt=Abstract&list_uids=11868156

- **Histopathology of the uvula and the soft palate in patients with mild, moderate, and severe obstructive sleep apnea.**
  Author(s): Berger G, Gilbey P, Hammel I, Ophir D.
  Source: The Laryngoscope. 2002 February; 112(2): 357-63.
  http://www.ncbi.nlm.nih.gov/entrez/query.fcgi?cmd=Retrieve&db=pubmed&dopt=Abstract&list_uids=11889397

- **Home diagnosis of sleep apnea: a systematic review of the literature. An evidence review cosponsored by the American Academy of Sleep Medicine, the American College of Chest Physicians, and the American Thoracic Society.**
  Author(s): Flemons WW, Littner MR, Rowley JA, Gay P, Anderson WM, Hudgel DW, McEvoy RD, Loube DI.
  Source: Chest. 2003 October; 124(4): 1543-79. Review.
  http://www.ncbi.nlm.nih.gov/entrez/query.fcgi?cmd=Retrieve&db=pubmed&dopt=Abstract&list_uids=14555592

- **Home oximetry studies for diagnosis of sleep apnea/hypopnea syndrome: limitation of memory storage capabilities.**
  Author(s): Wiltshire N, Kendrick AH, Catterall JR.
  Source: Chest. 2001 August; 120(2): 384-9.
  http://www.ncbi.nlm.nih.gov/entrez/query.fcgi?cmd=Retrieve&db=pubmed&dopt=Abstract&list_uids=11502633

- **Home sleep studies in the assessment of sleep apnea/hypopnea syndrome.**
  Author(s): Golpe R, Jimenez A, Carpizo R.
  Source: Chest. 2002 October; 122(4): 1156-61.
  http://www.ncbi.nlm.nih.gov/entrez/query.fcgi?cmd=Retrieve&db=pubmed&dopt=Abstract&list_uids=12377836

- **Home unattended vs hospital telemonitored polysomnography in suspected obstructive sleep apnea syndrome: a randomized crossover trial.**
  Author(s): Gagnadoux F, Pelletier-Fleury N, Philippe C, Rakotonanahary D, Fleury B.
  Source: Chest. 2002 March; 121(3): 753-8.
  http://www.ncbi.nlm.nih.gov/entrez/query.fcgi?cmd=Retrieve&db=pubmed&dopt=Abstract&list_uids=11888956

- **Hospital use in the treatment of sleep apnea.**
  Author(s): Petersen EJ, Reiter ER.
  Source: The Laryngoscope. 2004 March; 114(3): 460-6.
  http://www.ncbi.nlm.nih.gov/entrez/query.fcgi?cmd=Retrieve&db=pubmed&dopt=Abstract&list_uids=15091219

- **How, what, and why of sleep apnea. Perspectives for primary care physicians.**
  Author(s): Chung SA, Jairam S, Hussain MR, Shapiro CM.
  Source: Can Fam Physician. 2002 June; 48: 1073-80. Review.
  http://www.ncbi.nlm.nih.gov/entrez/query.fcgi?cmd=Retrieve&db=pubmed&dopt=Abstract&list_uids=12113194

- **Hyoid myotomy with suspension under local anesthesia for obstructive sleep apnea syndrome.**
  Author(s): Neruntarat C.
  Source: Eur Arch Otorhinolaryngol. 2003 May;260(5):286-90. Epub 2002 December 05.
  http://www.ncbi.nlm.nih.gov/entrez/query.fcgi?cmd=Retrieve&db=pubmed&dopt=Abstract&list_uids=12750922

- **Hypercapnia and ventilatory periodicity in obstructive sleep apnea syndrome.**
  Author(s): Ayappa I, Berger KI, Norman RG, Oppenheimer BW, Rapoport DM, Goldring RM.
  Source: American Journal of Respiratory and Critical Care Medicine. 2002 October 15; 166(8): 1112-5.
  http://www.ncbi.nlm.nih.gov/entrez/query.fcgi?cmd=Retrieve&db=pubmed&dopt=Abstract&list_uids=12379556

- **Hypertension and obstructive sleep apnea.**
  Author(s): Phillips BG, Somers VK.
  Source: Current Hypertension Reports. 2003 October; 5(5): 380-5. Review.
  http://www.ncbi.nlm.nih.gov/entrez/query.fcgi?cmd=Retrieve&db=pubmed&dopt=Abstract&list_uids=12948430

- **Identification and evaluation of obstructive sleep apnea prior to adenotonsillectomy in children: a survey of practice patterns.**
  Author(s): Weatherly RA, Mai EF, Ruzicka DL, Chervin RD.
  Source: Sleep Medicine. 2003 July; 4(4): 297-307.
  http://www.ncbi.nlm.nih.gov/entrez/query.fcgi?cmd=Retrieve&db=pubmed&dopt=Abstract&list_uids=14592302

- **Identification and evaluation of obstructive sleep apnea prior to adenotonsillectomy in children: is there a problem?**
Author(s): Rosen G.
Source: Sleep Medicine. 2003 July; 4(4): 273-4.
http://www.ncbi.nlm.nih.gov/entrez/query.fcgi?cmd=Retrieve&db=pubmed&dopt=Abstract&list_uids=14592298

- **Identification and treatment of obstructive sleep apnea in adults and children with epilepsy: a prospective pilot study.**
Author(s): Malow BA, Weatherwax KJ, Chervin RD, Hoban TF, Marzec ML, Martin C, Binns LA.
Source: Sleep Medicine. 2003 November; 4(6): 509-15.
http://www.ncbi.nlm.nih.gov/entrez/query.fcgi?cmd=Retrieve&db=pubmed&dopt=Abstract&list_uids=14607344

- **Impact of nasal continuous positive airway pressure therapy on the quality of life of bed partners of patients with obstructive sleep apnea syndrome.**
Author(s): Doherty LS, Kiely JL, Lawless G, McNicholas WT.
Source: Chest. 2003 December; 124(6): 2209-14.
http://www.ncbi.nlm.nih.gov/entrez/query.fcgi?cmd=Retrieve&db=pubmed&dopt=Abstract&list_uids=14665502

- **Improvement in neuropsychological performance following surgical treatment for obstructive sleep apnea syndrome.**
Author(s): Dahlof P, Norlin-Bagge E, Hedner J, Ejnell H, Hetta J, Hallstrom T.
Source: Acta Oto-Laryngologica. 2002 January; 122(1): 86-91.
http://www.ncbi.nlm.nih.gov/entrez/query.fcgi?cmd=Retrieve&db=pubmed&dopt=Abstract&list_uids=11876604

- **Improvement of metabolic function in sleep apnea: the power of positive pressure.**
Author(s): Punjabi NM.
Source: American Journal of Respiratory and Critical Care Medicine. 2004 January 15; 169(2): 139-40.
http://www.ncbi.nlm.nih.gov/entrez/query.fcgi?cmd=Retrieve&db=pubmed&dopt=Abstract&list_uids=14718227

- **Incidence of undiagnosed sleep apnea in patients scheduled for elective total joint arthroplasty.**
  Author(s): Harrison MM, Childs A, Carson PE.
  Source: The Journal of Arthroplasty. 2003 December; 18(8): 1044-7.
  http://www.ncbi.nlm.nih.gov/entrez/query.fcgi?cmd=Retrieve&db=pubmed&dopt=Abstract&list_uids=14658110

- **Increased upper airway collapsibility in children with obstructive sleep apnea during wakefulness.**
  Author(s): Gozal D, Burnside MM.
  Source: American Journal of Respiratory and Critical Care Medicine. 2004 January 15; 169(2): 163-7. Epub 2003 October 02.
  http://www.ncbi.nlm.nih.gov/entrez/query.fcgi?cmd=Retrieve&db=pubmed&dopt=Abstract&list_uids=14525806

- **Increases in leptin levels, sympathetic drive, and weight gain in obstructive sleep apnea.**
  Author(s): Phillips BG, Kato M, Narkiewicz K, Choe I, Somers VK.
  Source: American Journal of Physiology. Heart and Circulatory Physiology. 2000 July; 279(1): H234-7.
  http://www.ncbi.nlm.nih.gov/entrez/query.fcgi?cmd=Retrieve&db=pubmed&dopt=Abstract&list_uids=10899061

- **Inflammation and obstructive sleep apnea syndrome pathogenesis: a working hypothesis.**
  Author(s): Hatipoglu U, Rubinstein I.
  Source: Respiration; International Review of Thoracic Diseases. 2003 November-December; 70(6): 665-71. Review.
  http://www.ncbi.nlm.nih.gov/entrez/query.fcgi?cmd=Retrieve&db=pubmed&dopt=Abstract&list_uids=14732803

- **Inflammatory ideas about sleep apnea.**
  Author(s): Cherniack NS.
  Source: Respiration; International Review of Thoracic Diseases. 2004 January-February; 71(1): 20-1.
  http://www.ncbi.nlm.nih.gov/entrez/query.fcgi?cmd=Retrieve&db=pubmed&dopt=Abstract&list_uids=14872105

- **Insulin resistance and obstructive sleep apnea: is increased sympathetic stimulation the link?**
  Author(s): Chasens ER, Weaver TE, Umlauf MG.
  Source: Biological Research for Nursing. 2003 October; 5(2): 87-96. Review.
  http://www.ncbi.nlm.nih.gov/entrez/query.fcgi?cmd=Retrieve&db=pubmed&dopt=Abstract&list_uids=14531213

- **Integrating psychosocial and biomedical CPAP adherence models. A commentary on: "Improving CPAP use by patients with the sleep apnea/hypopnea syndrome (SAHS)" (HM Engleman & MR Wild).**
  Author(s): Krakow B, Melendrez D, Haynes P.
  Source: Sleep Medicine Reviews. 2003 October; 7(5): 441-4.
  http://www.ncbi.nlm.nih.gov/entrez/query.fcgi?cmd=Retrieve&db=pubmed&dopt=Abstract&list_uids=14573379

- **Interleukin-6 and tumor necrosis factor-alpha in patients with obstructive sleep apnea-hypopnea syndrome.**
  Author(s): Imagawa S, Yamaguchi Y, Ogawa K, Obara N, Suzuki N, Yamamoto M, Nagasawa T.
  Source: Respiration; International Review of Thoracic Diseases. 2004 January-February; 71(1): 24-9.
  http://www.ncbi.nlm.nih.gov/entrez/query.fcgi?cmd=Retrieve&db=pubmed&dopt=Abstract&list_uids=14872107

- **Interleukin-6, obstructive sleep apnea, and obesity.**
  Author(s): Inoue K, Takano H, Yoshikawa T.
  Source: Chest. 2003 October; 124(4): 1621-2; Author Reply 1622-3.
  http://www.ncbi.nlm.nih.gov/entrez/query.fcgi?cmd=Retrieve&db=pubmed&dopt=Abstract&list_uids=14555603

- **Investigation into the correlation in SIDS victims between Alzheimer precursor protein A4 in the brainstem and sleep apnea.**
  Author(s): Sawaguchi T, Patricia F, Kadhim H, Groswasser J, Sottiaux M, Nishida H, Sawaguchi A, Kahn A.
  Source: Early Human Development. 2003 December; 75 Suppl: S21-30.
  http://www.ncbi.nlm.nih.gov/entrez/query.fcgi?cmd=Retrieve&db=pubmed&dopt=Abstract&list_uids=14693388

- **Investigation of cardiac function in children with suspected obstructive sleep apnea.**
  Author(s): James AL, Runciman M, Burton MJ, Freeland AP.
  Source: The Journal of Otolaryngology. 2003 June; 32(3): 151-4.
  http://www.ncbi.nlm.nih.gov/entrez/query.fcgi?cmd=Retrieve&db=pubmed&dopt=Abstract&list_uids=12921132

- **Is obstructive sleep apnea syndrome associated with headache?**
  Author(s): Jensen R, Olsborg C, Salvesen R, Torbergsen T, Bekkelund SI.
  Source: Acta Neurologica Scandinavica. 2004 March; 109(3): 180-4.
  http://www.ncbi.nlm.nih.gov/entrez/query.fcgi?cmd=Retrieve&db=pubmed&dopt=Abstract&list_uids=14763954

- **Is there a rationale in modulating brainstem neurons in obstructive sleep apnea and is it clinically relevant?**
  Author(s): Horner RL.
  Source: Sleep. 2000 June 15; 23 Suppl 4: S179-81. No Abstract Available.
  http://www.ncbi.nlm.nih.gov/entrez/query.fcgi?cmd=Retrieve&db=pubmed&dopt=Abstract&list_uids=10893097

- **Is treatment of obstructive sleep apnea syndrome with auto-CPAP useful?**
  Author(s): Series F.
  Source: Sleep. 2000 June 15; 23 Suppl 4: S161-5.
  http://www.ncbi.nlm.nih.gov/entrez/query.fcgi?cmd=Retrieve&db=pubmed&dopt=Abstract&list_uids=10893094

- **Knowledge of sleep apnea in a sample grouping of primary care physicians.**
  Author(s): Chung SA, Jairam S, Hussain MR, Shapiro CM.
  Source: Sleep & Breathing = Schlaf & Atmung. 2001 September; 5(3): 115-21.
  http://www.ncbi.nlm.nih.gov/entrez/query.fcgi?cmd=Retrieve&db=pubmed&dopt=Abstract&list_uids=11868150

- **Lack of efficacy for a cervicomandibular support collar in the management of obstructive sleep apnea.**
  Author(s): Skinner MA, Kingshott RN, Jones DR, Taylor DR.
  Source: Chest. 2004 January; 125(1): 118-26.
  http://www.ncbi.nlm.nih.gov/entrez/query.fcgi?cmd=Retrieve&db=pubmed&dopt=Abstract&list_uids=14718430

- **Laryngomalacia causing sleep apnea in an osteogenesis imperfecta patient.**
  Author(s): Li HY, Fang TJ, Lin JL, Lee ZL, Lee LA.
  Source: American Journal of Otolaryngology. 2002 November-December; 23(6): 378-81.
  http://www.ncbi.nlm.nih.gov/entrez/query.fcgi?cmd=Retrieve&db=pubmed&dopt=Abstract&list_uids=12430132

- **Laser midline glossectomy and lingual tonsillectomy as treatments for sleep apnea syndrome.**
  Author(s): Yonekura A, Kawakatsu K, Suzuki K, Nishimura T.
  Source: Acta Otolaryngol Suppl. 2003; (550): 56-8.
  http://www.ncbi.nlm.nih.gov/entrez/query.fcgi?cmd=Retrieve&db=pubmed&dopt=Abstract&list_uids=12737344

- **Laser-assisted uvulopalatoplasty and tonsillectomy for the management of obstructive sleep apnea syndrome.**
  Author(s): Kern RC, Kutler DI, Reid KJ, Conley DB, Herzon GD, Zee P.
  Source: The Laryngoscope. 2003 July; 113(7): 1175-81.
  http://www.ncbi.nlm.nih.gov/entrez/query.fcgi?cmd=Retrieve&db=pubmed&dopt=Abstract&list_uids=12838016

- **Laser-assisted uvulopalatoplasty for the treatment of snoring and mild obstructive sleep apnea syndrome.**
  Author(s): Kyrmizakis DE, Chimona TS, Papadakis CE, Bizakis JG, Velegrakis GA, Schiza S, Siafakas NM, Helidonis ES.
  Source: The Journal of Otolaryngology. 2003 June; 32(3): 174-9.
  http://www.ncbi.nlm.nih.gov/entrez/query.fcgi?cmd=Retrieve&db=pubmed&dopt=Abstract&list_uids=12921136

- **Lateral pharyngoplasty: a new treatment for obstructive sleep apnea hypopnea syndrome.**
  Author(s): Cahali MB.
  Source: The Laryngoscope. 2003 November; 113(11): 1961-8.
  http://www.ncbi.nlm.nih.gov/entrez/query.fcgi?cmd=Retrieve&db=pubmed&dopt=Abstract&list_uids=14603056

- **Lateral position decreases collapsibility of the passive pharynx in patients with obstructive sleep apnea.**
  Author(s): Isono S, Tanaka A, Nishino T.
  Source: Anesthesiology. 2002 October; 97(4): 780-5.
  http://www.ncbi.nlm.nih.gov/entrez/query.fcgi?cmd=Retrieve&db=pubmed&dopt=Abstract&list_uids=12357140

- **Learning in children and sleep disordered breathing: findings of the Tucson Children's Assessment of Sleep Apnea (tuCASA) prospective cohort study.**
  Author(s): Kaemingk KL, Pasvogel AE, Goodwin JL, Mulvaney SA, Martinez F, Enright PL, Rosen GM, Morgan WJ, Fregosi RF, Quan SF.
  Source: Journal of the International Neuropsychological Society : Jins. 2003 November; 9(7): 1016-26.
  http://www.ncbi.nlm.nih.gov/entrez/query.fcgi?cmd=Retrieve&db=pubmed&dopt=Abstract&list_uids=14738283

- **Left ventricular dysfunction and sleep apnea syndrome: cause or consequence?**
  Author(s): Bendjelid K.
  Source: Chest. 2003 May; 123(5): 1774; Author Reply 1774-5.
  http://www.ncbi.nlm.nih.gov/entrez/query.fcgi?cmd=Retrieve&db=pubmed&dopt=Abstract&list_uids=12740306

- **Left ventricular hypertrophy and abnormal ventricular geometry in children and adolescents with obstructive sleep apnea.**
  Author(s): Amin RS, Kimball TR, Bean JA, Jeffries JL, Willging JP, Cotton RT, Witt SA, Glascock BJ, Daniels SR.
  Source: American Journal of Respiratory and Critical Care Medicine. 2002 May 15; 165(10): 1395-9.
  http://www.ncbi.nlm.nih.gov/entrez/query.fcgi?cmd=Retrieve&db=pubmed&dopt=Abstract&list_uids=12016102

- **Left ventricular hypertrophy is a common echocardiographic abnormality in severe obstructive sleep apnea and reverses with nasal continuous positive airway pressure.**
  Author(s): Cloward TV, Walker JM, Farney RJ, Anderson JL.
  Source: Chest. 2003 August; 124(2): 594-601.
  http://www.ncbi.nlm.nih.gov/entrez/query.fcgi?cmd=Retrieve&db=pubmed&dopt=Abstract&list_uids=12907548

- **Left ventricular systolic dysfunction in patients with obstructive sleep apnea syndrome.**
  Author(s): Laaban JP, Pascal-Sebaoun S, Bloch E, Orvoen-Frija E, Oppert JM, Huchon G.
  Source: Chest. 2002 October; 122(4): 1133-8.
  http://www.ncbi.nlm.nih.gov/entrez/query.fcgi?cmd=Retrieve&db=pubmed&dopt=Abstract&list_uids=12377833

- **Levels of vascular endothelial growth factor are elevated in patients with obstructive sleep apnea--hypopnea syndrome.**
  Author(s): Imagawa S, Yamaguchi Y, Higuchi M, Neichi T, Hasegawa Y, Mukai HY, Suzuki N, Yamamoto M, Nagasawa T.
  Source: Blood. 2001 August 15; 98(4): 1255-7.
  http://www.ncbi.nlm.nih.gov/entrez/query.fcgi?cmd=Retrieve&db=pubmed&dopt=Abstract&list_uids=11493479

- **Longitudinal follow-up of obstructive sleep apnea following Furlow palatoplasty in children with cleft palate: a preliminary report.**
  Author(s): Liao YF, Yun C, Huang CS, Chen PK, Chen NH, Hung KF, Chuang ML.
  Source: The Cleft Palate-Craniofacial Journal : Official Publication of the American Cleft Palate-Craniofacial Association. 2003 May; 40(3): 269-73.
  http://www.ncbi.nlm.nih.gov/entrez/query.fcgi?cmd=Retrieve&db=pubmed&dopt=Abstract&list_uids=12733955

- **Long-term changes in quality of life after surgery for pediatric obstructive sleep apnea.**
  Author(s): Mitchell RB, Kelly J, Call E, Yao N.
  Source: Archives of Otolaryngology--Head & Neck Surgery. 2004 April; 130(4): 409-12.
  http://www.ncbi.nlm.nih.gov/entrez/query.fcgi?cmd=Retrieve&db=pubmed&dopt=Abstract&list_uids=15096422

- **Long-term follow-up and mechanisms of obstructive sleep apnea (OSA) and related syndromes through infancy and childhood.**
  Author(s): Contencin P, Guilleminault C, Manach Y.
  Source: International Journal of Pediatric Otorhinolaryngology. 2003 December; 67 Suppl 1: S119-23.
  http://www.ncbi.nlm.nih.gov/entrez/query.fcgi?cmd=Retrieve&db=pubmed&dopt=Abstract&list_uids=14662182

- **Long-term surgical follow-up of sleep apnea syndrome.**
  Author(s): Kawakatsu K, Nishimura T.
  Source: Acta Otolaryngol Suppl. 2003; (550): 11-21.
  http://www.ncbi.nlm.nih.gov/entrez/query.fcgi?cmd=Retrieve&db=pubmed&dopt=Abstract&list_uids=12737335

- **Mandibular advancement devices in 630 men and women with obstructive sleep apnea and snoring: tolerability and predictors of treatment success.**
  Author(s): Marklund M, Stenlund H, Franklin KA.
  Source: Chest. 2004 April; 125(4): 1270-8.
  http://www.ncbi.nlm.nih.gov/entrez/query.fcgi?cmd=Retrieve&db=pubmed&dopt=Abstract&list_uids=15078734
- **Maxillomandibular advancement surgery for obstructive sleep apnea syndrome.**
  Author(s): Prinsell JR.
  Source: The Journal of the American Dental Association. 2002 November; 133(11): 1489-97; Quiz 1539-40. Review.
  http://www.ncbi.nlm.nih.gov/entrez/query.fcgi?cmd=Retrieve&db=pubmed&dopt=Abstract&list_uids=12462692

- **Measurement of changes in cytochrome oxidase redox state during obstructive sleep apnea using near-infrared spectroscopy.**
  Author(s): McGown AD, Makker H, Elwell C, Al Rawi PG, Valipour A, Spiro SG.
  Source: Sleep. 2003 Sep15; 26(6): 710-6.
  http://www.ncbi.nlm.nih.gov/entrez/query.fcgi?cmd=Retrieve&db=pubmed&dopt=Abstract&list_uids=14572124

- **Measurement of sleep apnea during obesity treatment.**
  Author(s): Billington CJ.
  Source: Obesity Research. 2002 November; 10 Suppl 1: 38S-41S. Review.
  http://www.ncbi.nlm.nih.gov/entrez/query.fcgi?cmd=Retrieve&db=pubmed&dopt=Abstract&list_uids=12446857

- **Mechanisms and treatment of obstructive sleep apnea.**
  Author(s): Lorber M.
  Source: Jama : the Journal of the American Medical Association. 2004 February 4; 291(5): 557; Author Reply 557-8.
  http://www.ncbi.nlm.nih.gov/entrez/query.fcgi?cmd=Retrieve&db=pubmed&dopt=Abstract&list_uids=14762028

- **Mechanisms and treatment of obstructive sleep apnea.**
Author(s): Hussain N, Karnath B.
Source: Jama : the Journal of the American Medical Association. 2004 February 4; 291(5): 557; Author Reply 557-8.
http://www.ncbi.nlm.nih.gov/entrez/query.fcgi?cmd=Retrieve&db=pubmed&dopt=Abstract&list_uids=14762027

- **Modafinil as adjunct therapy for daytime sleepiness in obstructive sleep apnea: a 12-week, open-label study.**
Author(s): Schwartz JR, Hirshkowitz M, Erman MK, Schmidt-Nowara W.
Source: Chest. 2003 December; 124(6): 2192-9.
http://www.ncbi.nlm.nih.gov/entrez/query.fcgi?cmd=Retrieve&db=pubmed&dopt=Abstract&list_uids=14665500

- **Modified maxillomandibular advancement for the treatment of obstructive sleep apnea: a preliminary report.**
Author(s): Goh YH, Lim KA.
Source: The Laryngoscope. 2003 September; 113(9): 1577-82.
http://www.ncbi.nlm.nih.gov/entrez/query.fcgi?cmd=Retrieve&db=pubmed&dopt=Abstract&list_uids=12972937

- **Molecular and physiologic basis of obstructive sleep apnea.**
Author(s): Veasey SC.
Source: Clinics in Chest Medicine. 2003 June; 24(2): 179-93. Review.
http://www.ncbi.nlm.nih.gov/entrez/query.fcgi?cmd=Retrieve&db=pubmed&dopt=Abstract&list_uids=12800777

- **Multilevel temperature-controlled radiofrequency therapy of soft palate, base of tongue, and tonsils in adults with obstructive sleep apnea.**
Author(s): Fischer Y, Khan M, Mann WJ.
Source: The Laryngoscope. 2003 October; 113(10): 1786-91.
http://www.ncbi.nlm.nih.gov/entrez/query.fcgi?cmd=Retrieve&db=pubmed&dopt=Abstract&list_uids=14520107

- **Narcolepsy-like symptoms in a patient with down syndrome and without obstructive sleep apnea.**
Author(s): Dominguez-Ortega L, Salin-Pascual RJ, Diaz-Gallego E.
Source: Sleep. 2003 May 1; 26(3): 285-6.
http://www.ncbi.nlm.nih.gov/entrez/query.fcgi?cmd=Retrieve&db=pubmed&dopt=Abstract&list_uids=12749546

- **Nasal breathing and continuous positive airway pressure (CPAP) in patients with obstructive sleep apnea (OSA).**
  Author(s): Hollandt JH, Mahlerwein M.
  Source: Sleep & Breathing = Schlaf & Atmung. 2003 June; 7(2): 87-94.
  http://www.ncbi.nlm.nih.gov/entrez/query.fcgi?cmd=Retrieve&db=pubmed&dopt=Abstract&list_uids=12861488

- **Nasal CPAP treatment for obstructive sleep apnea: developing a new perspective on dosing strategies and compliance.**
  Author(s): Stepnowsky CJ Jr, Moore PJ.
  Source: Journal of Psychosomatic Research. 2003 June; 54(6): 599-605. Review.
  http://www.ncbi.nlm.nih.gov/entrez/query.fcgi?cmd=Retrieve&db=pubmed&dopt=Abstract&list_uids=12781315

- **Neurobehavioral functioning in obstructive sleep apnea: differential effects of sleep quality, hypoxemia and subjective sleepiness.**
  Author(s): Naismith S, Winter V, Gotsopoulos H, Hickie I, Cistulli P.
  Source: J Clin Exp Neuropsychol. 2004 February; 26(1): 43-54.
  http://www.ncbi.nlm.nih.gov/entrez/query.fcgi?cmd=Retrieve&db=pubmed&dopt=Abstract&list_uids=14972693

- **Neuropsychological impairment and quality of life in obstructive sleep apnea.**
  Author(s): Sateia MJ.
  Source: Clinics in Chest Medicine. 2003 June; 24(2): 249-59. Review.
  http://www.ncbi.nlm.nih.gov/entrez/query.fcgi?cmd=Retrieve&db=pubmed&dopt=Abstract&list_uids=12800782

- **Nitric oxide (NO) and obstructive sleep apnea (OSA).**
  Author(s): Haight JS, Djupesland PG.
  Source: Sleep & Breathing = Schlaf & Atmung. 2003 June; 7(2): 53-62. Review.
  http://www.ncbi.nlm.nih.gov/entrez/query.fcgi?cmd=Retrieve&db=pubmed&dopt=Abstract&list_uids=12861485

- **Nocturia: a problem that disrupts sleep and predicts obstructive sleep apnea.**
  Author(s): Chasens ER, Umlauf MG.
  Source: Geriatric Nursing (New York, N.Y.). 2003 March-April; 24(2): 76-81, 105.
  http://www.ncbi.nlm.nih.gov/entrez/query.fcgi?cmd=Retrieve&db=pubmed&dopt=Abstract&list_uids=12714959

- **Nocturnal gastroesophageal reflux: symptom of obstructive sleep apnea syndrome in association with impaired swallowing.**
  Author(s): Teramoto S, Kume H, Ouchi Y.
  Source: Chest. 2002 December; 122(6): 2266-7; Author Reply 2267.
  http://www.ncbi.nlm.nih.gov/entrez/query.fcgi?cmd=Retrieve&db=pubmed&dopt=Abstract&list_uids=12475880

- **Nonpharmacologic care of heart failure: counseling, dietary restriction, rehabilitation, treatment of sleep apnea, and ultrafiltration.**
  Author(s): Colonna P, Sorino M, D'Agostino C, Bovenzi F, De Luca L, Arrigo F, de Luca I.
  Source: The American Journal of Cardiology. 2003 May 8; 91(9A): 41F-50F. Review.
  http://www.ncbi.nlm.nih.gov/entrez/query.fcgi?cmd=Retrieve&db=pubmed&dopt=Abstract&list_uids=12729849

- **Nonprescription treatments of snoring or obstructive sleep apnea: an evaluation of products with limited scientific evidence.**
  Author(s): Meoli AL, Rosen CL, Kristo D, Kohrman M, Gooneratne N, Aguillard RN, Fayle R, Troell R; Clinical Practice Review Committee, American Academy of Sleep Medicine.
  Source: Sleep. 2003 August 1; 26(5): 619-24. Review.
  http://www.ncbi.nlm.nih.gov/entrez/query.fcgi?cmd=Retrieve&db=pubmed&dopt=Abstract&list_uids=12938818

- **Obesity and obstructive sleep apnea.**
  Author(s): Gami AS, Caples SM, Somers VK.
  Source: Endocrinology and Metabolism Clinics of North America. 2003 December; 32(4): 869-94. Review.
  http://www.ncbi.nlm.nih.gov/entrez/query.fcgi?cmd=Retrieve&db=pubmed&dopt=Abstract&list_uids=14711066

- **Obesity, sleep apnea, and hypertension.**
  Author(s): Wolk R, Shamsuzzaman AS, Somers VK.
  Source: Hypertension. 2003 December; 42(6): 1067-74. Epub 2003 November 10. Review.
  http://www.ncbi.nlm.nih.gov/entrez/query.fcgi?cmd=Retrieve&db=pubmed&dopt=Abstract&list_uids=14610096

- **Obstructive sleep apnea and tonsillectomy: do we have a new indication for extended postoperative observation?**
  Author(s): Cote CJ, Sheldon SH.
  Source: Canadian Journal of Anaesthesia = Journal Canadien D'anesthesie. 2004 January; 51(1): 6-12. English, French.
  http://www.ncbi.nlm.nih.gov/entrez/query.fcgi?cmd=Retrieve&db=pubmed&dopt=Abstract&list_uids=14709453

- **Obstructive sleep apnea in a referral population in India.**
  Author(s): Vigg A, Vigg A, Vigg A.
  Source: Sleep & Breathing = Schlaf & Atmung. 2003 December; 7(4): 177-84.
  http://www.ncbi.nlm.nih.gov/entrez/query.fcgi?cmd=Retrieve&db=pubmed&dopt=Abstract&list_uids=14710337

- **Obstructive sleep apnea in children.**
  Author(s): Chan J, Edman JC, Koltai PJ.
  Source: American Family Physician. 2004 March 1; 69(5): 1147-54. Review.
  http://www.ncbi.nlm.nih.gov/entrez/query.fcgi?cmd=Retrieve&db=pubmed&dopt=Abstract&list_uids=15023015

- **Obstructive sleep apnea syndromes.**
  Author(s): Guilleminault C, Abad VC.
  Source: The Medical Clinics of North America. 2004 May; 88(3): 611-30, Viii. Review.
  http://www.ncbi.nlm.nih.gov/entrez/query.fcgi?cmd=Retrieve&db=pubmed&dopt=Abstract&list_uids=15087207

- **Obstructive sleep apnea, nasal congestion, and snoring: their systemic effects and impact on quality of life.**
  Author(s): Boyd EL, Philpot EE.
  Source: Allergy and Asthma Proceedings : the Official Journal of Regional and State Allergy Societies. 2004 January-February; 25(1): 43-51. Review.
  http://www.ncbi.nlm.nih.gov/entrez/query.fcgi?cmd=Retrieve&db=pubmed&dopt=Abstract&list_uids=15055562

- **Obstructive sleep apnea-hypopnea syndrome.**
  Author(s): Olson EJ, Moore WR, Morgenthaler TI, Gay PC, Staats BA.
  Source: Mayo Clinic Proceedings. 2003 December; 78(12): 1545-52. Review.
  http://www.ncbi.nlm.nih.gov/entrez/query.fcgi?cmd=Retrieve&db=pubmed&dopt=Abstract&list_uids=14661684

- **Oral airway resistance during wakefulness in eucapnic and hypercapnic sleep apnea syndrome.**
  Author(s): Lin CC, Wu KM, Chou CS, Liaw SF.
  Source: Respiratory Physiology & Neurobiology. 2004 January 15; 139(2): 215-24.
  http://www.ncbi.nlm.nih.gov/entrez/query.fcgi?cmd=Retrieve&db=pubmed&dopt=Abstract&list_uids=15123004

- **Oral continuous positive airway pressure for sleep apnea: effectiveness, patient preference, and adherence.**
  Author(s): Beecroft J, Zanon S, Lukic D, Hanly P.
  Source: Chest. 2003 December; 124(6): 2200-8.
  http://www.ncbi.nlm.nih.gov/entrez/query.fcgi?cmd=Retrieve&db=pubmed&dopt=Abstract&list_uids=14665501

- **Pathological data on apoptosis in the brainstem and physiological data on sleep apnea in SIDS victims.**
  Author(s): Sawaguchi T, Patricia F, Kadhim H, Groswasser J, Sottiaux M, Nishida H, Kahn A.
  Source: Early Human Development. 2003 December; 75 Suppl: S13-20.
  http://www.ncbi.nlm.nih.gov/entrez/query.fcgi?cmd=Retrieve&db=pubmed&dopt=Abstract&list_uids=14693387

- **Pituitary-gonadal function in men with obstructive sleep apnea. The effect of continuous positive airways pressure treatment.**
  Author(s): Luboshitzky R, Lavie L, Shen-Orr Z, Lavie P.
  Source: Neuroendocrinol Lett. 2003 December; 24(6): 463-7.
  http://www.ncbi.nlm.nih.gov/entrez/query.fcgi?cmd=Retrieve&db=pubmed&dopt=Abstract&list_uids=15073577

- **Planning adenotonsillectomy in children with obstructive sleep apnea: the role of overnight oximetry.**
  Author(s): Nixon GM, Kermack AS, Davis GM, Manoukian JJ, Brown KA, Brouillette RT.
  Source: Pediatrics. 2004 January; 113(1 Pt 1): E19-25.
  http://www.ncbi.nlm.nih.gov/entrez/query.fcgi?cmd=Retrieve&db=pubmed&dopt=Abstract&list_uids=14702490

- **Plasma cytokine levels in patients with obstructive sleep apnea syndrome: a preliminary study.**
  Author(s): Alberti A, Sarchielli P, Gallinella E, Floridi A, Floridi A, Mazzotta G, Gallai V.
  Source: Journal of Sleep Research. 2003 December; 12(4): 305-11.
  http://www.ncbi.nlm.nih.gov/entrez/query.fcgi?cmd=Retrieve&db=pubmed&dopt=Abstract&list_uids=14633242

- **Polysomnography vs self-reported measures in patients with sleep apnea.**
  Author(s): Weaver EM, Kapur V, Yueh B.
  Source: Archives of Otolaryngology--Head & Neck Surgery. 2004 April; 130(4): 453-8.
  http://www.ncbi.nlm.nih.gov/entrez/query.fcgi?cmd=Retrieve&db=pubmed&dopt=Abstract&list_uids=15096430

- **Practice parameters for the use of portable monitoring devices in the investigation of suspected obstructive sleep apnea in adults.**
  Author(s): Chesson AL Jr, Berry RB, Pack A; American Academy of Sleep Medicine; American Thoracic Society; American College of Chest Physicians.
  Source: Sleep. 2003 November 1; 26(7): 907-13.
  http://www.ncbi.nlm.nih.gov/entrez/query.fcgi?cmd=Retrieve&db=pubmed&dopt=Abstract&list_uids=14655928

- **Preventative risk management for obstructive sleep apnea.**
  Author(s): Strohl KP.
  Source: Sleep & Breathing = Schlaf & Atmung. 2003 December; 7(4): 197.
  http://www.ncbi.nlm.nih.gov/entrez/query.fcgi?cmd=Retrieve&db=pubmed&dopt=Abstract&list_uids=14710340

- **Pro: Sleep apnea causes cardiovascular disease.**
  Author(s): Lavie P.
  Source: American Journal of Respiratory and Critical Care Medicine. 2004 January 15; 169(2): 147-8; Discussion 150.
  http://www.ncbi.nlm.nih.gov/entrez/query.fcgi?cmd=Retrieve&db=pubmed&dopt=Abstract&list_uids=14718233

- **Pulmonary function and sleep apnea.**
  Author(s): Hoffstein V, Oliver Z.
  Source: Sleep & Breathing = Schlaf & Atmung. 2003 December; 7(4): 159-65.
  http://www.ncbi.nlm.nih.gov/entrez/query.fcgi?cmd=Retrieve&db=pubmed&dopt=Abstract&list_uids=14710335

- **Pulmonary hypertension and sleep apnea.**
  Author(s): Avnon LS, Heimer D.
  Source: Isr Med Assoc J. 2004 April; 6(4): 255; Author Reply 255. No Abstract Available.
  http://www.ncbi.nlm.nih.gov/entrez/query.fcgi?cmd=Retrieve&db=pubmed&dopt=Abstract&list_uids=15115271

- **Quality of life after adenotonsillectomy for obstructive sleep apnea in children.**
  Author(s): Mitchell RB, Kelly J, Call E, Yao N.
  Source: Archives of Otolaryngology--Head & Neck Surgery. 2004 February; 130(2): 190-4.
  http://www.ncbi.nlm.nih.gov/entrez/query.fcgi?cmd=Retrieve&db=pubmed&dopt=Abstract&list_uids=14967749

- **Quality of life in bed partners of patients with obstructive sleep apnea or hypopnea after treatment with continuous positive airway pressure.**
  Author(s): Parish JM, Lyng PJ.
  Source: Chest. 2003 September; 124(3): 942-7.
  http://www.ncbi.nlm.nih.gov/entrez/query.fcgi?cmd=Retrieve&db=pubmed&dopt=Abstract&list_uids=12970021

- **Quality of life in patients with obstructive sleep apnea: effect of nasal continuous positive airway pressure--a prospective study.**
  Author(s): D'Ambrosio C, Bowman T, Mohsenin V.
  Source: Chest. 1999 January; 115(1): 123-9.
  http://www.ncbi.nlm.nih.gov/entrez/query.fcgi?cmd=Retrieve&db=pubmed&dopt=Abstract&list_uids=9925072

- **Quantitative assessment of the pharyngeal airway by dynamic magnetic resonance imaging in obstructive sleep apnea syndrome.**
  Author(s): Ikeda K, Ogura M, Oshima T, Suzuki H, Higano S, Takahashi S, Kurosawa H, Hida W, Matsuoka H, Takasaka T.
  Source: The Annals of Otology, Rhinology, and Laryngology. 2001 February; 110(2): 183-9.
  http://www.ncbi.nlm.nih.gov/entrez/query.fcgi?cmd=Retrieve&db=pubmed&dopt=Abstract&list_uids=11219527

- **Quantitative magnetic resonance imaging demonstrates alterations of the lingual musculature in obstructive sleep apnea.**
  Author(s): Schotland HM, Insko EK, Schwab RJ.
  Source: Sleep. 1999 August 1; 22(5): 605-13.
  http://www.ncbi.nlm.nih.gov/entrez/query.fcgi?cmd=Retrieve&db=pubmed&dopt=Abstract&list_uids=10450595

- **Re: Kaneko Y, Hajek VE, Zivanovic V et al. Relationship of sleep apnea to functional capacity and length of hospitalization following stroke. SLEEP 2003;26(3):293-7.**
  Author(s): Morcos Z, Phadke J.
  Source: Sleep. 2003 Sep15; 26(6): 761; Author Reply 762. No Abstract Available.
  http://www.ncbi.nlm.nih.gov/entrez/query.fcgi?cmd=Retrieve&db=pubmed&dopt=Abstract&list_uids=14572132

- **Reactive oxygen metabolites (ROMs) as an index of oxidative stress in obstructive sleep apnea patients.**
  Author(s): Christou K, Markoulis N, Moulas AN, Pastaka C, Gourgoulianis KI.
  Source: Sleep & Breathing = Schlaf & Atmung. 2003 September; 7(3): 105-10.
  http://www.ncbi.nlm.nih.gov/entrez/query.fcgi?cmd=Retrieve&db=pubmed&dopt=Abstract&list_uids=14569521

- **Recent advances in understanding the pathogenesis of obstructive sleep apnea.**
  Author(s): Jordan AS, White DP, Fogel RB.
  Source: Current Opinion in Pulmonary Medicine. 2003 November; 9(6): 459-64. Review.
  http://www.ncbi.nlm.nih.gov/entrez/query.fcgi?cmd=Retrieve&db=pubmed&dopt=Abstract&list_uids=14534395

- **Recent developments in the treatment of obstructive sleep apnea.**
Author(s): Verse T, Pirsig W, Stuck BA, Hormann K, Maurer JT.
Source: American Journal of Respiratory Medicine : Drugs, Devices, and Other Interventions. 2003; 2(2): 157-68. Review.
http://www.ncbi.nlm.nih.gov/entrez/query.fcgi?cmd=Retrieve&db=pubmed&dopt=Abstract&list_uids=14720014

- **Recurrent hypoxemia in young children with obstructive sleep apnea is associated with reduced opioid requirement for analgesia.**
Author(s): Brown KA, Laferriere A, Moss IR.
Source: Anesthesiology. 2004 April; 100(4): 806-10; Discussion 5A.
http://www.ncbi.nlm.nih.gov/entrez/query.fcgi?cmd=Retrieve&db=pubmed&dopt=Abstract&list_uids=15087614

- **Resistant hypertension, obesity, sleep apnea, and aldosterone: theory and therapy.**
Author(s): Goodfriend TL, Calhoun DA.
Source: Hypertension. 2004 March; 43(3): 518-24. Epub 2004 January 19.
http://www.ncbi.nlm.nih.gov/entrez/query.fcgi?cmd=Retrieve&db=pubmed&dopt=Abstract&list_uids=14732721

- **Reversible obstructive sleep apnea and right heart failure due to massive tonsillar hypertrophy.**
Author(s): Atiq M, Masood F, Ikram M, Haqqee R.
Source: J Ayub Med Coll Abbottabad. 2004 January-March; 16(1): 66-8.
http://www.ncbi.nlm.nih.gov/entrez/query.fcgi?cmd=Retrieve&db=pubmed&dopt=Abstract&list_uids=15125187

- **Risk factors for obstructive sleep apnea in adults.**
Author(s): Young T, Skatrud J, Peppard PE.
Source: Jama : the Journal of the American Medical Association. 2004 April 28; 291(16): 2013-6. Review.
http://www.ncbi.nlm.nih.gov/entrez/query.fcgi?cmd=Retrieve&db=pubmed&dopt=Abstract&list_uids=15113821

- **Role of arousals in the pathogenesis of obstructive sleep apnea.**
Author(s): Younes M.
Source: American Journal of Respiratory and Critical Care Medicine. 2004 March 1; 169(5): 623-33. Epub 2003 December 18.
http://www.ncbi.nlm.nih.gov/entrez/query.fcgi?cmd=Retrieve&db=pubmed&dopt=Abstract&list_uids=14684560

- **Role of portable sleep studies for diagnosis of obstructive sleep apnea.**
Author(s): Boyer S, Kapur V.
Source: Current Opinion in Pulmonary Medicine. 2003 November; 9(6): 465-70. Review.
http://www.ncbi.nlm.nih.gov/entrez/query.fcgi?cmd=Retrieve&db=pubmed&dopt=Abstract&list_uids=14534396

- **Serotonergic receptors in the midbrain correlated with physiological data on sleep apnea in SIDS victims.**
Author(s): Sawaguchi T, Ozawa Y, Patricia F, Kadhim H, Groswasser J, Sottiaux M, Takashima S, Nishida H, Kahn A.
Source: Early Human Development. 2003 December; 75 Suppl: S65-74.
http://www.ncbi.nlm.nih.gov/entrez/query.fcgi?cmd=Retrieve&db=pubmed&dopt=Abstract&list_uids=14693393

- **Severe, but not mild, obstructive sleep apnea syndrome is associated with erectile dysfunction.**
Author(s): Margel D, Cohen M, Livne PM, Pillar G.
Source: Urology. 2004 March; 63(3): 545-9.
http://www.ncbi.nlm.nih.gov/entrez/query.fcgi?cmd=Retrieve&db=pubmed&dopt=Abstract&list_uids=15028455

- **Should women with obstructive sleep apnea syndrome be screened for hypothyroidism?**
Author(s): Miller CM, Husain AM.
Source: Sleep & Breathing = Schlaf & Atmung. 2003 December; 7(4): 185-8.
http://www.ncbi.nlm.nih.gov/entrez/query.fcgi?cmd=Retrieve&db=pubmed&dopt=Abstract&list_uids=14710338

- **Simultaneous use of antidepressant and antihypertensive medications increases likelihood of diagnosis of obstructive sleep apnea syndrome.**
Author(s): Farney RJ, Lugo A, Jensen RL, Walker JM, Cloward TV.
Source: Chest. 2004 April; 125(4): 1279-85.
http://www.ncbi.nlm.nih.gov/entrez/query.fcgi?cmd=Retrieve&db=pubmed&dopt=Abstract&list_uids=15078735

- **Sleep apnea and Down's syndrome.**
  Author(s): Dahlqvist A, Rask E, Rosenqvist CJ, Sahlin C, Franklin KA.
  Source: Acta Oto-Laryngologica. 2003 December; 123(9): 1094-7.
  http://www.ncbi.nlm.nih.gov/entrez/query.fcgi?cmd=Retrieve&db=pubmed&dopt=Abstract&list_uids=14710914

- **Sleep apnea in mice: a useful animal model for study of SIDS?**
  Author(s): Nakamura A, Kuwaki T.
  Source: Early Human Development. 2003 December; 75 Suppl: S167-74. Review.
  http://www.ncbi.nlm.nih.gov/entrez/query.fcgi?cmd=Retrieve&db=pubmed&dopt=Abstract&list_uids=14693402

- **Sleep apnea obstructive syndrome: a new complication previously undescribed in cirrhotic patients with ascites.**
  Author(s): Crespo J, Cifrian J, Pinto JA, Jimenez-Gomez A, Pons-Romero F.
  Source: The American Journal of Gastroenterology. 2003 December; 98(12): 2815-6.
  http://www.ncbi.nlm.nih.gov/entrez/query.fcgi?cmd=Retrieve&db=pubmed&dopt=Abstract&list_uids=14687850

- **Sleep apnea: a review for life insurance medical directors and underwriters.**
  Author(s): Richie RC.
  Source: J Insur Med. 2003; 35(1): 36-50. Review.
  http://www.ncbi.nlm.nih.gov/entrez/query.fcgi?cmd=Retrieve&db=pubmed&dopt=Abstract&list_uids=14694824

- **Staging of obstructive sleep apnea/hypopnea syndrome: a guide to appropriate treatment.**
  Author(s): Friedman M, Ibrahim H, Joseph NJ.
  Source: The Laryngoscope. 2004 March; 114(3): 454-9.
  http://www.ncbi.nlm.nih.gov/entrez/query.fcgi?cmd=Retrieve&db=pubmed&dopt=Abstract&list_uids=15091218

- **Substance P in the midbrains of SIDS victims and its correlation with sleep apnea.**
  Author(s): Sawaguchi T, Ozawa Y, Patricia F, Kadhim H, Groswasser J, Sottiaux M, Takashima S, Nishida H, Kahn A.
  Source: Early Human Development. 2003 December; 75 Suppl: S51-9.
  http://www.ncbi.nlm.nih.gov/entrez/query.fcgi?cmd=Retrieve&db=pubmed&dopt=Abstract&list_uids=14693391

- **The correlation between microtubule-associated protein 2 in the brainstem of SIDS victims and physiological data on sleep apnea.**
  Author(s): Sawaguchi T, Patricia F, Kadhim H, Groswasser J, Sottiaux M, Nishida H, Kahn A.
  Source: Early Human Development. 2003 December; 75 Suppl: S87-97.
  http://www.ncbi.nlm.nih.gov/entrez/query.fcgi?cmd=Retrieve&db=pubmed&dopt=Abstract&list_uids=14693395

- **The correlation between serotonergic neurons in the brainstem and sleep apnea in SIDS victims.**
  Author(s): Sawaguchi T, Patricia F, Kadhim H, Groswasser J, Sottiaux M, Nishida H, Kahn A.
  Source: Early Human Development. 2003 December; 75 Suppl: S31-40.
  http://www.ncbi.nlm.nih.gov/entrez/query.fcgi?cmd=Retrieve&db=pubmed&dopt=Abstract&list_uids=14693389

- **The correlation between tau protein in the brainstem and sleep apnea in SIDS victims.**
  Author(s): Sawaguchi T, Patricia F, Kadhim H, Groswasser J, Sottiaux M, Nishida H, Kahn A.
  Source: Early Human Development. 2003 December; 75 Suppl: S99-107.
  http://www.ncbi.nlm.nih.gov/entrez/query.fcgi?cmd=Retrieve&db=pubmed&dopt=Abstract&list_uids=14693396

- **The correlation between ubiquitin in the brainstem and sleep apnea in SIDS victims.**
  Author(s): Sawaguchi T, Patricia F, Kadhim H, Groswasser J, Sottiaux M, Nishida H, Kahn A.
  Source: Early Human Development. 2003 December; 75 Suppl: S75-86.
  http://www.ncbi.nlm.nih.gov/entrez/query.fcgi?cmd=Retrieve&db=pubmed&dopt=Abstract&list_uids=14693394

- **The presence of TATA-binding protein in the brainstem, correlated with sleep apnea in SIDS victims.**
Author(s): Sawaguchi T, Patricia F, Kadhim H, Groswasser J, Sottiaux M, Nishida H, Kahn A.
Source: Early Human Development. 2003 December; 75 Suppl: S109-18.
http://www.ncbi.nlm.nih.gov/entrez/query.fcgi?cmd=Retrieve&db=pubmed&dopt=Abstract&list_uids=14693397

- **The prevalence of glaucoma in patients with sleep apnea syndrome: same as in the general population.**
Author(s): Geyer O, Cohen N, Segev E, Rath EZ, Melamud L, Peled R, Lavie P.
Source: American Journal of Ophthalmology. 2003 December; 136(6): 1093-6.
http://www.ncbi.nlm.nih.gov/entrez/query.fcgi?cmd=Retrieve&db=pubmed&dopt=Abstract&list_uids=14644220

- **Transitory increased blood pressure after upper airway surgery for snoring and sleep apnea correlates with the apnea-hypopnea respiratory disturbance index.**
Author(s): Araujo MT, Ouayoun M, Poirier JM, Bayle MM, Vasquez EC, Fleury B.
Source: Brazilian Journal of Medical and Biological Research = Revista Brasileira De Pesquisas Medicas E Biologicas / Sociedade Brasileira De Biofisica. [et Al.]. 2003 December; 36(12): 1741-9. Epub 2003 November 17.
http://www.ncbi.nlm.nih.gov/entrez/query.fcgi?cmd=Retrieve&db=pubmed&dopt=Abstract&list_uids=14666260

- **Treatment of obstructive sleep apnea in primary care.**
Author(s): Victor LD.
Source: American Family Physician. 2004 February 1; 69(3): 561-8. Review.
http://www.ncbi.nlm.nih.gov/entrez/query.fcgi?cmd=Retrieve&db=pubmed&dopt=Abstract&list_uids=14971838

- **Treatment outcome of obstructive sleep apnea syndrome in a patient with schizophrenia: case report.**
  Author(s): Boufidis S, Kosmidis MH, Bozikas VP, Daskalopoulou-Vlahoyianni E, Pitsavas S, Karavatos A.
  Source: International Journal of Psychiatry in Medicine. 2003; 33(3): 305-10.
  http://www.ncbi.nlm.nih.gov/entrez/query.fcgi?cmd=Retrieve&db=pubmed&dopt=Abstract&list_uids=15089011

- **Two different degrees of mandibular advancement with a dental appliance in treatment of patients with mild to moderate obstructive sleep apnea.**
  Author(s): Tegelberg A, Walker-Engstrom ML, Vestling O, Wilhelmsson B.
  Source: Acta Odontologica Scandinavica. 2003 December; 61(6): 356-62.
  http://www.ncbi.nlm.nih.gov/entrez/query.fcgi?cmd=Retrieve&db=pubmed&dopt=Abstract&list_uids=14960007

- **Unexpected risks during administration of conscious sedation: previously undiagnosed obstructive sleep apnea.**
  Author(s): Sharma VK, Galli W, Haber A, Pressman MR, Stevenson R, Meyer TJ, Peterson DD, Zachariah JS, Mercogliano G, Greenspon L.
  Source: Annals of Internal Medicine. 2003 October 21; 139(8): 707-8. Erratum In: Ann Intern Med. 2003 November 18; 139(10): 873.
  http://www.ncbi.nlm.nih.gov/entrez/query.fcgi?cmd=Retrieve&db=pubmed&dopt=Abstract&list_uids=14568871

- **Update for nurse anesthetists. The Starling resistor: a model for explaining and treating obstructive sleep apnea.**
  Author(s): Stalford CB.
  Source: Aana Journal. 2004 April; 72(2): 133-8. Review.
  http://www.ncbi.nlm.nih.gov/entrez/query.fcgi?cmd=Retrieve&db=pubmed&dopt=Abstract&list_uids=15098527

- **Upper airway management of the adult patient with obstructive sleep apnea in the perioperative period--avoiding complications.**
  Author(s): Meoli AL, Rosen CL, Kristo D, Kohrman M, Gooneratne N, Aguillard RN, Fayle R, Troell R, Kramer R, Casey KR, Coleman J Jr; Clinical Practice Review Committee; American Academy of Sleep Medicine.
  Source: Sleep. 2003 December 15; 26(8): 1060-5.
  http://www.ncbi.nlm.nih.gov/entrez/query.fcgi?cmd=Retrieve&db=pubmed&dopt=Abstract&list_uids=14746392

- **Upper airway motion depicted at cine MR imaging performed during sleep: comparison between young Patients with and those without obstructive sleep apnea.**
  Author(s): Donnelly LF, Surdulescu V, Chini BA, Casper KA, Poe SA, Amin RS.
  Source: Radiology. 2003 April; 227(1): 239-45. Epub 2003 February 28.
  http://www.ncbi.nlm.nih.gov/entrez/query.fcgi?cmd=Retrieve&db=pubmed&dopt=Abstract&list_uids=12616001

- **Upper airway obstruction-related sleep apnea in a child with thalassemia intermedia.**
  Author(s): Kapelushnik J, Shalev H, Schulman H, Moser A, Tamary H.
  Source: Journal of Pediatric Hematology/Oncology : Official Journal of the American Society of Pediatric Hematology/Oncology. 2001 November; 23(8): 525-6.
  http://www.ncbi.nlm.nih.gov/entrez/query.fcgi?cmd=Retrieve&db=pubmed&dopt=Abstract&list_uids=11878781

- **Upper airway response to electrical stimulation of the genioglossus in obstructive sleep apnea.**
  Author(s): Oliven A, O'Hearn DJ, Boudewyns A, Odeh M, De Backer W, van de Heyning P, Smith PL, Eisele DW, Allan L, Schneider H, Testerman R, Schwartz AR.
  Source: Journal of Applied Physiology (Bethesda, Md. : 1985). 2003 November; 95(5): 2023-9.
  http://www.ncbi.nlm.nih.gov/entrez/query.fcgi?cmd=Retrieve&db=pubmed&dopt=Abstract&list_uids=14555669

- **Upper airway size analysis by magnetic resonance imaging of children with obstructive sleep apnea syndrome.**
  Author(s): Arens R, McDonough JM, Corbin AM, Rubin NK, Carroll ME, Pack AI, Liu J, Udupa JK.
  Source: American Journal of Respiratory and Critical Care Medicine. 2003 January 1; 167(1): 65-70. Epub 2002 October 11.
  http://www.ncbi.nlm.nih.gov/entrez/query.fcgi?cmd=Retrieve&db=pubmed&dopt=Abstract&list_uids=12406826

- **Upper airway surgery for obstructive sleep apnea.**
  Author(s): Sher AE.
  Source: Sleep Medicine Reviews. 2002 June; 6(3): 195-212. Review.
  http://www.ncbi.nlm.nih.gov/entrez/query.fcgi?cmd=Retrieve&db=pubmed&dopt=Abstract&list_uids=12531121

- **Utility of oxygen saturation and heart rate spectral analysis obtained from pulse oximetric recordings in the diagnosis of sleep apnea syndrome.**
  Author(s): Zamarron C, Gude F, Barcala J, Rodriguez JR, Romero PV.
  Source: Chest. 2003 May; 123(5): 1567-76.
  http://www.ncbi.nlm.nih.gov/entrez/query.fcgi?cmd=Retrieve&db=pubmed&dopt=Abstract&list_uids=12740275

- **Uvulopalatopharyngoplasty for sleep apnea in mentally retarded obese 14-year-old: an anaesthetic challenge.**
  Author(s): Govindarajan R, Bakalova T, Gerges M, Mendelsohn M, Michael R, Abadir A.
  Source: Acta Anaesthesiologica Scandinavica. 2003 March; 47(3): 366-8.
  http://www.ncbi.nlm.nih.gov/entrez/query.fcgi?cmd=Retrieve&db=pubmed&dopt=Abstract&list_uids=12648207

- **Validity of neural network in sleep apnea.**
  Author(s): el-Solh AA, Mador MJ, Ten-Brock E, Shucard DW, Abul-Khoudoud M, Grant BJ.
  Source: Sleep. 1999 February 1; 22(1): 105-11.
  http://www.ncbi.nlm.nih.gov/entrez/query.fcgi?cmd=Retrieve&db=pubmed&dopt=Abstract&list_uids=9989371

- **Value of clinical, functional, and oximetric data for the prediction of obstructive sleep apnea in obese patients.**
  Author(s): Herer B, Roche N, Carton M, Roig C, Poujol V, Huchon G.
  Source: Chest. 1999 December; 116(6): 1537-44.
  http://www.ncbi.nlm.nih.gov/entrez/query.fcgi?cmd=Retrieve&db=pubmed&dopt=Abstract&list_uids=10593773

- **Variation in the arousal pattern after obstructive events in obstructive sleep apnea.**
  Author(s): Stradling JR, Pitson DJ, Bennett L, Barbour C, Davies RJ.
  Source: American Journal of Respiratory and Critical Care Medicine. 1999 January; 159(1): 130-6.
  http://www.ncbi.nlm.nih.gov/entrez/query.fcgi?cmd=Retrieve&db=pubmed&dopt=Abstract&list_uids=9872830

- **Vascular dysfunction in sleep apnea: a reversible link to cardiovascular disease?**
  Author(s): Imadojemu VA, Sinoway LI, Leuenberger UA.
  Source: American Journal of Respiratory and Critical Care Medicine. 2004 February 1; 169(3): 328-9.
  http://www.ncbi.nlm.nih.gov/entrez/query.fcgi?cmd=Retrieve&db=pubmed&dopt=Abstract&list_uids=14739129

- **Vascular reactivity in obstructive sleep apnea syndrome.**
  Author(s): Duchna HW, Guilleminault C, Stoohs RA, Faul JL, Moreno H, Hoffman BB, Blaschke TF.
  Source: American Journal of Respiratory and Critical Care Medicine. 2000 January; 161(1): 187-91.
  http://www.ncbi.nlm.nih.gov/entrez/query.fcgi?cmd=Retrieve&db=pubmed&dopt=Abstract&list_uids=10619819

- **Velopharyngeal anatomy in snorers and patients with obstructive sleep apnea.**
  Author(s): Marien S, Schmelzer B.
  Source: Acta Otorhinolaryngol Belg. 2002; 56(2): 93-9. Review.
  http://www.ncbi.nlm.nih.gov/entrez/query.fcgi?cmd=Retrieve&db=pubmed&dopt=Abstract&list_uids=12092332

- **Ventilatory dynamics of transient arousal in patients with obstructive sleep apnea.**
  Author(s): Khoo MC, Shin JJ, Asyali MH, Kim TS, Berry RB.
  Source: Respiration Physiology. 1998 June; 112(3): 291-303.
  http://www.ncbi.nlm.nih.gov/entrez/query.fcgi?cmd=Retrieve&db=pubmed&dopt=Abstract&list_uids=9749952

- **Ventilatory response to CO2 in children with obstructive sleep apnea from adenotonsillar hypertrophy.**
  Author(s): Strauss SG, Lynn AM, Bratton SL, Nespeca MK.
  Source: Anesthesia and Analgesia. 1999 August; 89(2): 328-32.
  http://www.ncbi.nlm.nih.gov/entrez/query.fcgi?cmd=Retrieve&db=pubmed&dopt=Abstract&list_uids=10439742

- **Ventilatory-control abnormalities in familial sleep apnea.**
  Author(s): Redline S, Leitner J, Arnold J, Tishler PV, Altose MD.
  Source: American Journal of Respiratory and Critical Care Medicine. 1997 July; 156(1): 155-60.
  http://www.ncbi.nlm.nih.gov/entrez/query.fcgi?cmd=Retrieve&db=pubmed&dopt=Abstract&list_uids=9230740

- **Vocal tract resonance characteristics of adults with obstructive sleep apnea.**
  Author(s): Robb MP, Yates J, Morgan EJ.
  Source: Acta Oto-Laryngologica. 1997 September; 117(5): 760-3.
  http://www.ncbi.nlm.nih.gov/entrez/query.fcgi?cmd=Retrieve&db=pubmed&dopt=Abstract&list_uids=9349877

- **Websites on oral appliances for obstructive sleep apnea.**
  Author(s): Zwetchkenbaum SR, Avidan AY.
  Source: Sleep Medicine. 2003 January; 4(1): 77-8.
  http://www.ncbi.nlm.nih.gov/entrez/query.fcgi?cmd=Retrieve&db=pubmed&dopt=Abstract&list_uids=14592365

- **When does 'mild' obstructive sleep apnea/hypopnea syndrome merit continuous positive airway pressure treatment?**
  Author(s): Engleman HM.
  Source: American Journal of Respiratory and Critical Care Medicine. 2002 March 15; 165(6): 743-5.
  http://www.ncbi.nlm.nih.gov/entrez/query.fcgi?cmd=Retrieve&db=pubmed&dopt=Abstract&list_uids=11897636

- **When snoring is serious. Diagnosis and treatment of sleep apnea.**
  Author(s): Garcia JD.
  Source: Adv Nurse Pract. 2004 April; 12(4): 51-3. Review. No Abstract Available.
  http://www.ncbi.nlm.nih.gov/entrez/query.fcgi?cmd=Retrieve&db=pubmed&dopt=Abstract&list_uids=15101135

- **When to suspect obstructive sleep apnea syndrome. Symptoms may be subtle, but treatment is straightforward.**
  Author(s): Attarian HP, Sabri AN.
  Source: Postgraduate Medicine. 2002 March; 111(3): 70-6; Quiz 14. Review.
  http://www.ncbi.nlm.nih.gov/entrez/query.fcgi?cmd=Retrieve&db=pubmed&dopt=Abstract&list_uids=11912998

- **White coat hypertension and sleep apnea: is there a link?**
  Author(s): Ventura HO, Mehra MR.
  Source: Chest. 2004 March; 125(3): 805-7.
  http://www.ncbi.nlm.nih.gov/entrez/query.fcgi?cmd=Retrieve&db=pubmed&dopt=Abstract&list_uids=15006931

- **White coat hypertension in patients with obstructive sleep apnea-hypopnea syndrome.**
  Author(s): Garcia-Rio F, Pino JM, Alonso A, Arias MA, Martinez I, Alvaro D, Villamor J.
  Source: Chest. 2004 March; 125(3): 817-22.
  http://www.ncbi.nlm.nih.gov/entrez/query.fcgi?cmd=Retrieve&db=pubmed&dopt=Abstract&list_uids=15006937

- **Why are men more susceptible to sleep apnea?**
  Author(s): Bederka M.
  Source: Adv Nurse Pract. 2004 April; 12(4): 54. Review. No Abstract Available.
  http://www.ncbi.nlm.nih.gov/entrez/query.fcgi?cmd=Retrieve&db=pubmed&dopt=Abstract&list_uids=15101136

- **Will orthodontists become more involved in treating patients who have sleep apnea?**
  Author(s): Legan HL.
  Source: American Journal of Orthodontics and Dentofacial Orthopedics : Official Publication of the American Association of Orthodontists, Its Constituent Societies, and the American Board of Orthodontics. 2004 May; 125(5): 16A.
  http://www.ncbi.nlm.nih.gov/entrez/query.fcgi?cmd=Retrieve&db=pubmed&dopt=Abstract&list_uids=15151107

- **Willingness to pay for polysomnography in children with obstructive sleep apnea syndrome: a cost-benefit analysis.**
  Author(s): Tarasiuk A, Simon T, Regev U, Reuveni H.
  Source: Sleep. 2003 December 15; 26(8): 1016-21.
  http://www.ncbi.nlm.nih.gov/entrez/query.fcgi?cmd=Retrieve&db=pubmed&dopt=Abstract&list_uids=14746384

Vocabulary Builder

Adenoma: A benign tumor originating from, or having the appearance of, glandular epithelium; of endocrine or exocrine origin. [NIH]

Attenuated: Strain with weakened or reduced virulence. [NIH]

Attenuation: Reduction of transmitted sound energy or its electrical equivalent. [NIH]

Axonal: Condition associated with metabolic derangement of the entire neuron and is manifest by degeneration of the distal portion of the nerve fiber. [NIH]

Berger: A binocular loupe with the lenses mounted at the anterior end of a light-excluding chamber fitting over the eyes and held in place by an elastic headband. [NIH]

Bioengineering: The application of engineering principles to the solution of biological problems, for example, remote-handling devices, life-support systems, controls, and displays. [NIH]

Biophysics: The science of physical phenomena and processes in living organisms. [NIH]

Brachial: All the nerves from the arm are ripped from the spinal cord. [NIH]

Catecholamine: A group of chemical substances manufactured by the adrenal medulla and secreted during physiological stress. [NIH]

CDNA: Synthetic DNA reverse transcribed from a specific RNA through the action of the enzyme reverse transcriptase. DNA synthesized by reverse transcriptase using RNA as a template. [NIH]

Clamp: A u-shaped steel rod used with a pin or wire for skeletal traction in the treatment of certain fractures. [NIH]

Cofactor: A substance, microorganism or environmental factor that activates or enhances the action of another entity such as a disease-causing agent. [NIH]

Competency: The capacity of the bacterium to take up DNA from its surroundings. [NIH]

Confounder: A factor of confusion which blurs a specific connection between a disease and a probable causal factor which is being studied. [NIH]

Continuum: An area over which the vegetation or animal population is of constantly changing composition so that homogeneous, separate communities cannot be distinguished. [NIH]

Cortisol: A steroid hormone secreted by the adrenal cortex as part of the body's response to stress. [NIH]

Cytokine: Small but highly potent protein that modulates the activity of many cell types, including T and B cells. [NIH]

Deletion: A genetic rearrangement through loss of segments of DNA (chromosomes), bringing sequences, which are normally separated, into close proximity. [NIH]

Density: The logarithm to the base 10 of the opacity of an exposed and processed film. [NIH]

Discrete: Made up of separate parts or characterized by lesions which do not become blended; not running together; separate. [NIH]

EEG: A graphic recording of the changes in electrical potential associated with the activity of the cerebral cortex made with the electroencephalogram. [NIH]

Electrode: Component of the pacing system which is at the distal end of the lead. It is the interface with living cardiac tissue across which the stimulus is transmitted. [NIH]

Empirical: A treatment based on an assumed diagnosis, prior to receiving confirmatory laboratory test results. [NIH]

Estrogen: One of the two female sex hormones. [NIH]

Evoke: The electric response recorded from the cerebral cortex after stimulation of a peripheral sense organ. [NIH]

Excitatory: When cortical neurons are excited, their output increases and each new input they receive while they are still excited raises their output markedly. [NIH]

Expiratory: The volume of air which leaves the breathing organs in each expiration. [NIH]

Extraocular: External to or outside of the eye. [NIH]

Fat: Total lipids including phospholipids. [NIH]

Fatigue: The feeling of weariness of mind and body. [NIH]

Fold: A plication or doubling of various parts of the body. [NIH]

Forearm: The part between the elbow and the wrist. [NIH]

Generator: Any system incorporating a fixed parent radionuclide from which is produced a daughter radionuclide which is to be removed by elution or by any other method and used in a radiopharmaceutical. [NIH]

Genetics: The biological science that deals with the phenomena and mechanisms of heredity. [NIH]

Gestational: Psychosis attributable to or occurring during pregnancy. [NIH]

Glossectomy: Amputation of the tongue. [NIH]

Heterogeneity: The property of one or more samples or populations which implies that they are not identical in respect of some or all of their parameters, e. g. heterogeneity of variance. [NIH]

Impairment: In the context of health experience, an impairment is any loss or abnormality of psychological, physiological, or anatomical structure or function. [NIH]

Incisor: Anything adapted for cutting; any one of the four front teeth in each jaw. [NIH]

Infancy: The period of complete dependency prior to the acquisition of competence in walking, talking, and self-feeding. [NIH]

Initiation: Mutation induced by a chemical reactive substance causing cell changes; being a step in a carcinogenic process. [NIH]

Insight: The capacity to understand one's own motives, to be aware of one's own psychodynamics, to appreciate the meaning of symbolic behavior. [NIH]

Latency: The period of apparent inactivity between the time when a stimulus is presented and the moment a response occurs. [NIH]

Linkage: The tendency of two or more genes in the same chromosome to remain together from one generation to the next more frequently than expected according to the law of independent assortment. [NIH]

Loop: A wire usually of platinum bent at one end into a small loop (usually 4 mm inside diameter) and used in transferring microorganisms. [NIH]

Modification: A change in an organism, or in a process in an organism, that is acquired from its own activity or environment. [NIH]

Morphological: Relating to the configuration or the structure of live organs. [NIH]

MRNA: The RNA molecule that conveys from the DNA the information that is to be translated into the structure of a particular polypeptide molecule. [NIH]

Nuclei: A body of specialized protoplasm found in nearly all cells and containing the chromosomes. [NIH]

Nucleus: A body of specialized protoplasm found in nearly all cells and containing the chromosomes. [NIH]

Otology: The branch of medicine which deals with the diagnosis and treatment of the disorders and diseases of the ear. [NIH]

Outpatient: A patient who is not an inmate of a hospital but receives diagnosis or treatment in a clinic or dispensary connected with the hospital. [NIH]

Patch: A piece of material used to cover or protect a wound, an injured part, etc.: a patch over the eye. [NIH]

Pathologies: The study of abnormality, especially the study of diseases. [NIH]

Phenotypes: An organism as observed, i. e. as judged by its visually perceptible characters resulting from the interaction of its genotype with the environment. [NIH]

Plasticity: In an individual or a population, the capacity for adaptation: a) through gene changes (genetic plasticity) or b) through internal physiological modifications in response to changes of environment (physiological plasticity). [NIH]

Polymorphism: The occurrence together of two or more distinct forms in the same population. [NIH]

Pontine: A brain region involved in the detection and processing of taste. [NIH]

Postsynaptic: Nerve potential generated by an inhibitory hyperpolarizing stimulation. [NIH]

Potentiate: A degree of synergism which causes the exposure of the organism to a harmful substance to worsen a disease already contracted. [NIH]

Potentiation: An overall effect of two drugs taken together which is greater than the sum of the effects of each drug taken alone. [NIH]

Probe: An instrument used in exploring cavities, or in the detection and dilatation of strictures, or in demonstrating the potency of channels; an elongated instrument for exploring or sounding body cavities. [NIH]

Protocol: The detailed plan for a clinical trial that states the trial's rationale, purpose, drug or vaccine dosages, length of study, routes of administration, who may participate, and other aspects of trial design. [NIH]

Race: A population within a species which exhibits general similarities within itself, but is both discontinuous and distinct from other populations of that species, though not sufficiently so as to achieve the status of a taxon. [NIH]

Reliability: Used technically, in a statistical sense, of consistency of a test with itself, i. e. the extent to which we can assume that it will yield the same result if repeated a second time. [NIH]

Reticular: Coarse-fibered, netlike dermis layer. [NIH]

Retractor: An instrument designed for pulling aside tissues to improve exposure at operation; an instrument for drawing back the edge of a wound. [NIH]

Schizophrenia: A mental disorder characterized by a special type of disintegration of the personality. [NIH]

Secretory: Secreting; relating to or influencing secretion or the secretions. [NIH]

Segmental: Describing or pertaining to a structure which is repeated in similar form in successive segments of an organism, or which is undergoing segmentation. [NIH]

Segregation: The separation in meiotic cell division of homologous chromosome pairs and their contained allelomorphic gene pairs. [NIH]

Sensor: A device designed to respond to physical stimuli such as temperature, light, magnetism or movement and transmit resulting impulses for interpretation, recording, movement, or operating control. [NIH]

Spectrometer: An apparatus for determining spectra; measures quantities such as wavelengths and relative amplitudes of components. [NIH]

Splint: A rigid appliance used for the immobilization of a part or for the correction of deformity. [NIH]

Stimulus: That which can elicit or evoke action (response) in a muscle, nerve, gland or other excitable issue, or cause an augmenting action upon any function or metabolic process. [NIH]

Stromal: Large, veil-like cell in the bone marrow. [NIH]

Superoxide: Derivative of molecular oxygen that can damage cells. [NIH]

Synapse: The region where the processes of two neurons come into close contiguity, and the nervous impulse passes from one to the other; the fibers of the two are intermeshed, but, according to the general view, there is no direct contiguity. [NIH]

Synchrony: The normal physiologic sequencing of atrial and ventricular activation and contraction. [NIH]

TATA: One sequence thought to be important for the transcription initiation in eukaryotes was found in most of the yeast genes. It is an AT-rich region with the canonical sequence TATA/AATA usually located 25-32 bp upstream from the transcription initiation site. [NIH]

Temporal: One of the two irregular bones forming part of the lateral surfaces and base of the skull, and containing the organs of hearing. [NIH]

Therapeutics: The branch of medicine which is concerned with the treatment of diseases, palliative or curative. [NIH]

Threshold: For a specified sensory modality (e. g. light, sound, vibration), the lowest level (absolute threshold) or smallest difference (difference threshold, difference limen) or intensity of the stimulus discernible in prescribed conditions of stimulation. [NIH]

Tractus: A part of some structure, usually that part along which something passes. [NIH]

Translation: The process whereby the genetic information present in the linear sequence of ribonucleotides in mRNA is converted into a corresponding sequence of amino acids in a protein. It occurs on the ribosome and is unidirectional. [NIH]

Translational: The cleavage of signal sequence that directs the passage of the protein through a cell or organelle membrane. [NIH]

Transmitter: A chemical substance which effects the passage of nerve impulses from one cell to the other at the synapse. [NIH]

Tubercle: A rounded elevation on a bone or other structure. [NIH]

Ubiquitin: A highly conserved 76 amino acid-protein found in all eukaryotic cells. [NIH]

Vitro: Descriptive of an event or enzyme reaction under experimental investigation occurring outside a living organism. Parts of an organism or microorganism are used together with artificial substrates and/or conditions. [NIH]

CHAPTER 4. PATENTS ON SLEEP APNEA

Overview

You can learn about innovations relating to sleep apnea by reading recent patents and patent applications. Patents can be physical innovations (e.g. chemicals, pharmaceuticals, medical equipment) or processes (e.g. treatments or diagnostic procedures). The United States Patent and Trademark Office defines a patent as a grant of a property right to the inventor, issued by the Patent and Trademark Office.[21] Patents, therefore, are intellectual property. For the United States, the term of a new patent is 20 years from the date when the patent application was filed. If the inventor wishes to receive economic benefits, it is likely that the invention will become commercially available to patients with sleep apnea within 20 years of the initial filing. It is important to understand, therefore, that an inventor's patent does not indicate that a product or service is or will be commercially available to patients with sleep apnea. The patent implies only that the inventor has "the right to exclude others from making, using, offering for sale, or selling" the invention in the United States. While this relates to U.S. patents, similar rules govern foreign patents.

In this chapter, we show you how to locate information on patents and their inventors. If you find a patent that is particularly interesting to you, contact the inventor or the assignee for further information.

[21] Adapted from The U. S. Patent and Trademark Office:
http://www.uspto.gov/web/offices/pac/doc/general/whatis.htm.

Patents on Sleep Apnea

By performing a patent search focusing on sleep apnea, you can obtain information such as the title of the invention, the names of the inventor(s), the assignee(s) or the company that owns or controls the patent, a short abstract that summarizes the patent, and a few excerpts from the description of the patent. The abstract of a patent tends to be more technical in nature, while the description is often written for the public. Full patent descriptions contain much more information than is presented here (e.g. claims, references, figures, diagrams, etc.). We will tell you how to obtain this information later in the chapter. The following is an example of the type of information that you can expect to obtain from a patent search on sleep apnea:

- **Active implantable medical device for treating sleep apnea syndrome by electrostimulation**

  Inventor(s): Bonnet; Jean-Luc (Monrouge, FR)

  Assignee(s): Ela Medical S.A. (Montrouge, FR)

  Patent Number: 6,574,507

  Date filed: March 6, 2000

  Abstract: An active implantable medical device for electrostimulation in response to a determined **sleep apnea syndrome,** particularly a pacemaker. This device measures the respiratory activity of the patient, using for example, a minute ventilation sensor and/or a blood oxygen saturation sensor, and analyzes the sensor signal, to determine occurrence of an apnea according to the signal delivered by the sensor. The device also delivers an increase cardiiac pacing rate in the event of detection of apnea. The device also can deliver a neurological and/or cardiac stimulation so as to apply selectively to the patient an electric stimulus. The device also determines the patients's state of activity, according to predetermined criteria, such that the increased pacing rate is provided only during a sleep phase and otherwise inhibited. The analysis can in particular detect and occurrence of successive apnea during a phase of sleep and determine the occurrence of a **sleep apnea syndrome** when the number of apnea events detected during a given period of time exceeds a predetermined threshold.

  Excerpt(s): The present invention relates to the diagnosis of the syndrome of **sleep apnea** and more particularly, cardiac pacemakers able to detect **sleep apnea** and respond to the detection with electrostimulation.... The syndrome of **sleep apnea** ("SAS"), more precisely the syndrome of obstructive and non **central sleep apnea** ("SOAS") is an affliction having generally as its origin an obstruction of the respiratory tracts. It is likely to involve a certain number of disorders such as painful and/or insufficient breathing, an abnormal heartbeat, and hypertension. Various treatments of SAS have been proposed, including treatments involving surgery, medication, and maintenance of a positive pressure in the respiratory tract by means of a facial mask worn during sleep.... One technique, as discussed in EP-A-0 702 979 (to Medtronic) proposes to treat SAS by electrostimulation. This document describes an implanted pulse generator, controlled by a sensor, which may be a dynamic pressure sensor or a sensor of intrathoracic impedance, making it possible to follow (monitor) the patient's respiration rate and thus to detect the occurrence of an apnea. When an apnea is detected, the generator delivers a salvo (sequence) of pulses to a stimulation electrode implanted in the muscles controlling the patient's airway. This technique is not, however, in practice, completely satisfactory. This is because the stimulation which is systematically started in the event of an increase in the intratracheal pressure, whatever the cause of this increase in pressure, and whether it is due to an SAS or not, will include inappropriate stimulations.

Web site: http://www.delphion.com/details?pn=US06574507__

- **Apparatus and method for providing a breathing gas employing a bi-level flow generator with an AC synchronous motor**

  Inventor(s): Campbell; James L. (Plymouth, MN), Delache; Alain J. (Nice, FR), Emerson; Paul F. (St. Louis Park, MN), Souquet; Jacques (Nice, FR)

  Assignee(s): Mallinckrodt Inc. (St. Louis, MO)

  Patent Number: 6,644,310

  Date filed: September 29, 2000

  Abstract: An apparatus and method for treating **sleep apnea** includes a bilevel flow generator having an alternating current (AC) synchronous motor coupled to a low inertia centrifugal rotor/impeller. The process of acceleration and deceleration of the rotor involves moving from frequency A, amplitude A to frequency B, amplitude B in an optimal linear fashion using the so-called Bresenham algorithm. This is coupled with a tuned increase of the amplitude during the acceleration process which will produce the acceleration using minimum current allowing the use of smaller power supplies. During deceleration the process is accomplished in reverse fashion using a tuned decrease of the amplitude coupled with a special shunt circuit to prevent power supply voltage changes. These changes in amplitude overlay a current feedback mechanism used to prevent loss of synchronization of the motor by changing amplitude. Speed changes can also be timed so as to prevent desynchronization.

Excerpt(s): The present invention relates to an apparatus and method for delivering a breathing gas to a user at alternating levels of pressure as a treatment for respiratory conditions such as **sleep apnea**... The **sleep apnea syndrome** affects some 1% to 5% of the general population and is due to upper airway obstruction during sleep. The direct consequences of **sleep apnea** are sleep fragmentation, partial cessation of ventilation and oxyhemoglobin desaturation. These in turn translate into daytime somnolence, cardiac arrhythmia, congestive heart failure and a variety of other health as well as cognitive dysfunctions. All of these have secondary social and behavioral effects which can result in increased patient morbidity as well as possible mortality if they are engaged in activities which require alertness (such as driving a car).... The causes of upper airway obstruction are varied but may include anatomical changes leading to a narrowing of the pathway, loss of muscle tone and/or increased weight of the structures. Age and obesity appear to be risk factors suggesting that an excess of soft tissue in the neck may provide sufficient pressure on internal structures to compromise the patency of the airway.

Web site: http://www.delphion.com/details?pn=US06644310__

- **Apparatus and methods for treatment of conditions including obstructive sleep apnea and snoring**

  Inventor(s): Palmisano; Richard George (8/9 Guilfoyle Ave., Double Bay, New South Wales 2028, AU)

  Assignee(s): none reported

  Patent Number: 6,536,439

  Date filed: September 30, 1997

  Abstract: Apparatus and methods for the treatment of conditions including **obstructive sleep apnea** and/or snoring resulting from excessive nasal airway resistance are disclosed. A rapid maxillary expansion device (10) is fitted to teeth (12, 14) of the upper jaw, and by operation of the jack screw (20), the maxilla is expanded such that, usually, the intermaxillary suture opens. The expansion is maintained until the maxilla stabilizes, for example by new bone growth along the suture. In this way the minimum cross-sectional area of the nasal cavity increases, reducing nasal airway resistance and curing, or at least ameliorating, **obstructive sleep apnea** and/or snoring.

Excerpt(s): This invention relates to apparatus and methods for the treatment of conditions including **obstructive sleep apnea** (OSA) and snoring. The invention is believed also to relate to the treatment of other upper respiratory conditions.... The preferred clinical treatment for OSA is Continuous Positive Airway Pressure (CPAP) which acts to alleviate the occurrence of apneas and hypopneas during sleep. CPAP is the technique of pneumatically splinting the airway open by supplying air at a pressure elevated above atmospheric pressure to the nose, or to the nose and mouth. It is not, however, a curative treatment.... Surgical techniques are also known, however they are radical treatments that have generally been disappointing as a curative.

Web site: http://www.delphion.com/details?pn=US06536439__

- **Combined cryotherapy and hyperthermia method for the treatment of airway obstruction or prostrate enlargement**

  Inventor(s): Beyar; Motti (Herzliya, IL), DeRowe; Ari (Mosahav Salit, IL)

  Assignee(s): American Medical Systems, Inc. (Minnetonka, MN)

  Patent Number: 6,378,525

  Date filed: January 29, 1998

  Abstract: A method of reducing tissue volume for treatment of airway obstruction, **obstructive sleep apnea,** snoring, prostate tumor, and other pathologies comprising: applying a cryoprobe with a diameter preferably less than about 2 mm and with a sharp tip to first freeze the affected interstitial tissue of the soft palate, base of the tongue, tonsils or adenoids, singularly or in combination, or to the prostate, or other tissue, and then applying the same cryoprobe to heat the treated tissue.

  Excerpt(s): The present invention relates to a method of reducing tissue volume by applying a unique cryoprobe. The invention is especially useful in reducing pharyngeal tissues, including tonsils and soft palate, in treating upper airway obstruction, such as exists in **obstructive sleep apnea,** and/or snoring, or in treating an enlarged prostate, and is described below with respect to such applications, but it will be appreciated that the invention could advantageously be used in other applications as well, such as, in treating abundant vascular tissue in the uterus, as found in menometrorrhagia, or in treating hypertrophic inferior turbinates in nasal obstruction.... Obstructive **Sleep Apnea** is of unknown etiology, but it is generally accepted that it results from the combination of a structurally small upper airway and a normal or abnormal loss of physiologic muscle tone during sleep. Patterns of pharyngeal narrowing and collapse suggest that 30-50% of patients with

obstructive sleep apnea have obstruction at the level of the upper pharynx or in the retropalatal segment. This can be due to abundant tissue of the palate or tonsillar hypertrophy. An even higher percentage of snorers have the soft palate as the source of the vibrations of snoring.... Obstructive **Sleep Apnea** is a potentially life threatening disorder, which affects up to 2 to 4% of the adult population. Even when not life threatening, it is annoying to a bed mate. **Obstructive Sleep Apnea** is associated with snoring, which is believed to affect 20% of adults.

Web site: http://www.delphion.com/details?pn=US06378525__

- **Continuous positive airway pressure headgear**

  Inventor(s): Jestrabek-Hart; Bernadette (Meridian, ID)

  Assignee(s): Creations by B J H, LLC (Meridian, ID)

  Patent Number: 6,470,886

  Date filed: March 23, 2000

  Abstract: The present invention is a CPAP Headgear for assisting in the treatment of **sleep apnea.** The present invention uses a standard CPAP respiratory mask with air supplied under pressure by an air blower or other source. The present invention generally includes an improved Headgear, preferably having a head cover, a Lip Strap, and Clips and/or Extenders to hold the CPAP respiratory mask in place. The head cover designed with two side portions, each encircling an ear with an open area where the ear will fit and thereby stay a distance from the ear with material that goes upwards toward the top of the head, one side separating into 2 straps that connect across the top of the head to the second side. Another strap comes from the back of the left side that encircles the ear and around the nape of the neck to the right side that encircles the right ear, up and through, and back over toward the left, connecting upon itself, thereby connecting the two headpieces together across the nape of the neck. The Lip Strap extends from both lower sides in front of the ears and is attached from one side of the Headgear to the other, and is placed below and on the lower lip cooperating to help keep the wearer's lower lip against the teeth, thereby inhibiting the escape of air from the wearer's mouth, while allowing the chin to relax, and allowing the teeth to be apart as the wearer sleeps. The Clip is a bent hook that attaches to the side strap from the headgear to the respiratory mask attachment and allows the headgear to be removed and replaced easily without losing the adjustments. The Extenders are attachments that are part of a mask or can be or a bent wire attached to an existing respiratory mask. The Extenders drop/lower the attachment where the

Headgear is to fasten to the respiratory mask to an area blow the mask. The Extenders primary function is to make the respiratory mask more comfortable to wear, and they may take the place of the Clip. The open Extender allows the Headgear to be removed and replaced easily without losing adjustments.

Excerpt(s): The present invention generally relates to medical equipment. More specifically, the present invention relates to headgear used in the treatment of **sleep apnea**... Sleep apnea is a breathing disorder characterized by brief interruptions of breathing during sleep. Certain mechanical and structural problems in the airway of a person cause the interruptions in breathing during sleep. In some people, apnea occurs when the throat muscles and tongue relax during sleep and partially block the opening of the airway. When the muscles of the soft palate at the base of the tongue and the uvula (the small fleshy tissue hanging from the center of the back of the throat) relax and sag, the airway becomes blocked, making breathing labored and noisy and even stopping it all together. **Sleep apnea** also can occur in obese people when an excess amount of tissue in the airway causes it to be narrowed. With a narrowed airway, the person continues his or her efforts to breathe, but air cannot easily flow into or out of the nose or mouth. Unknown to the person, this results in heavy snoring, periods of no breathing, and frequent arousals (causing abrupt changes from deep sleep to light sleep). Source: Facts About **Sleep Apnea,** National Institute of Health, Publication No. 95-3798, September 1995.... During the apneic event, the person is unable to breathe in oxygen and to exhale carbon dioxide, resulting in low levels of oxygen and increased levels of carbon dioxide in the blood. The reduction in oxygen and increase in carbon dioxide alert the brain to resume breathing and cause an arousal. With each arousal, a signal is sent from the brain to the upper airway muscles to open the airway; breathing is resumed, often with a loud snort or gasp. Frequent arousals, although necessary for breathing to restart, prevent the patient from getting enough restorative, deep sleep. Id.

Web site: http://www.delphion.com/details?pn=US06470886__

- **Control member for a valve and method for determining fluid flow rate through a valve**

  Inventor(s): Bullock; Denis (Ryde, AU), McAuliffe; Patrick John (Carlingford, AU), Smith; Ian Malcolm (Westleigh, AU), Wickham; Peter John Deacon (Five Dock, AU)

  Assignee(s): ResMed Limited (North Ryde, AU)

  Patent Number: 6,357,463

  Date filed: June 21, 2000

  Abstract: The present invention has been developed primarily for a flow diverting valve used in controlling the pressure and flow rate, and measuring the flow rate, of a breathable gas supplied to the airways of a patient by a breathable gas supply apparatus during, for example, nasal Continuous Positive Airway Pressure (CPAP) treatment of **Obstructive Sleep Apnea** (OSA) and ventilatory assistance treatments such as non-invasive positive pressure ventilation (NIPPV).

  Excerpt(s): The present invention relates to a control member for a valve and method for determining fluid flow rate through a valve.... The invention has been developed primarily for a flow diverting valve used in controlling the pressure and flow rate, and measuring the flow rate, of a breathable gas supplied to the airways of a patient by a breathable gas supply apparatus during, for example, nasal Continuous Positive Airway Pressure (CPAP) treatment of **Obstructive Sleep Apnea** (OSA) and ventilatory assistance treatments such as non-invasive positive pressure ventilation (NIPPV). However, it will be appreciated that the invention is not limited to these particular uses and is equally applicable to controlling and measuring the flow of any fluid (ie. gas or liquid) passing a control member of a valve.... It is also known for the level of treatment pressure to vary during a period of treatment accordance with patient need, that form of CPAP being known as automatically adjusting nasal CPAP treatment, as described in U.S. Pat. No. 5,245,995.

  Web site: http://www.delphion.com/details?pn=US06357463__

- **Dental appliance for treatment of snoring and obstructive sleep apnea**

  Inventor(s): Halstrom; Leonard Wayne (Lions Bay, CA)

  Assignee(s): Silent Knights Ventures Inc. (Vancouver, CA)

  Patent Number: 6,729,335

  Date filed: March 27, 2000

Abstract: A dentally retained intra-oral appliance worn at night for treatment of snoring and **obstructive sleep apnea.** The appliance maintains the patient's mandible in an anterior, protruded position to prevent obstruction of the pharyngeal airway. The appliance allows a limited degree of lateral movement of the mandible relative to the upper jaw in the protruded position to prevent aggravation of the patient's tempromandibular joint and associated muscles and ligaments. The appliance preferably consists of an upper bite block conforming to the patient's maxillary dentition, a lower bite block conforming to the patient's mandibular dentition, and a connecting assembly secured to an anterior region of the upper and lower bite blocks for adjustably coupling the upper and lower bite blocks together.

Excerpt(s): This application relates to a dentally retained intra-oral appliance worn at night for treatment of snoring and **obstructive sleep apnea.** The appliance maintains the patient's mandible in an anterior, protruded position to prevent obstruction of the pharyngeal airway. The appliance allows a limited degree of lateral movement of the mandible relative to the upper jaw in the protruded position to prevent aggravation of the tempromandibular joint and associated muscles and ligaments.... Snoring and **obstructive sleep apnea** are typically caused by complete or partial obstruction of an individual's pharyngeal airway during sleep. Usually airway obstruction results from the apposition of the rear portion of the tongue or soft palate with the posterior pharyngeal wall. **Obstructive sleep apnea** is a potentially lethal disorder in which breathing stops during sleep for 10 seconds or more, sometimes up to 300 times per night. Snoring occurs when the pharyngeal airway is partially obstructed, resulting in vibration of the oral tissues during respiration. These sleep disorders tend to become more severe as patients grow older, likely due to a progressive loss of muscle tone in the patient's throat and oral tissues.... Habitual snoring and **sleep apnea** have been associated with other potentially serious medical conditions, such as hypertension, ischemic heart disease and strokes. Accordingly, early diagnosis and treatment is recommended. One surgical approach, known as uvulopalatopharyngoplasty, involves removal of a portion of the soft palate to prevent closure of the pharyngeal airway during sleep. However, this operation is not always effective and may result in undesirable complications, such as nasal regurgitation.

Web site: http://www.delphion.com/details?pn=US06729335__

- **ECG derived respiratory rhythms for improved diagnosis of sleep apnea**

  Inventor(s): Bebehani; Khosrow (Arlington, TX), Burk; John R. (Aledo, TX), Lucas; Edgar A. (Fort Worth, TX)

  Assignee(s): Board of Regents the University of Texas System (Arlington, TX)

  Patent Number: 6,415,174

  Date filed: November 5, 1999

  Abstract: Respiratory rhythms of a subject are derived from measured ECG signals utilizing leads placed for significant influence of chest movement on the ECG signals. The QRS pulses within ECG signals measured in two substantially orthogonal planes are located by applying a sequence of filters. The knot and period of the QRS pulses are then determined, with adjustments made during a learning phase of data sampling. The QRS pulse areas in both planes is then calculated. These pulse areas are employed to determine the angle of orientation of the depolarization wave's mean electrical axis (MEA) at the QRS pulse locations. Cubic spline interpolation of the data points for the MEA angle provides a smooth breathing curve, which may be scored for sleep disordered breathing events. The ECG-derived respiratory (EDR) signal may be employed in lieu of airflow measurements where such measurements are not available, or may be employed in conjunction with airflow measurements and/or measured cardiac activity data to discriminate between arrhythmias associated with disordered breathing versus those associated with cardiac malfunction, reducing misdiagnosis. The additional processing of ECG data required for derivation of respiratory rhythms may be easily automated and implemented at nominal incremental cost per unit.

  Excerpt(s): The present invention relates generally to diagnosis of sleep disordered breathing and in particular to diagnosis of sleep disordered breathing utilizing electrocardiographic measurements. Still more particularly, the present invention relates to derivation of respiratory data from electrocardiographic measurements for determining either the presence of sleep disordered breathing causing or aggravating cardiac symptoms or the absence of sleep disordered breathing influence on cardiac symptoms due to cardiac pathology.... Sleep disordered breathing is a significant problem for a large portion of the population. **Sleep apnea,** an intrinsic dyssomnia involving cessation of breathing during sleep and resulting in complete or partial arousal from sleep, is one of the most prevalent forms of sleep disordered breathing. Symptoms of the disorder include daytime sleepiness, fatigue or tiredness, and irritability, which may seriously impair the performance of the individual.... Sleep apnea is typically defined as the cessation of air exchange (breathing) from the nostrils or mouth lasting at least 10 seconds. Partial or complete arousal from sleep is considered a defensive mechanism most likely stimulated by rising carbon dioxide levels in the blood during the apneic event to reestablish ventilation and prevent death in the sleeping subject. Three established categorized of **sleep apnea** include: **obstructive sleep apnea,** obstruction of the upper airway; **central sleep apnea,** cessation of ventilatory effort; and mixed apnea, a combination of both upper airway obstruction and cessation of ventilatory effort.

Web site: http://www.delphion.com/details?pn=US06415174__

- **Electrode and method for measuring muscle activity in the pharyngeal airways**

  Inventor(s): Lindenthaler; Werner (Oberperfuss, AT)

  Assignee(s): MED-EL. Elektromedizinische Gerate Ges.m.b.H. (Innsbruck, AT)

  Patent Number: 6,361,494

  Date filed: May 18, 1999

  Abstract: An electrode for placement in a human mouth for the measurement of muscle activity in the pharyngeal airway. The electrode includes at least one leg extending from a planer face so as to make electrical contact with the genioglossus muscle. The electrode permits a reduction in the number of patients requiring overnight polysomnography to prediagnose people with **sleep apnea.**

  Excerpt(s): The present invention relates to an electrode and method for measuring muscle activity in the pharyngeal airways and, in particular, to diagnosing **sleep apnea** in wakeful patients.... An estimated 2% to 4% of the population are believed to suffer from **sleep apnea syndrome.**. **Sleep apnea** is a condition that results from a reduction in air intake through the air passage of sleeping individuals. This problem arises as a result of weak muscle tone in the throat and although compensated for during waking hours, gives rise to symptoms of fatigue during the day, poor quality sleep at night, and heavy snoring during sleep. Diagnosis of **sleep apnea** has been carried out in sleep laboratories where the patient is monitored at night during sleep in a process called nocturnal polysomnography. This diagnostic test is expensive, time consuming, and must be administered by highly trained technicians. Consequently, availability of the test is limited.... The monitoring of **sleep apnea** traditionally took the form of electromyographic (EMG) analyses of the genioglossus muscle. The analysis relied on intramuscular electrode recordings which were made by inserting a needle or wire electrode into the body of the muscle just below the teeth. With the needle electrodes it is not possible to make quantative comparisons to the EMG recordings if the electrode is moved or replaced because the tip of the needle cannot be placed at exactly the same position within the muscle. Consequently, the needle electrodes measure activities from different anatomical and architectural organizations and different fiber types.

Web site: http://www.delphion.com/details?pn=US06361494__

- **Flow diverter for controlling the pressure and flow rate in a CPAP device**

  Inventor(s): Bullock; Denis L. (Milton, AU), McAuliffe; Patrick J. (Carlingford, AU)

  Assignee(s): ResMed Limited (North Ryde, AU)

  Patent Number: 6,745,770

  Date filed: January 8, 2002

  Abstract: A flow diverter valve is used in controlling the pressure and/or flow rate of a breathable gas supplied to the airways of a patient by a breathable gas flow generator supply apparatus during, for example, ventilatory assistance treatments such as non-invasive positive pressure ventilation and nasal Continuous Positive Airway Pressure (CPAP) treatment of **Obstructive Sleep Apnea.** The flow diverter valve includes a vane and a housing. The housing has an inlet port, an outlet port, and an exhaust port. The exhaust port opens to atmosphere, and the inlet port is in fluid communication with the flow generator. The outlet port is in fluid communication with a patient mask via a conduit. The vane is configured with respect to the housing such that a blower associated with the CPAP apparatus remains substantially unchoked, regardless of whether the vane is in the open or closed position.

  Excerpt(s): The present invention relates to a ventilatory assistance apparatus, and in particular, a ventilatory assistance apparatus including a flow diverter valve in fluid communication with a flow generator.... Non-Invasive Positive Pressure Ventilation (NIPPV) is a form of treatment for breathing disorders which can involve a relatively higher pressure of air or other breathable gas being provided to the entrance of a patient's airways via a patient mask during the inspiratory phase of respiration, and a relatively lower pressure or atmospheric pressure being provided in the patient mask during the expiratory phase of respiration. In other NIPPV modes the pressure can be made to vary in a complex manner throughout the respiratory cycle. For example, the pressure at the mask during inspiration or expiration can be varied through the period of treatment.... Continuous Positive Airway Pressure (CPAP) treatment is commonly used to treat breathing disorders including **Obstructive Sleep Apnea** (OSA). CPAP treatment continuously provides pressurized air or other breathable gas to the entrance of a patient's airways via a patient mask at a pressure elevated above atmospheric pressure, typically in the range 3-20 cm H.sub.2 O. CPAP treatment can act as a pneumatic splint of a patient's upper airway.

Web site: http://www.delphion.com/details?pn=US06745770__

- **Garment with pouch for medical monitor**

  Inventor(s): Adlard; Terry K. (164 Borad St. South, Monmouth, OR 97361), Edwards; Patricia A. (640 "J" St., Springfield, OR 97477)

  Assignee(s): none reported

  Patent Number: 6,681,404

  Date filed: March 25, 2003

  Abstract: Patients are sometimes required to carry various medical appliances such as cardiac, gastric, or **sleep apnea** monitors, or medication injectors (either infusion pumps or other intravenous injectors). To carry these devices comfortably, a garment is worn having a pouch and shoulder straps. The pouch can be worn on the chest or back of the patient. The shoulder straps extend over the shoulders and are affixed to secure the garment to the wearer. In one embodiment, the ends of the straps are attached to a region near the bottom of the pouch. In a second embodiment, a back strap is passed around the patient's lower torso and the ends affixed to a region near the bottom of the pouch, and the shoulder straps affixed to the back strap.

  Excerpt(s): Not applicable.

  Web site: http://www.delphion.com/details?pn=US06681404__

- **Integrated sleep apnea screening system**

  Inventor(s): Hadas; Noam (Tel Aviv, IL)

  Assignee(s): S.L.P. Ltd. (Tel Aviv, IR)

  Patent Number: 6,368,287

  Date filed: June 14, 2000

Abstract: This invention is a method, and device, suitable for use without professional medical supervision, for screening for **sleep apnea.** All elements of the device are housed in a small, flexible, plastic housing which is placed on the user's philtrum. A thermistor acquires data describing the respiratory pattern. A processor analyzes the respiratory pattern in real time and outputs a study result, describing the occurrence of any episodes of apnea, to a non-volatile colored marker on the plastic housing. A flashing LED display informs the user when placement of the device is appropriate. A lithium battery, which powers all elements of the device, is activated by a pull-tab removed by the user.

Excerpt(s): The present invention relates to medical monitoring devices and, in particular, it relates to a monitor for the detection of **sleep apnea**... It is known that sleep related breathing disorders are a common medical problem. Two common sleep pathology syndromes are **Obstructive Sleep Apnea** (OSA) and **Central Sleep Apnea** (CSA).... Obstructive **Sleep Apnea** (OSA) occurs when the upper airway (the nose, mouth or throat) become obstructed in some way during sleep, and is usually accompanied by a decrease in the oxygen saturation of the blood (SpO.sub.2). Snoring indicates an intermittent obstruction, which at times may become complete, stopping air flow. Apnea (the cessation of breathing) may occur hundreds of times during one night of sleep, leading to severe sleep disruption and excessive daytime somnolence. As such, the patient may easily fall asleep during working hours, such as when the patient is driving a car or a truck. Many commercial trucking firms thus require that their drivers undergo sleep studies to determine if they suffer from OSA. Furthermore, OSA may cause heart problems such as cardiac arrhythmias and Cor Pulmonale.

Web site: http://www.delphion.com/details?pn=US06368287__

- **Medical equipment warning device**

Inventor(s): Most, Jr.; Clark (1909 S. Badour Rd., Midland, MI 48640)

Assignee(s): none reported

Patent Number: 6,392,555

Date filed: November 16, 1999

Abstract: The medical equipment warning device is employed in combination with a power operated medical treatment machine such as a **sleep apnea** treatment machine. The warning device includes a DC relay with contacts that are open when the relay is connected to an AC source. A signal generator is connected to a battery by the DC relay when the AC source is interrupted and contacts close the DC circuit. The signal generator produces an audible, visual or physical signal that warns a person that the AC power source has failed. Restoration of the AC power source activates the DC relay and opens the DC circuit thereby deactivating the signal generator.

Excerpt(s): This invention relates to a medical equipment warning device and more particularly to a warning device that provides an audible warning if a medical device such as a **sleep apnea** treatment device fails or the devices power source fails.... Sleep apnea is a transient cessation of respiration while a person is sleeping. The symptoms are varied and the cause of **sleep apnea** is unknown. Some individuals with **sleep apnea** may merely snore. Others reduce air intake and the oxygen level in their hemoglobin decreases. A reduction in hemoglobin oxygen level may be fatal if it is not corrected quickly.... Apnea is associated with restriction of the upper passages of the human respiratory system. The methodology for treating **sleep apnea** is to supply air to the respiratory system under pressure. The air under pressure tends to expand the air passages and thereby increase the flow of oxygen to the lungs. The air under pressure may be supplied by elaborate machines in a hospital for treatment of **sleep apnea.** The air under pressure may also be supplied to some individuals in their homes any time they sleep. The machines used in hospitals may supply air during inspiration at one pressure and during expiration at a lower pressure. These machines have central processing units that sense air flow rates, leakage, pressure, humidity and vibrations due to snoring. The measurements sensed may be recorded in the central processing unit. Some processing units make appropriate adjustments in air flow and pressure after each breath. The recorded measurements and the adjustments help doctors determine future treatment. These elaborate machines are relatively expensive. Individuals that require pressurized air when sleeping use less elaborate machines. Such machines are much less expensive. However, they are modified as required to meet the requirements of each individual with **sleep apnea** that requires such a machine. Some individuals for example, cannot tolerate pressurized air during expiration. Such individuals require a machine that supplies air at a lower pressure during expiration.

Web site: http://www.delphion.com/details?pn=US06392555__

- **Method and apparatus for closed-loop stimulation of the hypoglossal nerve in human patients to treat obstructive sleep apnea**

  Inventor(s): Durand; Dominique (36765 Valley Forge Dr., Solon, OH 44122), Haxhiu; Musa A. (3683 Meadowbrook Blvd., University Heights, OH 44118), Sahin; Mesut (711 S. Vienna, Ruston, LA 71270)

  Assignee(s): none reported

  Patent Number: 6,587,725

  Date filed: March 26, 2001

  Abstract: This invention is a fully implanted functional electrical stimulator (20) apparatus, a method for treatment of **obstructive sleep apnea** that provides for both reliable detection/prediction or airway occlusion that relieves, and/or prevents same by selective, direct electrical stimulation of the hypoglossal nerve (HG). The method, and apparatus sense hypoglossal nerve electro-neurogram activity for purposes of detecting or predicting **obstructive sleep apnea.** The sensed hypoglossal nerve activity, itself, is used to trigger functional electrical stimulation of the hypoglossal nerve in order to improve upper airway patency. Further, an improved hypoglossal nerve stimulation electrode (10) interface (IC) is provided that allows for simultaneous hypoglossal nerve activity sensing, and stimulation by eliminating stimulation artifacts that would otherwise trigger further erroneous stimulation.

  Excerpt(s): The present invention relates generally to the functional electrical stimulation (FES) arts. More particularly, the present invention relates to a method and apparatus for sensing hypoglossal nerve activity in human patients to detect **obstructive sleep apnea,** and using the sensed hypoglossal nerve activity to trigger selective functional electrical stimulation of the hypoglossal nerve, itself, for purposes of improving upper airway patency and, thus, treating **obstructive sleep apnea.** Further, the present invention relates to an improved hypoglossal nerve stimulation electrode interface that allows for simultaneous hypoglossal nerve activity sensing and nerve stimulation by eliminating stimulation artifacts that would otherwise trigger further, erroneous stimulation.... Obstructive **sleep apnea** (OSA) is the recurrent occlusion of the upper airways of human patients during sleep. In these patients, the upper airways obstruct as often as several times a minute with each episode lasting as long as 20-30 seconds. Each apneic episode ends with a brief arousal from sleep. Consequently, arterial oxyhemoglobin saturation decreases drastically. Complications include excessive daytime sleepiness, restless sleep, morning headache, job-related accidents, impaired short-term memory, polycythema, hypertension, right-sided congestive heart failure, decreased libido, and the like. Personality disorder and other psychological problems may also develop over time. **Obstructive sleep apnea** is found in 2 to 4 percent of the population, primarily in adult men and post-menopausal women.... In humans, the hypoglossal nerve innervates the intrinsic and extrinsic muscles of the tongue and the geniohyoid muscle. Of these muscles innervated by the hypoglossal nerve, the genioglossus and the geniohyoid muscles are the primary muscles involved in dilating the upper airways (UAWS). Contraction of the genioglossus muscle provides tongue protrusion and, hence, dilates the airways.

Web site: http://www.delphion.com/details?pn=US06587725__

- **Method and apparatus for diagnosing sleep breathing disorders while a patient in awake**

  Inventor(s): Katz; Richard A. (East Lyme, CT), Lawee; Michael S. (Marblehead, MA), Newman; Anthony Kiefer (Woburn, MA)

  Assignee(s): The United States of America as represented by the Secretary of the Navy (Washington, DC)

  Patent Number: 6,580,944

  Date filed: November 28, 2000

  Abstract: An apparatus and method for identifying the timing of the onset of and duration of an event characteristic of sleep breathing disorder while a patient is awake. Chaotic processing techniques analyze data concerning a cardio-respiratory function, such as nasal air flow. Excursions of the resulting signal beyond a threshold provide markers for delivering the average repetition rate for such events that is useful in the diagnosis of obstructed **sleep apnea** and other respiratory dysfunctions.

  Excerpt(s): The invention described herein may be manufactured and used by or for the Government of the United States of America for governmental purposes without the payment of any royalties thereon or therefor.... This invention is generally related to methods and apparatus for performing medical diagnoses and particularly to a method and apparatus for enabling the diagnosis of sleep breathing disorders or other physiological respiratory dysfunction while the patient is awake.... Sleep breathing disorders and other physiological respiratory dysfunctions in humans constitute an area requiring diagnosis. One such area is called **obstructive sleep apnea** or sleep disorder breathing. Within the pediatric, infant and newborn population the incidence of apparent life threatening events, sudden infant death syndrome and sleep disorder breathing have all been well documented. **Sleep apnea** also affects over 25% of apparently healthy adults age 55 and older. **Sleep apnea** contributes to daytime fatigue, increased work place accidents and a number of cardiovascular disorders. The need for a relatively easily implemented procedure exists to provide efficient methods and procedures for diagnosing these various physiological respiratory dysfunctions.

Web site: http://www.delphion.com/details?pn=US06580944__

- **Method and apparatus for providing variable positive airway pressure**

  Inventor(s): Hill; Peter D. (Monroeville, PA)

  Assignee(s): Respironics, Inc. (Murrysville, PA)

  Patent Number: 6,752,151

  Date filed: September 20, 2001

  Abstract: A method and apparatus for treating a breathing disorder and, more particularly, a method and apparatus for providing a pressurized air flow to an airway of a patient to treat congestive heart failure in combination with Cheyne-Stokes respiration and/or **sleep apnea** or other breathing disorders. A positive airway pressure ventilator is utilized in combination with an algorithm that adjusts IPAP and EPAP in order to counter a Cheyne-Stokes breathing pattern. Cheyne-Stokes respiration is detected by monitoring a peak flow of the patient.

  Excerpt(s): The present invention relates generally to a method and apparatus for providing a positive pressure therapy particularly suited treat a patient suffering from congestive heart failure, and, more particularly, to a method and apparatus for providing a pressurized flow of breathing gas to an airway of a patient to treat Cheyne-Stokes respiration, **sleep apnea,** or other breathing disorders commonly associated with congestive heart failure.... Relatively recent developments in the treatment of **sleep apnea** includes the use of continuous positive airway pressure (CPAP), which is the application of a constant pressure to the airway of a patient. This type of positive airway pressure therapy has been applied not only to the treatment of breathing disorders, but also to the treatment of CHF. In using CPAP on a CHF patient, the effect of the CPAP is to raise the pressure in the chest cavity surrounding the heart, which allows cardiac output to increase.... Bi-level positive airway pressure therapy is a form of positive airway pressure therapy that has been advanced in the treatment of **sleep apnea** and other breathing and cardiac disorders. In a bi-level pressure support therapy, pressure is applied to the airway of a patient alternately at relatively higher and lower pressure levels so that the therapeutic pressure is alternately administered at a larger and smaller magnitude force. The higher and lower magnitude positive prescription pressure levels are known as IPAP (inspiratory positive airway pressure) and EPAP (expiratory positive airway pressure), and are synchronized with the patient's inspiratory cycle and expiratory cycle, respectively.

Web site: http://www.delphion.com/details?pn=US06752151__

- **Method and apparatus useful in the diagnosis of obstructive sleep apnea of a patient**

  Inventor(s): Lynch; Christopher (North Ryde, AU), Sullivan; Colin Edward (Sydney, AU)

  Assignee(s): ResMed Limited (North Ryde, AU)

  Patent Number: 6,635,021

  Date filed: September 19, 1997

  Abstract: Patients may operate a CPAP system to deliver appropriate airway pressure at their home. A patient's apnea problem can be diagnosed at home without supervision with a CPAP device which delivers a continuously minimum appropriate pressure for substantially the entire period of therapy.

  Excerpt(s): The present invention relates to the diagnosis and treatment of partial or complete upper airway occlusion, a condition where the upper airway collapses, particularly under the reduced pressure generated by inhalation. This is most likely to happen during unconsciousness, sleep or anaesthesia.... A particular application of the present invention is to the diagnosis and/or treatment of snoring and **sleep apnea. Sleep apnea** is characterized by complete occlusion of the upper airway passage during sleep while snoring is characterized by partial occlusion. **Obstructive sleep apnea** sufferers repeatedly choke on their tongue and soft palate throughout an entire sleep period resulting in lowered arterial blood oxygen levels and poor quality of sleep. It should be realized that although the following specification discusses **sleep apnea** in detail, the present invention also applies to the diagnosis and treatment of other forms of upper airway disorders.... Reference to international patent publication WO 82/03548 will show that the application of continuous positive airway pressure (CPAP) has been used as a means of treating the occurrence of **obstructive sleep apnea.** The patient is connected to a positive pressure air supply by means of a nose mask or nasal prongs. The air supply breathed by the patient, is at all times, at slightly greater than atmospheric pressure. For example, gauge pressures will typically be within the range of 2 cm to 25 cm. It has been found that the application of continuous positive airway pressure provides what can be described as a "pneumatic splint", supporting and stabilizing the upper airway and thus eliminating the occurrence of upper airway occlusions. It is effective in eliminating both snoring and **obstructive sleep apnea** and in many cases, is effective in treating central and mixed apnea.

Web site: http://www.delphion.com/details?pn=US06635021__

- **Method and combination for treating sleep apnea using a cantilever mask attachment device**

  Inventor(s): Bloom; Nicole Denise (San Francisco, CA), Bordewick; Steven S. (Shoreview, MN), Hansen; Gary L. (Eden Prairie, MN)

  Assignee(s): Mallinckrodt, Inc. (St. Louis, MO)

  Patent Number: 6,516,802

  Date filed: May 2, 2001

  Abstract: A continuous positive airway pressure (CPAP) system in combination with a device for positioning a breathing apparatus over a breathing orifice in the head of a person, the person having an occipital lobe and an axis of symmetry, the device including an occipital anchor for anchoring against the head of the person beneath the occipital lobe of the person. The device further including a forward anchor for anchoring against a forward portion of the person's head. A spring connector connects the forward anchor and the occipital anchor, and biases the occipital anchor against the head of the person beneath the occipital lobe and the forward anchor against the corresponding portion of the person's head so as to attach the device to the person's head. The occipital anchor, the forward anchor and the spring connector are substantially aligned along the axis of symmetry of the person's head. The mount is connected to the spring connector for mounting the apparatus so as to locate the apparatus over the orifice.

  Excerpt(s): The present invention relates to the field of devices and methods for holding breathing devices and the like in place on a person's head.... Breathing devices, such as masks and the like, typically are held in place on a person's face by a harness including one or more straps extending around the person's head and along the side of the person's face.... Known devices have a variety of drawbacks. If the strap system is complex, it may not be obvious to the prospective wearer how to properly use the system, and elderly patients may struggle with putting on a mask when help is not present.

  Web site: http://www.delphion.com/details?pn=US06516802__

- **Method of treating obstructive sleep apnea using implantable electrodes**

  Inventor(s): Loeb; Gerald E. (South Pasadena, CA), Richmond; Frances J. R. (South Pasadena, CA)

  Assignee(s): Advanced Bionics Corporation (Sylmar, CA)

  Patent Number: 6,345,202

  Date filed: March 20, 2001

  Abstract: Electrodes are implanted at strategic locations within a patient and are then controlled in a manner so as to stimulate muscle and nerve tissue in a constructive manner which helps open blocked airways. In a preferred method, at least one microstimulator treats **sleep apnea** in an open loop fashion by providing electrical stimulation pulses in a rhythm or cycle having a period corresponding approximately to the natural respiratory rhythm of the patient. Such open loop stimulation entrains the patient's respiratory rate to follow the pattern set by the microstimulator so that stimulation is applied to open the airway during a period of inspiration by the patient.

  Excerpt(s): The present invention relates to a system and method for treating **sleep apnea,** and more particularly to a system and method for treatment of **obstructive sleep apnea** using implantable microstimulators.... Unfortunately, the muscles that control the airway and the nerves that supply them are, for the most part, located deep in the neck and oropharynx, adjacent to many vital and delicate structures. The present invention describes an approach in which very small electronic devices can be implanted with minimal surgical intervention in order to control these muscles to prevent or interrupt **sleep apnea** without disturbing the sleeping patient.... Obstructive **sleep apnea** (OSA) is characterized by frequent periods of airway occlusion during sleep, with concomitant obstruction of inspiratory airflow, drop in blood oxygen and interruption of sleep when the patient awakes to use voluntary muscle contraction to open the airway and take a few deep breaths. The mechanical locations and structural causes of obstruction are multiple. The most frequent mechanisms include settling of the tongue, uvula, soft palate or other tissues against the airway during the negative pressure associated with inspiration. This may be related to adipose tissue accumulation, lack of muscle tone or inadequate central respiratory drive to the tongue and/or other accessory respiratory muscles around the oropharyngeal airway.

  Web site: http://www.delphion.com/details?pn=US06345202__

- **Monitoring the occurrence of apneic and hypopneic arousals**

  Inventor(s): Brydon; John William Ernest (Waverton, AU), Colla; Gregory Alan (North Sydney, AU)

  Assignee(s): ResMed Limited (North Ryde, AU)

  Patent Number: 6,363,270

  Date filed: December 16, 1999

  Abstract: The occurrence of an arousal in a patient associated with an apneic or hypopneic episode car be determined. Sensors are placed on a patient to obtain signals representative of at least two physiological variables, for example skin conductance, heart rate and blood oxygen concentration. The signals are conditioned by conditioning circuitry, then processed by a processor to correlate at least two thereof. A coincident change in at least two of the processed signals is indicative of the occurrence of an arousal, that in turn indicates an apneic or hypopneic episode has occurred. A patient thus can be diagnosed as suffering conditions such as **obstructive sleep apnea.**

  Excerpt(s): This invention relates to methods and apparatus for the determination or monitoring of arousals that are indicative of an apneic or hypopneic episode. An "A/H episode", as used hereafter, is to be understood as including both obstructive apneas (lack of breathing) or hypopneas (reduction in breathing) occurring during sleep.... People suffering from **Obstructive Sleep Apnea** (OSA) and related conditions experience many A/H episodes during sleep. The conventional treatment for OSA is the well known Continuous Positive Airway Pressure (CPAP) treatment. An A/H episode often has an associated arousal, which is a nervous system response to low blood oxygen level and/or high blood carbon dioxide level.... The condition of OSA normally is diagnosed by laboratory based polysomnography (PSG). PSG involves the measurement of sleep and respiratory variables including EEG, EOG, chin EMG, ECG, respiratory activity, nasal airflow, chest and abdominal movements, abdominal effort and oxygen saturation. The data gathered leads to a calculation of the Respiratory Disturbance Index (RDI) which is the average number of arousals per hour due to respiratory disturbance. PSG is uncomfortable for a patient due to the placement of numerous electrodes on the patient's head or face and the wearing of a mask or nasal prongs. PSG is an expensive procedure and has the inconvenience of requiring the patient to attend a sleep clinic for a whole night requiring continuous technician attendance.

  Web site: http://www.delphion.com/details?pn=US06363270__

- **Oral orthesis to reduce snoring and sleep apnea symptoms**

  Inventor(s): Tielemans; W. M. J. (Maaseik, BE)

  Assignee(s): TNV Research and Development (NL)

  Patent Number: 6,408,852

  Date filed: January 11, 2001

  Abstract: An oral orthesis for reduction of snoring and **sleep apnea** symptoms.

  Excerpt(s): The invention relates to an oral orthesis for reducing snoring and **sleep apnea** symptoms comprising a maxilla pallatum plate (1) and, attached thereon, fixing means (2) to fix the plate in the oral cavity and a tongue positioning device (3). Snoring results from the blocking of the airway by the tongue causing the vibrations when air is passed through. In serious occasions, the blocking can cause a temporary lack of oxygen supply to the brain and unconsciousness which may be life threatening.... The disadvantage of the known oral orthesis is that it does not sufficiently prevent the blocking of the airway in all circumstances. The object of the present invention therefor is to provide an improved oral orthesis that better prevents snoring and **sleep apnea**... This object is achieved, according to the invention, in that the plate 1 extents to cover and support also the soft tissue (1b) of the palate moll.

  Web site: http://www.delphion.com/details?pn=US06408852__

- **Sleep apnea avoidance process and apparatus**

  Inventor(s): Zuberi; Najeeb (391 Augustine Ct., Oviedo, FL 32765)

  Assignee(s): none reported

  Patent Number: 6,671,907

  Date filed: April 15, 2003

  Abstract: A **sleep apnea** avoidance process includes selecting a pillow having a pair of sides, angled at a predetermined angle and shaped to hold a person's head face down on one side thereof. The selected pillow has a pair of arm openings thereunder to position a person's arm to assist in holding a person's head face down on the pillow angle side such that the user can use one or the other arms when placing the head on one or the other angled side of the pillow. The process includes resting on one of the pillow's angled sides with one arm placed through the arm opening whereby jaw movement and **sleep apnea** are avoided.

Excerpt(s): The present invention relates to a **sleep apnea** avoidance process and apparatus and especially to a **sleep apnea** avoidance process utilizing a pillow shaped to hold the face of a person resting on the pillow facing downwards at a predetermined angle.... There are several types of **sleep apnea** but in each type people with untreated **sleep apnea** stop breathing repeatedly during their sleep. In **sleep apnea,** a person's brain will briefly arouse the person from sleep in order for them to resume breathing. This results in a fragmented and poor quality sleep. An untreated **sleep apnea** can cause cardiovascular disease, memory problems, weight gain, stroke, headaches and high blood pressure. **Sleep apnea** is very common in the U.S. and can occur at any age but special risk factors include being male, overweight, and over forty years old.... In the past, there have been a great variety of pillow shapes for positioning a person's head in a predetermined position for a variety of reasons. The U.S. Patent to Shaffer No. 6,128,797 is for a face down tanning and massage pad made of an inflatable plastic or rubber material or solid foam material with a center opening and ventilation for holding a person's head in a downward position. The Armstrong U.S. Pat. No. 4,118,813 is a sleep training pillow for the prevention of snoring and is designed to train a person to sleep in a position which prevents snoring. The pillow has a pillow support surface and a face support surface. The face support surface is inclined downward from a high end to a low end and a relief cavity is cut out near the low end of the pillow. In the Tommaney U.S. Pat. No. 5,579,551, an arched shape pillow apparatus is provided with an ear accommodation. In the Hartunian U.S. Pat. No. 5,269,035, a head support for a person lying in a prone position is provided which supports the patient's head at the chin and forehead and includes a side opening for an anesthetist to view a patient's face for passage of an endotracheal or other tube used during surgery. The Treace U.S. Pat. No. 3,694,831 shows a medical head support for a variety of uses in hospitals. The pillow has two inwardly angled portions along with a cutout and a hole to position the head facing upward or downward or to one side. A variety of U.S. design patents include many different shaped pillows, many with angled sides including the Larsen patent No. D215,536 for a Pillow and the Winston patent No. D236,062 for a Face Pillow and the Righini patent No. D282,803 for a Head Rest. Other U.S. design patents include the McDonald D340,380 for a Pillow for Separating Knees and the Pierce et al. design patent D343,754 for a Pyramid Shaped Pillow Set and the Marrone, II et al. design patent D414,974 for a Face Down Cushion. Other U.S. design patents include the Blackhurst patent No. D441,823 for a Practice Platform and the Miller U.S. Patent D442,006 for an Assembly of Pregnancy Support Pillows.

Web site: http://www.delphion.com/details?pn=US06671907__

- **Sleep apnea detection system and method**

  Inventor(s): Greene; Leonard M. (White Plains, NY)

  Assignee(s): Safe Flight Instrument Corporation (White Plains, NY)

  Patent Number: 6,454,724

  Date filed: October 25, 2000

  Abstract: An apnea monitor and alarm for monitoring the breathing of an individual and for sounding an alarm in response to an interruption in the cyclical rhythm of breathing is disclosed. The monitor and alarm includes a respiration detector, an alarm and a signal processor and analyzer. The signal processor and analyzer is programmed to arm the alarm after a preselected time of cyclical breathing. The signal processor and analyzer is also programmed to sense an interruption in the breathing cycle and to actuate the alarm after a preselected period of interrupted breathing. The monitor and alarm may also include a deactivation system that recycles the program back to an initial part of the program so that the alarm is once again armed after a preselected time of continuous breathing.

  Excerpt(s): The invention relates to a **sleep apnea** detection system and method for detecting apnea and respiratory arrest and more particularly to systems wherein a detector is used in conjunction with an alarm to wake an individual or to summon help to restore a normal an breathing cycle.... Breathing is normally characterized by a regular rhythm of inhaling and exhaling. However, in many individuals apnea or cessation of respiratory airflow causes an interruption in the breathing cycle which can be hazardous to an individual's health. At times such interruption may result in a complete arrest of breathing.... Apnea may be caused by a number of different mechanisms including obstructive episodes in upper airway, by neurologic or disease-medicated lack of diaphragmatic motion, and by a combination of these factors. Some individuals are particularly vulnerable to apnea after general anesthesia. Others receiving epidural narcotics and local anesthetics are at an increased risk of apnea and respiratory arrest.

  Web site: http://www.delphion.com/details?pn=US06454724__

- **Snore and teeth grinding prevention and treatment**

  Inventor(s): Pivovarov; Alexander R. (10189 W. Sample Rd., Coral Springs, FL 33065)

  Assignee(s): none reported

  Patent Number: 6,675,804

  Date filed: April 28, 2003

  Abstract: An apparatus adapted for partial insertion within the user's mouth for preventing snoring, teeth grinding, and light forms of **sleep apnea** is disclosed. The apparatus includes a multi-lobed tongue receiving structure, an undulating connector for connecting the multi-lobed structure to an inner lip plate, a hollow tube connecting the lip plate to a dome-shaped structure formed on an outer shield. The device is inserted within the oral cavity of the user in an operative configuration such that movement of the tongue is restrained within the multi-lobed structure, and the teeth clamp down upon the undulating connector with the lip plate positioned between the teeth and the inner portions of the upper and lower lips. As a result of proper application of the apparatus breathing at night is normalized, while snoring, grinding of the teeth, and apnea are prevented.

  Excerpt(s): A portion of the disclosure of this patent document contains material that is subject to copyright protection. The copyright owner has no objection to the facsimile reproduction by anyone of the patent document or patent disclosure as it appears in the Patent and Trademark Office patent file or records, but otherwise reserves all copyrights.... The present invention relates to devices for preventing snoring, teeth grinding, and light forms of **sleep apnea,** and more particularly, to mouth piece for personal use for the treatment and prevention of uncomplicated snoring, light forms of obstructive apnea syndrome, and grinding of the teeth during sleep.... Snoring is caused by vibration of the uvula or the soft palate in the interior of the mouth when a person breathes through his/her mouth while sleeping. The act of snoring results in an irritating sound capable of disturbing sleep patterns of many, including the person snoring. In addition to the irritating snoring sound, many consider mouth breathing to be unhealthy as it contributes to dry mouth syndrome, as well as contributing to the development of gum disease.

  Web site: http://www.delphion.com/details?pn=US06675804__

- **System and method for detecting the onset of an obstructive sleep apnea event**

  Inventor(s): Halleck; Michael E. (Longmont, CO), Lehrman; Michael L. (Washington, DC)

  Assignee(s): East River Ventures, LP (New York, NY)

  Patent Number: 6,666,830

  Date filed: August 17, 2000

  Abstract: There is disclosed a system and method for detecting the onset of an **obstructive sleep apnea** event before the **obstructive sleep apnea** event fully develops and before the cessation of breathing occurs. The system comprises one or more microphones capable of detecting breathing sounds within an airway of a person. The microphones generate signals representative of the breathing sounds and send the signals to a controller. The controller identifies at least one signal pattern that is associated with a breathing pattern of the person that occurs at the onset of an **obstructive sleep apnea** event. The controller may also identify at least one signal pattern that is associated with a partially occluded breathing pattern of the person. The controller identifies the signal patterns by using digital signal processing techniques to analyze the signals representative of breathing sounds. The method involves detecting breathing sounds within an airway of a person, generating signals representative of the breathing sounds, and identifying at least one signal pattern that is associated with a breathing pattern of the person that occurs at the onset of an **obstructive sleep apnea** event.

  Excerpt(s): The present invention is directed to a system and method for detecting the onset of an **obstructive sleep apnea** event before cessation of breathing occurs.... Apnea is the cessation of breathing. **Sleep apnea** is the cessation of breathing during sleep. **Sleep apnea** is a common sleep disorder that affects over twelve million (12,000,000) people in the United States. Persons with **sleep apnea** may stop and start breathing several times an hour while sleeping. Each individual episode of the cessation of breathing is referred to as a **sleep apnea** event.... When a person stops breathing during sleep the person's brain soon senses that oxygen levels in the blood are low and carbon dioxide levels in the blood are high. The brain then sends emergency signals to the body to cause the body to try to increase gas exchange in the lungs to increase the amount of oxygen and to decrease the amount of carbon dioxide. The body's autonomic physiological reflexes initiate survival reactions such as gasping for air, the production of enzymes to constrict arteries to increase blood pressure, and the production of enzymes to increase heart rate. The person will then usually gasp for air and thereby restore the effective gas exchange of oxygen and carbon dioxide in the lungs. This causes the **sleep apnea** event to end.

Web site: http://www.delphion.com/details?pn=US06666830__

- **System and method for monitoring and controlling a plurality of polysomnographic devices**

  Inventor(s): Berquin; Yves (Brussels, BE), Haberland; Ben (Palm City, FL), Michel; Didier (Linkebeek, BE)

  Assignee(s): Respironics, Inc. (Pittsburgh, PA)

  Patent Number: 6,425,861

  Date filed: December 3, 1999

  Abstract: A polysomnographic system is provided for use in conjunction with a communications network to simultaneously perform sleep studies on a plurality of patients. The polysomnographic system includes a first remote polysomnographic unit for collecting physiological data from a first patient and a second remote polysomnographic unit for collecting physiological data from a second patient. The first and second remote polysomnographic units communicate with a host unit which allows for remote observation and manipulation of sensors and therapeutic devices unit via a communication network. An affiliated pressure support device is controlled if **obstructive sleep apnea** is present.

  Excerpt(s): This invention generally relates to a method and apparatus for monitoring and treating sleep disorders, and, more particularly, to a computerized polysomnographic system for simultaneously monitoring a plurality of patients undergoing respective sleep studies and for controlling a pressure support device for each individual patient, either treating a patient or for determining a prescription for treatment of a patient having a breathing disorder, such as **sleep apnea...** There are three recognized types of **sleep apnea. Central sleep apnea** is characterized by the suspension of all respiratory movement and is generally believed to be neurological in origin. **Obstructive sleep apnea** is characterized by the collapse of the upper airways during sleep. The third type of **sleep apnea** is a combination of central and **obstructive sleep apnea** and is known as mixed apnea. Individuals having **sleep apnea** often are only able to sleep for short periods of time before interruption by apneic episodes and, therefore, are only able to obtain fragmented and intermittent sleep. As a result, **sleep apnea** can cause a host of secondary symptoms, such as general fatigue and daytime sleepiness, high blood pressure, cognitive dysfunction, cardiac arrhythmia, and even congestive heart failure. It is estimated that between 1% and 5% of the general population are afflicted with some level of **sleep apnea**... Treatments for **sleep apnea** have included a number of pharmacological agents and several surgical procedures such as tracheostomy or the removal of excess muscle and tissue from the tongue or airway walls. However, pharmacological treatments for **sleep apnea** have been generally ineffective and may have adverse side effects. Furthermore, the surgical procedures involve major surgery which may cause extreme discomfort and may involve significant risk of postoperative complications.

Web site: http://www.delphion.com/details?pn=US06425861__

- **Ventilatory stabilization technology**

  Inventor(s): Hajduk; Eric A. (7531 Fountain Road SE., Calgary Alberta, CA T2H 0W9), Platt; Ronald S. (3413 Eighth Street SE., Calgary Alberta, CA T2G 3A4), Remmers; John E. (Box 12, Site 23, R.R. 12, Calgary Alberta, CA T3E 6W3)

  Assignee(s): none reported

  Patent Number: 6,752,150

  Date filed: February 3, 2000

  Abstract: A system for reducing **central sleep apnea** (CSA) is described in which certain methods of increasing a patient's rebreathing during periods of the sleep cycle are used. By increasing rebreathing during periods of overbreathing, the over-oxygenation which typically results from the overbreathing period can be reduced, thus reducing the compensating underbreathing period and effectively reducing the loop gain associated with the **central sleep apnea.**

  Excerpt(s): Central **sleep apnea** is a type of sleep-disordered breathing that is characterized by a failure of the sleeping brain to generate regular, rhythmic bursts of neural activity. The resulting cessation of rhythmic breathing, referred to as apnea, represents a disorder of the respiratory control system responsible for regulating the rate and depth of breathing, i.e. overall pulmonary ventilation. **Central sleep apnea** should be contrasted with **obstructive sleep apnea,** where the proximate cause of apnea is obstruction of the pharyngeal airway despite ongoing rhythmic neural outflow to the respiratory muscles. The difference between **central sleep apnea** and **obstructive sleep apnea** is clearly established, and the two can co-exist. While **central sleep apnea** can occur in a number of clinical settings, it is most commonly observed in association with heart failure or cerebral vascular insufficiency. An example of **central sleep apnea** is Cheyne-Stokes respiration.... This normal regulation of arterial blood gases is accomplished by a stable ventilatory output of the respiratory central pattern generator. By contrast, **central sleep apnea** represents an instability of the respiratory control system. The instability can arise from one of two mechanisms, namely: (1) intrinsic failure of the respiratory central pattern generator in the face of adequate stimulation by respiratory chemoreceptors; or (2) lack of adequate stimulation of the central pattern generator by respiratory chemoreceptors. The former is referred to as the "intrinsic instability" and the latter is referred to as the "chemoreflex instability." Theoretically, both mechanisms can co-exist. The common form of **central sleep apnea** is thought to be caused by the chemoreflex instability mechanism.... The chemoreflex control of breathing might exhibit instability either because the delay of the negative feedback signal is excessively long or because the gain of the system is excessively high. Current evidence indicates that the latter constitutes the principal derangement in **central sleep apnea** caused by heart failure. Specifically, the overall response of the control system to a change in arterial P.sub.CO2 is three-fold higher in heart-failure patients with **central sleep apnea** than in those having no sleep-disordered breathing. This increased gain probably resides within the central chemoreflex loop; however, high gain of the peripheral chemoreflex loop cannot be excluded. Accordingly, the fundamental mechanism of **central sleep apnea** is taken to be high loop gain of the control system, which results in feedback instability during sleep.

Web site: http://www.delphion.com/details?pn=US06752150__

Patent Applications on Sleep Apnea

As of December 2000, U.S. patent applications are open to public viewing.[22] Applications are patent requests which have yet to be granted (the process to achieve a patent can take several years). The following patent applications have been filed since December 2000 relating to sleep apnea:

- **Active medical device for the diagnosis of the sleep apnea syndrome**

  Inventor(s): Poezevera, Yann; (Courcouronne, FR)

  Correspondence: Robert M. Isackson, Esq.; ORRICK, HERRINGTON & SUTCLIFFE LLP; 666 Fifth Avenue; New York; NY; 10103-0001; US

  Patent Application Number: 20030130589

  Date filed: December 16, 2002

[22] This has been a common practice outside the United States prior to December 2000.

Abstract: An active medical device have an improved diagnosis of a **sleep apnea syndrome.**. This device measures the respiratory activity of the patient, determines a state of activity, this state being likely to take, according to satisfaction of predetermined criteria, a value representative of a state of sleep of the patient, and analyzes a detected signal corresponding to the respiratory activity to detect, when the aforementioned state is a state of sleep, the presence of respiratory pauses, and thereby to produce an indicating signal of **sleep apnea** in the event of the occurrence of a respiratory pause of duration longer than a first predetermined duration. The analysis also includes inhibiting the production of the aforesaid indicating signal, or a treatment to resolve an apnea, when the duration of the detected respiratory pause is longer than a second predetermined duration, typically of at least one minute.

Excerpt(s): The present invention relates to the diagnosis of the respiratory disorders, more particularly the diagnosis of the **sleep apnea syndrome.**.... The **sleep apnea syndrome** (SAS), more precisely the syndrome of obstructive apnea of sleep (SOAS) (as contrasted with the syndrome of central sleep apnea) is an affection generally caused by an obstruction of the respiratory tracts. It is susceptible to cause a certain number of disorders such as painful and insufficient breathing, heartbeat disturbance, and hypertension.... Various treatments of SOAS have been proposed including, for example, surgery, medications or maintenance of a positive pressure in the respiratory tracts by means of a facial mask applied during the sleep. It also has been proposed to treat SAS by neuro-muscular electric stimulation of the muscles controlling the air routes of the patient, as described in the U.S. Pat. No. 5,485,851 (to Medtronic, Inc.), and, more recently, by a particular stimulation of the myocardium (the so-called "electro-cardiac" stimulation) in the event of a detected SAS, as described, for example, in the U.S. Pat. No. 6,126,611 (to Medtronic, Inc.) and European patent application EO-A-0 970 713 and its corresponding U.S. patent application No.______ (attorney docket no. 8707.2148; 152 Detection Sommeil) (to Ela Mdical). EP-A-0 970 713 (and U.S. application______) has the advantage of operating a discrimination between phases of awakening and sleep, in order to apply a therapy only during a phase of sleep, and to inhibit any treatment if the detected apnea occurs during a phase of awakening, because in this case it is normally not a pathological affection.

Web site: http://appft1.uspto.gov/netahtml/PTO/search-bool.html

- **Adenosine derivatives**

  Inventor(s): Bays, David Edmund; (Ware, GB), Cousins, Richard Peter Charles; (Stevenage, GB), Dyke, Hazel Joan; (Cambridge, GB), Eldred, Colin David; (Stevenage, GB), Judkins, Brian David; (Stevenage, GB), Pass, Martin; (Macclesfield, GB), Pennell, Andrew Michael Kenneth; (San Carlos, CA)

  Correspondence: BACON & THOMAS, PLLC; 625 SLATERS LANE; FOURTH FLOOR; ALEXANDRIA; VA; 22314

  Patent Application Number: 20030096788

  Date filed: August 13, 2002

  Abstract: A method of treating a patient suffering from or susceptible to ischemic heart disease, peripheral vascular disease or stroke or which subject is suffering pain, a CNS disorder or **sleep apnea** which comprises administering a therapeutically effective amount of an adenosine derivative which is an agonist at the adenosine A1 receptor and which exhibits little or no agonist activity of the A3 receptor. The adenosine derivative has a general formula (I) as follows: 1

  Excerpt(s): The present invention relates to novel adenosine derivatives, to processes for their preparation, to pharmaceutical compositions containing them and to their use in medicine.... Publications in this area include WO 98/16539 (Novo Nordisk A/S) which describes adenosine derivatives for the treatment of myocardial and cerebral ischaemia and epilepsy; WO 98/04126 (Rhone-Poulenc Rorer Pharmaceuticals Inc.) which relates to adenosine derivatives possessing antihypertensive, cardioprotective, anti-ischaemic and antilipolytic properties; and WO 98/01459 (Novo Nordisk A/S) which describes N,9-disubstituted adenine derivatives which are substituted in the 4' position by unsubstituted oxazolyl or isoxazolyl and the use of such compounds for the treatment of disorders involving cytokines in humans.... R.sup.3 represents H, phenyl (optionally substituted by halogen), a 5 or 6 membered heteroaryl group, C.sub.1-6 alkoxy, C.sub.1-6 alkylO(CH.sub.2).sub.n where n is 0-6, C.sub.3-7 cycloalkyl, C.sub.1-6 hydroxyalkyl, halogen or a C.sub.1-6 straight or branched alkyl, C.sub.1-6 alkenyl or C.sub.1-6 alkynyl group optionally substituted by one or more halogens.

  Web site: http://appft1.uspto.gov/netahtml/PTO/search-bool.html

- **Alkylaryl polyether alcohol polymers for treatment and prophylaxis of snoring, sleep apnea, sudden infant death syndrome and for improvement of nasal breathing**

  Inventor(s): Hofmann, Thomas; (Seattle, WA)

  Correspondence: HANA VERNY; PETERS, VERNY, JONES & SCHMITT, LLP; SUITE 6; 385 SHERMAN AVENUE; PALO ALTO; CA; 94306; US

  Patent Application Number: 20030053956

  Date filed: January 23, 2002

  Abstract: A method and composition for treatment and prophylaxis of snoring, **sleep apnea** or sudden infant death syndrome and for improvement of nasal breathing in mammals by nasal and/or pharyngeal administration of tyloxapol or a related alkylaryl polyether alcohol polymer. A spray, liquid or solid composition comprising from about 0.01 to about 20% (w/v), equivalent to about 100.mu.g/ml to about 200 mg/ml, of tyloxapol or another alkylaryl polyether alcohol polymer alone or in admixture with pharmaceutically acceptable excipients and additives. The composition is administered as a spray, liquid, liquid drops, lozenges or powder suitable for nasal and/or pharyngeal application.

  Excerpt(s): This application is based on and claims priority of the provisional application Ser. No. 60/264,166 filed on Jan. 24, 2001.... The current invention concerns a method and composition for treatment and prophylaxis of snoring, **sleep apnea** or sudden infant death syndrome and for improvement of nasal breathing in mammals by nasal and/or pharyngeal administration of tyloxapol or a related alkylaryl polyether alcohol polymer. In particular, the present invention provides a spray, liquid or solid composition comprising from about 0.01 to about 20% (w/v), equivalent to about 100.mu.g/ml to about 200 mg/ml, of tyloxapol or another selected alkylaryl polyether alcohol polymer alone, in combination, or in admixture with pharmaceutically acceptable excipients and additives. The composition is administered as a spray, liquid, liquid drops, lozenges or powder suitable for nasal and/or pharyngeal application.... Snoring and related **sleep apnea** are amongst the most troublesome sleeping impairments. Snoring is not only a nuisance for other people, but it has been shown, similarly to **sleep apnea,** to correlate with increased daytime sleepiness and decreased alertness and work performance.

  Web site: http://appft1.uspto.gov/netahtml/PTO/search-bool.html

- **Analysis of sleep apnea**

  Inventor(s): Sheldon, Stephen H.; (Chicago, IL)

  Correspondence: JAECKLE FLEISCHMANN & MUGEL, LLP; 39 State Street; Rochester; NY; 14614-1310; US

  Patent Application Number: 20030139680

  Date filed: January 22, 2003

  Abstract: A non-intrusive and quantitative method and apparatus for diagnosing **sleep apnea** and detecting apnea events by monitoring during sleep abdominal effort and thoracic effort, determining the phase of each effort, determining the difference in phase between each type of effort, and then determining the rate of phase angle change and standard deviation over time. Also provided may be treatment when apnea events are detected to trigger therapy apparatus such as airway positive pressure apparatus.

  Excerpt(s): This application claims the benefit of U.S. Provisional Application Ser. No. 60/350,770, filed Jan. 22, 2002.... Obstructive **Sleep Apnea** one of the most common disorders in the U.S. Lower oxygen levels associated with **Obstructive Sleep Apnea** (OSA) is now known to be a major cause of cardiovascular morbidity including heart attack and stroke. At present expensive polysomnography is used to identify these patients but not on a sufficient scale to provide diagnosis as a practical matter. The development of a diagnostic system which can allow simplified diagnosis of **obstructive sleep apnea** by the primary care physician would be a major step. The prevention of hundreds of thousands of annual excess deaths, stroke and heart attacks associated with **obstructive sleep apnea** through simplified recognition of this disorder is the most important purpose of the present invention. These excess deaths are occurring annually in a great part due to the lack of availability of this technology resulting in a vast pool of undiagnosed cases of **Sleep Apnea** and other breathing disorders. Despite the fact that **obstructive sleep apnea** is easily treated, both the patient and the family are often completely unaware of the presence of this dangerous disease, thinking the patient just a "heavy snorer".... Obstructive **sleep apnea** often develops insidiously as a patient enters middle age and begins to snore. The major cause is an increase in fat deposition (often age related) in the neck which results in narrowing of the airway. (In fact the probability that a 40 year Id has **sleep apnea** is directly related to his or her neck circumference). When the muscle tone of the upper airway diminishes during sleep coupled with negative pressure associated with inspiration through this somewhat narrow airway results in collapse of the upper airway in a manner analogous to the collapse of a cellophane straw. This results in airway obstruction and, effectively chokes off all air movement The choking patient (still asleep) begins to struggle and inhales more forcibly, thereby, further lowering upper airway pressure and causing further collapse of the upper airway. During this time, substantially no air movement into the chest occurs and the patient experiences a progressive fall in oxygen (similar to the fall occurring early in drowning). The fall in oxygen produces central nervous system stimulation contributing to hypertension and potential heart and blood vessel injury and finally results in arousal. Upon arousal, increase in airway muscle tone opens the airway and the patient rapidly inhales and ventilates quickly to correct the low oxygen levels. Generally, the arousal is brief and the patient is not aware of the arousal (or of the choking since this occurs during sleep). Once oxygen levels have been restored, the patient begins again to sleep more deeply, upper airway tone again diminishes, the upper airway collapses and the cycle is repeated stressing the heart with low oxygen in a repetitive fashion. Often this repeating cycle over many years eventually results in damage to the heart muscle and/or the coronary arteries. As the patient ages, the consequences of undiagnosed **obstructive sleep apnea** is often either a progressive decline in heart muscle function (and eventual heart failure) or heart infarction.

Web site: http://appft1.uspto.gov/netahtml/PTO/search-bool.html

- **Apparatus for detecting sleep apnea using electrocardiogram signals**

  Inventor(s): Chazal, Phillip de; (Sutton, AU), Heneghan, Conor; (Dublin, IE), sheridan, Elaine; (Crossdoney, IE)

  Correspondence: Patrick R. Scanlon; Pierce Atwood; One Monument Square; Portland; ME; 04101; US

  Patent Application Number: 20030055348

  Date filed: September 14, 2001

  Abstract: There is provided a method of determining a diagnostic measure of **sleep apnea** including the following steps: acquiring an electrocardiogram signal, calculating a set of RR intervals and electrocardiogram-derived respiratory signal from said electrocardiogram, and hence calculating a set of spectral and time-domain measurements over time periods including power spectral density, mean, and standard deviation. These measurements are processed by a classifier model which has been trained on a pre-existing data base of electrocardiogram signals to provide a probability of a specific time period containing apneic episodes or otherwise. These probabilities can be combined to form an overall diagnostic measure. The system also provides a system and apparatus for providing a diagnostic measure of **sleep apnea.**

Excerpt(s): This invention relates to cardio-respiratory monitoring and analysis, and more particularly to methods for diagnosing sleep disorders. More specifically, the present invention is aimed at detection of **sleep apnea** using the electrocardiogram. The invention can be embodied in a form suitable for use in a dedicated medical setting, or in the home.... Sleep apnea is a significant public health problem. Current estimates are that approximately 4% of the male middle-aged population, and 2% of the female middle-aged population suffer from **sleep apnea.** Patients suffering from **sleep apnea** are more prone to hypertension, heart disease, stroke, and irregular heart rhythms. Continued interruption of quality sleep is also associated with depression, irritability, loss of memory, lack of energy, and a higher risk of car and workplace accidents.... Current techniques for detection and diagnosis of **sleep apnea** rely upon hospital-based polysomnography. A polysomnogram simultaneously records multiple physiologic signals from the sleeping patient. A typical polysomnogram includes measurements of blood oxygen saturation level, blood pressure, electroencephalogram, electrocardiogram, electrooculogram, electromyogram, nasal and/or oral airflow chest effort, and abdominal effort. Typically, signals are recorded from a full night's sleep and then a diagnosis is reached following a clinical review of recorded signals. In some patients a second night's recording is required. Because of the number and variety of measurements made, this test can be uncomfortable for the patient and also has a relatively high cost. In general, it is only performed in a dedicated medical facility.

Web site: http://appft1.uspto.gov/netahtml/PTO/search-bool.html

- **BI/PAP mask for sleep apnea and other related clinical uses**

  Inventor(s): Moone, Samuel Joseph; (Pickerington, OH)

  Correspondence: Samuel Joseph Moone; 13450 Falmouth Ave.; Pickerington; OH; 43147; US

  Patent Application Number: 20020144684

  Date filed: April 6, 2001

  Abstract: The introduction of gas/air flow tubes molded/inserted from the top gas/air flow channel to the front area below the nasal area will generate additional air flow to the user's nose below the nasal openings. The gas/air flow tubes will allow users of breathing masks to become accustomed to masks that will be providing gas/air for various purposes.

In this instance the mask will be providing comforting simulated breathing for a BIPAP user with **sleep apnea,** eliminating the feeling of insufficient airflow to the nasal area. This will eliminate user discomfort with current masks that cause discontinued cooperation by patients with the sleeping regimen. By inserting a plug in the bottom of the gas/air flow tube top the mask will convert from a BIPAP mask, to a CPaP mask. This mask can be used in a variety of hospital/healthcare settings where gas/air is used by patients.

Excerpt(s): A variety of respiratory masks are known which have flexible seals that cover the nose and/or mouth of a human user and are designed to create a continuous seal against the user's face.... Because of the sealing effect that is created, the user may provide gases/air at a positive/simulated breathing pressure within the mask for consumption. The uses for such a mask would range from high altitude breathing (i.e., aviation applications) to mining and fire fighting applications, to various medical diagnostic and therapeutic applications.... One requisite of such respiratory masks has been that they provide an effective seal against the user's face to prevent leakage of the gas/air being supplied. Commonly, in mask configurations, a good mask-to-face seal has been attained in many instances only with considerable discomfort for the user. This problem is most crucial in those applications, especially medical applications, which require the user to wear such a mask continuously for hours or perhaps even days. In such situations, the user will not tolerate the mask for long duration's and optimum therapeutic or diagnostic objectives thus will not be achieved, or will be achieved with great difficulty and considerable user discomfort.

Web site: http://appft1.uspto.gov/netahtml/PTO/search-bool.html

- **Breathing gas delivery method and apparatus**

  Inventor(s): Estes, Mark; (Sylmar, CA), Sanders, Mark H.; (Wexford, PA), Zdrojkowski, Ronald J.; (Pittsburgh, PA)

  Correspondence: MICHAEL W. HAAS, INTELLECTUAL PROPERTY COUNSEL; RESPIRONICS, INC.; 1010 MURRY RIDGE LANE; MURRYSVILLE; PA; 15668; US

  Patent Application Number: 20030145856

  Date filed: March 3, 2003

  Abstract: An improved methodology and systems for delivery of breathing gas such as for the treatment of **obstructive sleep apnea** through application of alternating high and low level positive airway pressure within the airway of the patient with the high and low airway pressure being coordinated with the spontaneous respiration of the patient, and improved methods and apparatus for triggering and for leak management in such systems.

Excerpt(s): The **sleep apnea syndrome,** and in particular **obstructive sleep apnea,** afflicts an estimated 4% to 9% of the general population and i due to episodic upper airway obstruction during sleep. Those afflicted with **obstructive sleep apnea** experience sleep fragmentation and intermittent, complete or nearly complete cessation of ventilation during sleep with potentially severe degrees of oxyhemoglobin unsaturation. These features may be translated clinically into debilitating daytime sleepiness, cardiac disrhythmias, pulmonary-artery hypertension, congestive heart failure and cognitive dysfunction. Other sequelae of **sleep apnea** include right ventricular dysfunction with cor pulmonale, carbon dioxide retention during wakefulness as well as during sleep, and continuous reduced arterial oxygen tension. Hypersomnolent **sleep apnea** patients may be at risk for excessive mortality from these factors as well as from an elevated risk for accidents such as while driving or operating other potentially dangerous equipment.... Although details of the pathogenesis of upper airway obstruction in **sleep apnea** patients have not been fully defined, it is generally accepted that the mechanism includes either anatomic or functional abnormalities of the upper airway which result in increased air flow resistance. Such abnormalities may include narrowing of the upper airway due to suction forces evolved during inspiration, the effect of gravity pulling the tongue back to appose the pharyngeal wall, and/or insufficient muscle tone in the upper airway dilator muscles. It has also been hypothesized that a mechanism responsible for the known association between obesity and **sleep apnea** is excessive soft tissue in the anterior and lateral neck which applies sufficient pressure on internal structures to narrow the airway.... The treatment of **sleep apnea** has included such surgical interventions as uvalopalatopharyngoplasty, gastric surgery for obesity, and maxillo-facial reconstruction. Another mode of surgical intervention used in the treatment of **sleep apnea** is tracheostomy. These treatments constitute major undertakings with considerable risk of post-operative morbidity if not mortality. Pharmacologic therapy has in general been disappointing, especially in patients with more than mild **sleep apnea.** In addition, side effects from the pharmacologic agents that-have been used are frequent. Thus, medical practitioners continue to seek non-invasive modes of treatment for **sleep apnea** with high success rates and high patient compliance including, for example in cases relating to obesity, weight loss through a regimen of exercise and regulated diet.

Web site: http://appft1.uspto.gov/netahtml/PTO/search-bool.html

- **Centralized hospital monitoring system for automatically detecting upper airway instability and for preventing and aborting adverse drug reactions**

  Inventor(s): Lynn, Eric N.; (Villa Ridge, MO), Lynn, Lawrence A.; (Columbus, OH)

  Correspondence: Lawrence A. Lynn; 1507 CHAMBERS RD.; COLUMBUS; OH; 43212; US

  Patent Application Number: 20030000522

  Date filed: May 17, 2002

  Abstract: A system and method for the automatic diagnosis of **obstructive sleep apnea** in a centralized hospital critical care monitoring system for the monitoring of a plurality of patients in at least one of a critical care, step down, and cardiac ward by telemetry. The system includes a central processor having a display, and a plurality of telemetry units for mounting with patients, each of the telemetry units has a plurality of sensors for connection with each patient, the telemetry unit is capable of the transmission of multiple signals derived from the sensors to the central processor, in one preferred embodiment the method comprising steps of programming the system to analyze the signals and to automatically identify the presence and severity of **obstructive sleep apnea** and to provide an indication of the identification.

  Excerpt(s): This application claims priority of provisional application Nos. 60/291,691 and 60/291,687, both filed May 17, 2001 and provisional application No. 60/295,484 filed Jun. 10, 2001, the disclosures and contents of each of which is incorporated by reference as if completely disclosed herein.... This invention relates to centralized hospital monitoring systems and particular to the organization, analysis, and automatic detection of patterns indicative of upper airway instability during sleep, deep sedation, and analgesia.... This failure of conventional hospital based patient monitors to timely and/or automatically detect cluster patterns indicative of airway instability can be seen as a major health care deficiency indicative of a long unsatisfied need. Because **obstructive sleep apnea,** a condition derived from airway instability, is so common, the consequence of the failure of conventional hospital monitors to routinely recognize upper airway instability clusters means that many of patients with this disorder will never be diagnosed in their lifetime. For these patients, the diagnostic opportunity was missed and the health implications and risk of complications associated with undiagnosed airway instability and **sleep apnea** will persist in this group throughout the rest of their life. A second group of patients will have a complication in the hospital due to the failure to timely recognize airway instability. Without recognition of the inherent instability, a patient may be extubated too early after surgery or given too much narcotic (the right drug, the right patient, the ordered dose but unknowingly a "relative drug excess"). Indeed until clusters indicative of airway instability are routinely recognized by hospital monitors, the true incidence of respiratory failure, arrest, and/or death related to the administration of IV sedation and narcotics to patients in the hospital with airway instability will never be known but the number is probably in the tens of thousands each year and airway instability is just one example of the types of physiologic instability which are not automatically characterized by central hospital systems.

Web site: http://appft1.uspto.gov/netahtml/PTO/search-bool.html

- **Combination treatment for sleep disorders including sleep apnea**

  Inventor(s): Howard, Harry R. JR.; (Bristol, CT)

  Correspondence: PFIZER INC; 150 EAST 42ND STREET; 5TH FLOOR - STOP 49; NEW YORK; NY; 10017-5612; US

  Patent Application Number: 20020183306

  Date filed: February 13, 2002

  Abstract: The present invention relates to a method of treating sleep disorders including **sleep apnea** in a mammal, including a human, by administering to the mammal a 5HT1a antagonist or an alpha-2-adrenergic antagonist in combination with an SRI antidepressant agent with improvement in efficacy. It also relates to pharmaceutical compositions containing a pharmaceutically acceptable carrier, a 5HT1a antagonist or an alpha-2-adrenergic antagonist, and an SRI antidepressant agent.

  Excerpt(s): The present invention relates to a method of treating sleep disorders including **sleep apnea** with improved efficacy in a mammal, including a human, by administering to the mammal a 5HT1a antagonist or an alpha-2-adrenergic antagonist in combination with a serotonin reuptake inhibitor (SRI). It also relates to pharmaceutical compositions containing a pharmaceutically acceptable carrier, a serotonin 5HT1a antagonist or an alpha-2-adrenergic antagonist and a serotonin reuptake inhibitor (SRI).... Sleep disorders including **sleep apnea** which are to be treated according to the present invention are of a psychiatric nature, and are to be diagnosed, and the treatment prescribed, by psychiatrists and other physicians. It will be understood that the patient and doctor cannot expect that such treatment will effect a cure in all cases. However, treatment according to the present invention, perhaps combined with other treatments such as psychiatric consultation and analysis, lifestyle modification, and perhaps other treatments for concomitant disorders, will be found to alleviate the disorder of sleep, producing a substantial benefit to the patient. In some cases, the benefit will be in the form of an alleviation of the unpleasant symptoms of the disorders, and in other cases substantial or even complete diminution of the symptoms will be obtained, amounting to complete cure of the disorder.... Serotonin Selective Reuptake Inhibitors (SSRIs) currently provide efficacy in the treatment of major depressive disorder (MDD) and are generally perceived by psychiatrists and primary care physicians as effective, well-tolerated and easily administered. However, they are associated with undesirable features, such as high incidence of sexual dysfunction, delayed onset of action and a level of non-responsiveness estimated to be as high as 30% (see M. J. Gitlin, Journal of Clinical Psychiatry, 1994, 55, 406-413 and R. T. Segraves, Journal of Clinical Psychiatry, 1992, 10(2), 4-10). Preclinical and clinical evidence has indicated that the sexual dysfunction associated with SSRI therapy can be reduced through the use of serotonin reuptake inhibitors (SRI) and dopamine reuptake inhibitors (DRIs), such as bupropion (see A. K. Ashton, Journal of Clinical Psychiatry, 1998, 59(3), 112-115). Furthermore, the combination of SRI and DRI may hasten the onset of action as well as offering relief to refractory patients, possibly through a synergistic mechanism (see R. D. Marshall et al, Journal of Psychopharmacology, 1995, 9(3), 284-286) and prove beneficial in the treatment of substance abuse and attention deficit hyperactivity disorder (ADHD) according to Barrickman et al, Journal of the American Academy of Child and Adolescent Psychology, 1995, 34(5), 649 and Shekim et al, Journal of Nervous and Mental Disease, 1989, 177(5), 296. Psychology, 1995, 34(5), 649 and Shekim et al, Journal of Nervous and Mental Disease, 1989, 177(5), 296.

Web site: http://appft1.uspto.gov/netahtml/PTO/search-bool.html

- **Detecting, assessing, and diagnosing sleep apnea**

  Inventor(s): Beckman, Luke; (Arlington, VA), Beckman, Robert; (Arlington, VA), Crutchfield, Kevin E.; (Potomac, MD), Mozayeni, B. Robert; (Rockville, MD)

  Correspondence: HOGAN & HARTSON LLP; IP GROUP, COLUMBIA SQUARE; 555 THIRTEENTH STREET, N.W.; WASHINGTON; DC; 20004; US

  Patent Application Number: 20030176788

  Date filed: January 28, 2003

Abstract: The present invention comprises methods for detecting, assessing, diagnosing, and pre-diagnosing **sleep apnea,** and for assessing the efficacy of a treatment for **sleep apnea.** Methods for the detection, assessment, diagnosis and pre-diagnosis (screening) of **sleep apnea** and the assessment of a treatment for **sleep apnea** according to the present invention may be performed in the absence of a sleep study. The patients subject to these methods may remain awake during their performance. The invention may be applied to other vascular conditions besides **sleep apnea,** wherein the **sleep apnea** methods described herein are example methods for the application of the present invention to the detection, assessment, diagnosis and pre-diagnosis (screening) of other vascular conditions.

Excerpt(s): This application claims priority under 35 U.S.C..sctn. 119(e) to U.S. Provisional Patent Application No. 60/351,411, filed Jan. 28, 2002 and incorporated herein by reference.... The invention relates to a system and method for assessing, diagnosing, and pre-diagnosing **sleep apnea** and assessing treatment of **sleep apnea.** Specifically, the invention relates to a system and method for identifying critical variables, through a Dynamic Vascular Assessment (DVA) of vascular Doppler data including transcranial Doppler (TCD) data, which distinguish patients suffering from **sleep apnea** and the normal population.... Sleep apnea is a breathing disorder characterized by brief interruptions of breathing during sleep. **Sleep apnea** is usually caused by blockage in the lower portion of the throat, or by lack of impulse from the brain to control air passage in the respiratory system. **Sleep apnea** is often misdiagnosed as heart and lung problems.

Web site: http://appft1.uspto.gov/netahtml/PTO/search-bool.html

- **Device for preventing sleep apnea**

  Inventor(s): Masayoshi, Furuya; (Nagano-shi, JP), Narihiko, Matsuda; (Kobe-shi, JP)

  Correspondence: BIRCH STEWART KOLASCH & BIRCH; PO BOX 747; FALLS CHURCH; VA; 22040-0747; US

  Patent Application Number: 20030056785

  Date filed: September 26, 2002

  Abstract: The present invention provides a device which prevents loud snoring and apnea during sleep so as not to cause discomfort to a user as much as possible. Stoppers 4 such as belts or straps having predetermined elasticity are attached to both right and left sides of a lower jaw fitting piece 3 which fits the both sides of the lower jaw, the lower jaw 2 is pushed forward via the lower jaw fitting piece 3 by setting and hanging the stoppers 4 on the nose or head of the face side, whereby occurrence of apnea and loud snoring during sleep is prevented.

Excerpt(s): The present invention relates to a device for preventing **sleep apnea** in the field of oral medical treatment.... There are surprisingly many people who snore during sleep, and some of them suffer from **sleep apnea**... Snoring is caused by muscle relaxation during sleep, and when the jaw muscle relaxes, the lower jaw moves rearward and moves the tongue to the rear side of the oral cavity, whereby the breathing airway of the pharynx is narrowed, the breathing airflow eddies, the velum and the surrounding soft muscle vibrates and causes a sound phenomenon called snoring.

Web site: http://appft1.uspto.gov/netahtml/PTO/search-bool.html

- **Headwear for use by a sleep apnea patient**

Inventor(s): Payne,, Charles E. JR.; (Charlotte, NC)

Correspondence: Adams, Schwartz & Evans, P.A.; 2180 Two Wachovia Center; Charlotte; NC; 28282; US

Patent Application Number: 20040025885

Date filed: August 9, 2002

Abstract: Headwear is adapted for use by a patient to position airway tubes of a nasal interface operatively connected to a positive airway pressure device. The headwear includes an elongated head strap for being worn around a head of the patient. First and second tube holders are attached to the head strap, and adapted for engaging and holding respective airway tubes of the nasal interface to retain the tubes in a desired position during use. Each of the tube holders includes an elastic strip extending along a longitudinal dimension of the head strap. The elastic strip cooperates with the head strap to form an eye for receiving an airway tube of the nasal interface.

Excerpt(s): This application relates to headwear for use by a **sleep apnea** patient. The invention serves to position airway tubes of a nasal interface operatively connected to a positive airway pressure device used in the treatment of **sleep apnea.** The invention is especially applicable for use with the NASAL-AIRE.RTM. interface sold by Innomed Technologies of Boca Raton, Fla. In alternative applications, the invention may be used in combination with any other medical device, such as that designed to provide mechanical respiration assistance in the treatment of congestive heart failure, emphysema, and other respiratory conditions.... Sleep apnea is a serious, potentially life-threatening breathing disorder characterized by brief interruptions of breathing during sleep. In a given night, the number of involuntary breathing pauses or "apneic events" may be as high as 20 to 30 or more per hour. These breathing pauses are almost always accompanied by snoring between apnea episodes, although not everyone who snores has this condition. **Sleep apnea** can also be characterized by choking sensations. The frequent interruptions of deep, restorative sleep often lead to early morning headaches and excessive daytime sleepiness.... Certain mechanical and structural problems in the airway cause the interruptions in breathing during sleep. In some people, apnea occurs when the throat muscles and tongue relax during sleep and partially block the opening of the airway. When the muscles of the soft palate at the base of the tongue and the uvula relax and sag, the airway becomes blocked, making breathing labored and noisy and even stopping it altogether. **Sleep apnea** also can occur in obese people when an excess amount of tissue in the airway causes it to be narrowed. With a narrowed airway, the person continues his or her efforts to breathe, but air cannot easily flow into or out of the nose or mouth. Unknown to the person, this results in heavy snoring, periods of no breathing, and frequent arousals causing abrupt changes from deep sleep to light sleep.

Web site: http://appft1.uspto.gov/netahtml/PTO/search-bool.html

- **Method and apparatus for optimizing the continuous positive airway pressure for treating obstructive sleep apnea**

  Inventor(s): Gruenke, Roger A.; (Overland Park, KS), Norman, Robert G.; (New Windsor, NY), Rapoport, David M.; (New York, NY)

  Correspondence: FULWIDER PATTON LEE & UTECHT, LLP; HOWARD HUGHES CENTER; 6060 CENTER DRIVE; TENTH FLOOR; LOS ANGELES; CA; 90045; US

  Patent Application Number: 20030055346

  Date filed: November 7, 2002

  Abstract: A diagnostic device having a nose fitting used without connection to a breathing gas supply for obtaining flow data values at ambient pressure. The nose fitting is connected to a pressure or flow sensor that supplies data values to a micro-processor. The detection and measurement of breathing gas flow is made from a tight sealing nose fitting (mask or prongs) configured with a resistive element inserted in the flow stream as breathing gas exits from and enters into the fitting. The nasal fitting is further provided with a port for connection to a flow or pressure transducer. The resistive element causes a pressure difference to occur between the upstream side and the downstream side when air flows through the element. The data values may be stored in computer memory to be analyzed for flow limitations.

Excerpt(s): This application is a continuation of U.S. Ser. No. 09/602,158, filed Jun. 22, 2000, which is a continuation of U.S. application Ser. No. 08/644,371, filed May 10, 1996 (U.S. Pat. No. 6,299,581), which is a continuation of U.S. application Ser. No. 08/482,866, filed Jun. 7, 1995 (U.S. Pat. No. 5,535,739), which is a division of U.S. application Ser. No. 08/246,964, filed May 20, 1994 (U.S. Pat. No. 5,490,502), which is a continuation-in-part of U.S. application Ser. No. 07/879,578, filed May 7, 1992 (U.S. Pat. No. 5,335,654), the contents of which are hereby incorporated herein by reference.... This invention relates to a method and apparatus for adjusting the positive airway pressure of a patient to an optimum value in the treatment of **obstructive sleep apnea,** and more particularly to a breathing device which maintains constant positive airway pressure and method of use which analyzes an inspiratory flow waveform to titrate such a pressure value.... Obstructive **sleep apnea syndrome** (OSAS) is a well recognized disorder which may affect as much as 1-5% of the adult population. OSAS is one of the most common causes of excessive daytime somnolence. OSAS is most frequent in obese males, and it is the single most frequent reason for referral to sleep disorder clinics.

Web site: http://appft1.uspto.gov/netahtml/PTO/search-bool.html

- **Method and apparatus for providing positive airway pressure to a patient**

Inventor(s): Estes, Mark C.; (Sylmar, CA), Fiore, John; (Monroeville, PA), Kepler, Jeff; (Pittsburgh, PA), Mechlenburg, Douglas M.; (Murrysville, PA), Ressler, Heather; (New Alexandria, PA)

Correspondence: MICHAEL W. HAAS, INTELLECTUAL PROPERTY COUNSEL; RESPIRONICS, INC.; 1010 MURRY RIDGE LANE; MURRYSVILLE; PA; 15668; US

Patent Application Number: 20030121519

Date filed: November 26, 2002

Abstract: A system including methods and apparatus for treatment of a medical disorder such as **obstructive sleep apnea** or congestive heart failure. The system involves applying a gain to flow rate of pressurized gas delivered to a patient during inspiratory and/or expiratory phases of a respiratory cycle to deliver the pressurized gas in proportion to the respective gains during inspiration and/or expiration. A base pressure may be applied in addition to the gain-modified pressures and an elevated pressure profile may be employed to assist or control inspiration. The system may be fully automated responsive to feedback provided by a flow sensor that determines the estimated patient flow rate. A leak computer can be included to instantaneously calculate gas leakage from the system. The system may be utilized in connection with conventional continuous positive airway pressure treatments, such as CPAP or bi-level positive airway pressure equipment to effect various beneficial treatment applications.

Excerpt(s): This is a continuation-in-part of U.S. patent application Ser. No. 09/610,733 filed Jul. 6, 2000, which is a continuation of U.S. patent application Ser. No. 09/041,195 filed Mar. 12, 1998, now U.S. Pat. No. 6,105,575, which is a continuation-in-part of U.S. patent application Ser. No. 08/679,898 filed Jul. 15, 1996, which is a continuation-in-part of application Ser. No. 08/253,496 filed Jun. 3, 1994, now U.S. Pat. No. 5,535,738.... The present invention relates generally to methods and apparatus for treating breathing and/or cardiac disorders and, more particularly, to methods and apparatus for providing a pressure to an airway of a patient during at least a portion of the breathing cycle to treat **obstructive sleep apnea** syndrome, chronic obstructive pulmonary disease, congestive heart failure, and other respiratory and/or breathing disorders.... During **obstructive sleep apnea** syndrome (OSAS), the airway is prone to narrowing and/or collapse while the patient sleeps. Continuous positive airway pressure (CPAP) therapy seeks to avoid this narrowing by supplying pressure to splint the airway open. With CPAP, this splinting pressure is constant and is optimized during a sleep study to be sufficient in magnitude to prevent narrowing of the airway. Providing a constant splinting pressure, i.e., CPAP, is a simple solution to the problem posed by the collapsing airway. However, this approach exposes the patient to pressures that are higher than the pressures needed to support the airway for most of the breathing cycle.

Web site: http://appft1.uspto.gov/netahtml/PTO/search-bool.html

- **Method and apparatus for the treatment of central sleep apnea using biventricular pacing**

  Inventor(s): Burnes, John E.; (Andover, MN), Cho, Yong K.; (Maple Grove, MN)

  Correspondence: MEDTRONIC, INC.; 710 MEDTRONIC PARKWAY NE; MS-LC340; MINNEAPOLIS; MN; 55432-5604; US

  Patent Application Number: 20030195571

  Date filed: April 12, 2002

  Abstract: An apparatus and method for treating **sleep apnea** includes a control unit in electrical communication with a lead. The control unit is capable of outputting a **sleep apnea** interruption pulse to stimulate at least one of a phrenic nerve and a diaphragm. Specifically, an implanted medical device (IMD) such as an ICD or a pacemaker paces the heart and a mode switch algorithm changes the pacing output to stimulate at least one of a phrenic nerve and diaphragm when **sleep apnea** is detected by the control unit. The method includes determining if the patient is experiencing **sleep apnea** and outputting a **sleep apnea** interruption pulse to the at least one of a phrenic nerve and a diaphragm. The control unit may be incorporated with the IMD. In another embodiment, the control unit may be in wireless communication with the IMD and positioned outside a patient's body.

  Excerpt(s): The present invention generally relates to implantable medical devices. Specifically, the invention relates to the prevention of hypopnia during **sleep apnea** by stimulating the phrenic nerve with implanted cardiac leads, when the onset of **sleep apnea** is detected. More specifically, the invention relates to a biventricular pacemaker adapted to provide an automatically adjustable output via a lead preferably located in the coronary sinus.... Sleep apnea is generally associated with the cessation of breathing during sleep. The medical characteristics of **sleep apnea** have been known for some time. **Sleep apnea** is terminated by the subject's arousal, followed by hyperventilation. Such arousals from sleep are generally associated with increased sympathetic nervous system activity and blood pressure, which may contribute to the worsening of a patient's cardiac condition.... Generally, there are two types of **sleep apnea.** The first is **central sleep apnea,** which relates to the failure of the body to automatically generate the neuro-muscular stimulation necessary to initiate and control the respiratory cycle at the proper time. The second **sleep apnea syndrome** is known as **obstructive sleep apnea.** This generally relates to an obstructive apnea that includes reduction of the size of the superior airways, an increase in their compliance and reduction in the activity of the dilator muscles.

Web site: http://appft1.uspto.gov/netahtml/PTO/search-bool.html

- **Method and apparatus to detect and monitor the frequency of obstructive sleep apnea**

  Inventor(s): Cho, Yong K.; (Maple Grove, MN), Condie, Catherine R.; (Shoreview, MN), Jensen, Donald N.; (Derwood, MD)

  Correspondence: MEDTRONIC, INC.; 710 MEDTRONIC PARKWAY NE; MS-LC340; MINNEAPOLIS; MN; 55432-5604; US

  Patent Application Number: 20030204213

  Date filed: April 30, 2002

  Abstract: The present invention provides a method and apparatus for detecting and monitoring **obstructive sleep apnea.** The apparatus includes an intracardiac impedance sensor to measure intracardiac impedance, a movement sensor to measure an amount of movement of a patient, and a controller operatively coupled to said intracardiac impedance sensor and said movement sensor, said controller adapted to receive at least one of an intracardiac impedance and the amount of movement of the patient and detect **obstructive sleep apnea** based upon said intracardiac impedance and said movement.

  Excerpt(s): This invention relates generally to implantable medical devices, and more particularly, to a method and apparatus to automatically detect and monitor the frequency of **obstructive sleep apnea**... Although the function of sleep is not well understood, one consequence of an inadequate quantity or poor quality of sleep is an inability to maintain adequate wakefulness. The amount of sleep an individual needs is thought to be neurologically determined and is generally stable over time. Among other factors, an insufficient amount of sleep (i.e., quantity of sleep) or a disruption of sleep continuity (i.e., quality of sleep) will result in increased daytime sleepiness. Increased sleepiness in a person may cause a plethora of problems to that person as well as others. Increased sleepiness is a major cause of accidents because people who are sleepy are generally not fully aware of their surroundings. Additionally, because of this decreased awareness, a person who does not receive the adequate quantity and quality of sleep at night may also be prone to decreased efficiency at home and at work. A sleepy person may also require frequent naps during the day to recuperate, thereby reducing productivity in the office as well as in the chores of daily life. As a result, it is important for people generally to receive a good night's rest. However, many people have medical conditions that prevent them from receiving a good night's rest. One such condition is **sleep apnea**... Sleep apnea is generally defined as the cessation of breathing during sleep. One type of a **sleep apnea, obstructive sleep apnea** ("OSA"), is caused by repetitive upper airway obstruction during sleep as a result of narrowing of the respiratory passages. Partial obstruction of the passageways may simply lead to hypopnea. Prolonged obstruction of the passageways, however, may lead to nocturnal arousals.

Web site: http://appft1.uspto.gov/netahtml/PTO/search-bool.html

- **Method and apparatus to treat conditions of the naso-pharyngeal area**

  Inventor(s): Conrad, Timothy R.; (Eden Prairie, MN), Knudson, Mark B.; (Shoreview, MN), Tweden, Katherine S.; (Mahtomedi, MN)

  Correspondence: MERCHANT & GOULD PC; P.O. BOX 2903; MINNEAPOLIS; MN; 55402-0903; US

  Patent Application Number: 20020170564

  Date filed: July 3, 2002

  Abstract: A patient's upper airway condition such as snoring and **sleep apnea** is treated by selecting a particulate material selected for limited migration within tissue and for encouraging a fibrotic response of tissue to the material. A bolus of the particulate material is injected into the tissue area to structurally stiffen the tissue.

  Excerpt(s): This invention is directed to methods and apparatuses for treating conditions of the naso-pharyngeal area such as snoring and **sleep apnea.** More particularly, this invention pertains to method and apparatus to stiffen tissue of the naso-pharyngeal area.... Snoring has received increased scientific and academic attention. One publication estimates that up to 20% of the adult population snores habitually. Huang, et al., "Biomechanics of Snoring", Endeavour, p. 96-100, Vol. 19, No. 3 (1995). Snoring can be a serious cause of marital discord. In addition, snoring can present a serious health risk to the snorer. In 10% of habitual snorers, collapse of the airway during sleep can lead to **obstructive sleep apnea** syndrome. Id.... Notwithstanding numerous efforts to address snoring, effective treatment of snoring has been elusive. Such treatment may include mouth guards or other appliances worn by the snorer during sleep. However, patients find such appliances uncomfortable and frequently discontinue use (presumably adding to marital stress).

  Web site: http://appft1.uspto.gov/netahtml/PTO/search-bool.html

- **Method and device for addressing sleep apnea and related breathing disorders**

  Inventor(s): Britt, Walter; (Wayland, MI), Heeke, David W.; (East Lansing, MI)

  Correspondence: Denise M. Glassmeyer; Dierker & Glassmeyer, P.C.; 3331 W. Big Beaver, Suite 109; Troy; MI; 48084; US

  Patent Application Number: 20030015198

  Date filed: June 14, 2002

  Abstract: A device which is removably insertable in the mouth for facilitating breathing while sleeping which provides a clear unobstructed airway by protrusive positioning of the mandible and/or delivery of pressurized air to the back of the mouth. The device has upper and lower tooth-contacting members and an airway defined between them.

  Excerpt(s): This application claims the benefit of U.S. Provisional Applications S. No. 60/298,997, filed Jun. 18, 2001. The invention relates to oral appliances and methods for making same. More particularly the present invention relates to oral appliances which can facilitate breathing while sleeping.... Difficulty breathing while sleeping often manifests itself as snoring or, the more serious condition, **obstructive sleep apnea.** Snoring is a condition affecting approximately 40% of the adult population, while **obstructive sleep apnea** affects approximately 7% of the adult population. Although snoring can occur as a result of a physical anomaly, such as enlarged tonsils or adenoids, generally, snoring occurs during sleep because the muscles of the upper throat relax. As a person breathes, the turbulence of the air causes a flutter valve effect on the soft tissues of the upper throat. The vibration resulting from the flutter valve effect of the soft tissues of the upper throat causes snoring sounds.... Airway occlusion during sleep may cause cessation of breathing (apnea) and can lead to undesirable physiological symptoms. **Sleep apnea** is due to the obstruction of the upper airway which produces short episodes of breathing stoppage that characterizes apnea. Frequent arousals during the night occur when the user awakens in order to overcome the airway blockage. As a result, **sleep apnea** can contribute to excessive daytime sleepiness as well as high blood pressure, strokes or cardiac arrest.

  Web site: http://appft1.uspto.gov/netahtml/PTO/search-bool.html

- **Method and system for treating sleep apnea**

  Inventor(s): Deem, Mark E.; (Woodside, CA), French, Ron; (Santa Clara, CA)

  Correspondence: TOWNSEND AND TOWNSEND AND CREW, LLP; TWO EMBARCADERO CENTER; EIGHTH FLOOR; SAN FRANCISCO; CA; 94111-3834; US

  Patent Application Number: 20030216789

  Date filed: May 6, 2003

  Abstract: Systems and apparatus for treating **obstructive sleep apnea** comprise an external generator and an implantable stimulator. The implantable stimulator includes an electrode which is placed in a target muscle or nerve which when stimulated will alleviate the symptoms of **sleep apnea.** The generator produces a radiofrequency or microwave signal which is broadcast to an antenna within the implanted stimulator. The implanted stimulator produces a stimulatory output, preferably without any other energy source.

  Excerpt(s): The present application is a non-provisional of U.S. Patent Application Serial No. 60/380,657 (Attorney Docket No. 020979-001200US), filed May 14, 2002, the full disclosure of which is incorporated herein by reference.... The present invention relates generally to medical apparatus and methods. More particularly, the present invention relates to methods and apparatus for alleviating **sleep apnea.**.. Sleep apnea is a condition characterized by the temporary but reoccurring suspension of breathing during sleep. The condition affects those who are overweight, who have obstructions in their upper airways, or who have a neurological disorder. In those who have airway obstructions, the disease is generally referred to as "obstructive **sleep apnea.**" **Sleep apnea** can be a very serious condition in some patients, and a number of treatment approaches have been evolved over the years.

  Web site: http://appft1.uspto.gov/netahtml/PTO/search-bool.html

- **Microprocessor system for the simplified diagnosis of sleep apnea**

  Inventor(s): Lynn, Eric N.; (Columbus, OH), Lynn, Lawrence A.; (Columbus, OH)

  Correspondence: Lawrence A. Lynn; 1507 Chambers Rd.; Columbus; OH; 43212; US

  Patent Application Number: 20020173707

  Date filed: April 24, 2002

Abstract: A method of evaluating a patient with **sleep apnea** includes monitoring a patient to produce at least one timed waveform of at least one physiologic parameter, identifying along the waveform a first waveform variation indicative of an apnea, identifying along the waveform a second waveform variation indicative of another apnea, determining the interval intermediate at least one portion of the first waveform variation and at least one portion of the second waveform, and assessing the severity of **sleep apnea** based on at least the determining. A device for determining the severity of **sleep apnea** comprises a monitor capable of generating a signal indicative of at least one physiologic parameter and a processor capable of processing the signal, the processor operating to generate a timed waveform of the parameter and to identify a plurality of sequential waveform variations indicative of a corresponding plurality of sequential apneas, the sequential waveform variations having temporal and spatial relationships between the waveform variations and along the waveform, the processor further operating to determine at least one of the temporal and the spatial relationships and displaying the determining so that the determining can be used to assess the severity of **sleep apnea.**

Excerpt(s): This application claims the benefit of U.S. Provisional Application No. 60/052,438, filed Jul. 14, 1997, the contents of which are hereby incorporated herein by reference and the benefit of U.S. Provisional Application No. 60/052,439, filed Jul. 14, 1997, the contents of which are hereby incorporated herein by reference.... This application is a continuation-in-part of U.S. application Ser. No. 08/789,460, filed Jan. 27, 1997, which is a continuation of U.S. patent application Ser. No. 08/391,811, filed Feb. 21, 1995, now U.S. Pat. No. 5,605,151, which is a continuation of U.S. patent application Ser. No. 08/151,901 filed Nov. 15, 1993, now U.S. Pat. No. 5,398,682, which is a continuation-in-part of U.S. patent application Ser. No. 08/931,976, filed Aug. 19, 1992, now abandoned. The contents of application Ser. Nos. 08/789,460, 08/391,811, 08/151,901, 08/931,976, and PCT/US 93/97726, and of U.S. Pat. Nos. 5,605,151 and 5,398,682 are all hereby incorporated herein by reference, the contents of which are incorporated herein by reference.... Obstructive **Sleep Apnea** is now recognized as one of the most common disorders in the US. The lower oxygen levels associated with **Obstructive Sleep Apnea** is now known to be a major cause of cardiovascular morbidity including heart attack and stroke. A crisis exists in the U.S. in that traditional expensive polysomnography cannot be used to identify these patients on a sufficient scale. The situation is analogous to having a disease as common and subtle as insulin dependent diabetes without an inexpensive and widely implementable and simple mechanism to diagnose the disorder (such as exists for diabetes). Millions of patients remain undiagnosed. The development of a diagnostic system which can allow simplified diagnosis of **obstructive sleep apnea** by the primary care physician is a national healthcare priority of substantial scale. The prevention of hundreds of thousands of annual excess deaths, stroke and heart attacks associated with **obstructive sleep apnea** through simplified recognition of this disorder is the most important purpose of the present invention. These excess deaths are occurring annually in a great part due to the lack of availability of this technology resulting in a vast pool of undiagnosed cases of **Sleep Apnea.**. Despite the fact that **obstructive sleep apnea** is easily treated, both the patient and the family are often completely unaware of the presence of this dangerous disease, thinking the patient just a "heavy snorer".

Web site: http://appft1.uspto.gov/netahtml/PTO/search-bool.html

- **Mouthpiece, nasal seal, head appliance, apparatus, and methods of treating sleep apnea**

  Inventor(s): Klemperer, Walter G.; (Champaign, IL)

  Correspondence: Frank S. Rosenberg; 18 Echo Hill Lane; Moraga; CA; 94556; US

  Patent Application Number: 20030183227

  Date filed: March 26, 2002

  Abstract: A CPAP device and a method for treating **sleep apnea** use a head appliance with an oral adaptor comprising a tube partially inserted in a person's mouth and a diaphragm applied over the tube against the mouth, such that the lips are formed into a tight seal with the tube. A nasal seal is described comprising two rollers to which a strap is attached, so that the nasal seal is easily put in place, adjusted and maintained by rolling the rollers on the nose sides or pulling the straps.

  Excerpt(s): Sleep apnea is a common sleep ailment that affects as many as five percent of the population worldwide. Persons with **sleep apnea** stop breathing for short durations many times during sleep, so that the depth and quality of their sleep is reduced. As a result, persons with **sleep apnea** suffer from a profound sleepiness, which can impair their ability and performance at work and in other activities.... Sleep apnea often results from a collapse of the person's throat tissues during sleep, which reduces or suppresses the air flow to the lungs. Lowered oxygen levels and increased carbon dioxide levels in blood alert the person's brain and breathing resumes, but each occurrence arouses the person and interrupts restorative sleep.... Surgery is a possible treatment but surgical procedures are complex and success rates are often low. A more common treatment for **sleep apnea** is to force air inside the person's throat during sleep with a respirator apparatus. Apparatuses of this type use continuous positive airway pressure or CPAP.

Web site: http://appft1.uspto.gov/netahtml/PTO/search-bool.html

- **Multipurpose device for preventing and treating snoring and sleep apnea and/or preventing gnashing of teeth**

  Inventor(s): Alekseevich, Ryazanov Evgeniy; (Moscow, RU), Ivanovich, Bredov Vladimir; (Moscow, RU)

  Correspondence: McDERMOTT, WILL & EMERY; 600 13th Street, N.W.; Washington; DC; 20005-3096; US

  Patent Application Number: 20020144685

  Date filed: March 22, 2002

  Abstract: The invention pertains to the medical devices and may be used as the method for prophylaxis and treating snoring and **sleep apnea,** and also for preventing gnashing of teeth during a sleep. The device contains joined through the connecting element the cup-shaped fixture and outer and inner restrictive petals with the holes. The petals are set up on the connecting element with an opportunity of moving along it and fixing on it.The cup-shaped fixture has the section in the form of the arc in the surface of the longitudinal axis section of the connecting element in the area of its adjoining to the fixture, symmetrical to the planes of the petals of the fixture, and the section in the form of the parabola in the surface of the axis section, perpendicular to the identified.

  Excerpt(s): The invention pertains to medical devices and is intended for treating snoring, **sleep apnea syndrome** (short pauses in breathing during a sleep), and also for preventing gnashing of teeth during a sleep.... During a sleep a human often can produce non-articulate sounds called snoring, caused by resonant vibrations during the oral cavity tissues and airflow interaction, when the airflow is going through between the palatine curtain and the tongue, and also between the route of the tongue and the posterior wall of the larynx. In the first case these sounds are caused most often by hypotonia of the muscles of the palatine curtain, in the second case, by tongue retraction.... Snoring **sleep apnea** is of great discomfort for the people around and for the snoring person it leads to appearing and developing of different diseases caused by breathing impairment. **Sleep apnea** can continue from several seconds to two minutes, the total time of such apneas may reach 4 hours during the night. The sequels of the multiple stops of breathing are blood and tissue gas disturbances (less saturation by oxygen) and of oxidation-reduction reactions in the tissues and organs of the organism. As a result those who snore do not have a good sleep and experience some sorts of malaise during the day.

Web site: http://appft1.uspto.gov/netahtml/PTO/search-bool.html

- **Pharmacological treatment for sleep apnea**

  Inventor(s): Carley, David W.; (Evanston, IL), Radulovacki, Miodrag; (Chicago, IL)

  Correspondence: MARSHALL, GERSTEIN & BORUN; 6300 SEARS TOWER; 233 SOUTH WACKER; CHICAGO; IL; 60606-6357; US

  Patent Application Number: 20030130266

  Date filed: October 31, 2002

  Abstract: The present invention relates generally to pharmacological methods for the prevention of amelioration of sleep-related breathing disorders via administration of agents or combinations of agents that possess serotonin-related pharmacological activity.

  Excerpt(s): Priority is claimed to U.S. patent application Ser. No. 10/016,901, filed Dec. 14, 2001, which claims priority to U.S. patent application Ser. No. 09/622,823, filed Aug. 23, 2000, now U.S. Pat. No. 6,331,536 issued Dec. 18, 2001, which claims priority International Patent Appl. No. PCT/US99/04347, filed Feb. 26, 1999, which claims priority to U.S. Provisional Pat. App. Ser. No. 60/076,216, all of which are incorporated herein by reference in their entirety.... This invention generally relates to methods for the pharmacological treatment of breathing disorders and, more specifically, to the administration of agents or compositions having serotonin-related receptor activity for the alleviation of **sleep apnea** (central and obstructive) and other sleep-related breathing disorders.... Over the past several years much effort has been devoted to the study of a discrete group of breathing disorders that occur primarily during sleep with consequences that may persist throughout the waking hours in the form of sleepiness, thereby manifesting itself into substantial economic loss (e.g., thousands of lost man-hours) or employment safety factors (e.g., employee non-attentiveness during operation of heavy-machinery). Sleep-related breathing disorders are characterized by repetitive reduction in breathing (hypopnea), periodic cessation of breathing (apnea), or a continuous or sustained reduction in ventilation.

  Web site: http://appft1.uspto.gov/netahtml/PTO/search-bool.html

- **Sleep apnea device and method thereof**

  Inventor(s): Wyckoff, Robert; (Smith River, CA)

  Correspondence: MYERS & KAPLAN, INTELLECTUAL; PROPERTY LAW, L.L.C.; 1827 POWERS FERRY ROAD; BUILDING 3, SUITE 200,; ATLANTA; GA; 30339; US

  Patent Application Number: 20030167018

  Date filed: March 4, 2002

  Abstract: A neck-worn device and a method thereof, wherein a plate having a generally arcuate configuration is placed securely and removably on the neck of a user, wherein a substantially airtight zone is created between the device and the neck of a user, and wherein a valve is provided to allow the escape of air from the airtight zone in response to soft neck tissue respiratory movements, thus enabling the creation of a negative pressure or vacuum and thereby effectively drawing open the air passages of a user. The present invention is particularly suited for, although not limited to, utilization as a **sleep apnea** device enabling a user to alleviate the bothersome and potentially detrimental effects of **sleep apnea** without utilizing costly equipment requiring electrical or battery power.

  Excerpt(s): The present invention relates generally to air pathway clearance devices and, more specifically, to a neck-worn device and a method thereof, wherein a generally negative pressure is created on the exterior surface of a user's neck, thereby effectively holding open the air pathways. The present invention is particularly suited for, although not limited to, utilization as a **sleep apnea** device enabling a user to alleviate the bothersome and potentially detrimental effects of **sleep apnea** without utilizing costly equipment requiring electrical or battery power.... Sleep apnea affects millions of individuals, causing each to experience a variety of symptoms while sleeping. These symptoms often decrease feelings of restfulness and reduce health benefits derived from adequate rapid eye movement (rem) sleep sessions. While the degree of effect varies between individuals, most **sleep apnea** sufferers with **obstructive sleep apnea** experience collapse and closure of the soft tissues which form the anterior and lateral walls of the pharynx causing erratic cessations of natural breathing cycles and airflow, disruptive snoring behaviors and drops in oxygen saturation, potentially leading to periodic stoppages and/or interruptions of heart rhythms and blood flow, increased cardiovascular disease risk, hypertension, and in extreme cases, even death.... The most popular, presently available, non-surgical treatment method for **sleep apnea** relies on an electrical instrument, or Continuous Positive Airway Pressure (CPAP) machine. The basic premise behind the CPAP machine and its ability to counteract the affects of **sleep apnea** rests in the creation of a closed respiratory system for the user, wherein a generally constant and positive pressure forces the airways to remain open. This closed, positive pressure system utilizes a powered generator to blow a stream of air into the user's face through a mask typically worn over the users nose. The complexity of the electronic CPAP instrument makes the device costly to purchase, thus eliminating its availability to many **sleep apnea** sufferers.

Web site: http://appft1.uspto.gov/netahtml/PTO/search-bool.html

- **Sleep apnea therapy device using dynamic overdrive pacing**

  Inventor(s): Bornzin, Gene A.; (Simi Valley, CA), Falkenberg, Eric; (Simi Valley, CA), Levine, Paul A.; (Santa Clarita, CA), Park, Euljoon; (Stevenson Ranch, CA)

  Correspondence: PACESETTER, INC.; 15900 Valley View Court; Sylmar; CA; 91392-9221; US

  Patent Application Number: 20030153954

  Date filed: February 14, 2002

  Abstract: A cardiac stimulation device uses dynamic overdrive pacing to prevent **sleep apnea.** In another aspect, the device can use dynamic overdrive pacing to terminate **sleep apnea** after detection. An implantable cardiac stimulation device comprises a sensor and one or more pulse generators. The sensor senses intrinsic cardiac electrical phenomena. The pulse generators can generate cardiac pacing pulses with timing based on the sensed intrinsic cardiac electrical phenomena to dynamically overdrive the intrinsic cardiac electrical phenomena. The timed cardiac pacing pulses can prevent a **sleep apnea** condition.

  Excerpt(s): This application is related to copending, commonly-assigned U.S. patent application Ser. No.______, titled CARDIAC STIMULATION DEVICE INCLUDING **SLEEP APNEA** PREVENTION AND TREATMENT; and U.S. patent application Ser. No.______, tilted STIMULATION DEVICE FOR **SLEEP APNEA** PREVENTION, DETECTION AND TREATMENT; both applications filed concurrently herewith.... The present invention relates to techniques for providing therapy to patients who suffer from **sleep apnea...** Sleep apnea is the cessation of breathing for a short time while sleeping. **Sleep apnea** has multiple classifications based on source of dysfunction. **Obstructive sleep apnea** results from mechanical blockage of the airway, for example due to weight of fatty neck tissue compressing the trachea. **Central sleep apnea** results from neurological dysfunction. Mixed **sleep apnea** has a combination of mechanical and neurological cause.

Web site: http://appft1.uspto.gov/netahtml/PTO/search-bool.html

- **Sleep apnea treatment apparatus**

  Inventor(s): Cattano, Janice M.; (South Boston, VA), Estes, Mark C.; (Northridge, CA)

  Correspondence: MICHAEL W. HAAS, INTELLECTUAL PROPERTY COUNSEL; RESPIRONICS, INC.; 1010 MURRY RIDGE LANE; MURRYSVILLE; PA; 15668; US

  Patent Application Number: 20040016433

  Date filed: July 18, 2003

  Abstract: Improved methodology and apparatus for the clinical study and treatment of **sleep apnea** which incorporates one or more of the following features: (1) application of mono-level, alternating high and low level, or variable positive airway pressure generally within the airway of the patient with the mono-level, high and low level, or variable airway pressure generally being coordinated with and/or responsive to the spontaneous respiration of the patient, (2) usage of adjustably programmable pressure ramp circuitry capable of producing multiple pressure ramp cycles of predetermined duration and pattern whereby the ramp cycles may be customized to accommodate the specific needs of an individual **sleep apnea** patient so as to ease the patient's transition from wakefulness to sleep, (3) remote control or patient-sensed operation of the apparatus, (4) employment of safety circuitry, reset circuitry and minimum system leak assurance circuitry, controls and methods, and (5) utilization of clinical control circuitry whereby sleep disorder data may be compiled and appropriate therapy implemented during a one-night sleep study.

  Excerpt(s): This application is a continuation-in-part of pending U.S. patent application Ser. No. 07/768,269, filed Nov. 1, 1991, of the same title, which is a continuation-in-part of U.S. patent application Ser. No. 07/411,012, filed Sep. 22, 1989, entitled METHOD AND APPARATUS FOR MAINTAINING AIRWAY PATENCY TO TREAT **SLEEP APNEA** AND OTHER DISORDERS, now U.S. Pat. No. 5,148,802, issued Sep. 22, 1992.... The present invention relates generally to methodology and apparatus for treatment of **sleep apnea** and, more particularly, to mono-level, bi-level and variable positive airway pressure apparatus, as well as feedback type versions thereof, including circuitry for enabling a patient to selectively actuate one or more pressure ramp cycles wherein, during each ramp cycle, available airway pressure increases with time from a predetermined minimum pressure value to a prescription pressure, thereby facilitating the patient's transition from a waking to a sleeping state.... The **sleep apnea syndrome** afflicts an estimated 1% to 5% of the general population and is due to episodic upper airway obstruction during sleep. Those afflicted with **sleep apnea** experience sleep fragmentation and intermittent, complete or nearly complete cessation of ventilation during sleep with potentially severe degrees of oxyhemoglobin desaturation. These features may be translated clinically into extreme daytime sleepiness, cardiac arrhythmias, pulmonary-artery hypertension, congestive heart failure and/or cognitive dysfunction. Other sequelae of **sleep apnea** include right ventricular dysfunction with cor pulmonale, carbon dioxide retention during wakefulness as well as during sleep, and continuous reduced arterial oxygen tension. Hypersomnolent **sleep apnea** patients may be at risk for excessive mortality from these factors as well as by an elevated risk for accidents while driving and/or operating potentially dangerous equipment.

Web site: http://appft1.uspto.gov/netahtml/PTO/search-bool.html

- **Split-night sleep diagnostic system**

  Inventor(s): Bowman, Bruce R.; (Eden Prairie, MN), Hansen, Gary L.; (Eden Prairie, MN)

  Correspondence: ROTHWELL, FIGG, ERNST & MANBECK, P.C.; 1425 K STREET, N.W.; SUITE 800; WASHINGTON; DC; 20005; US

  Patent Application Number: 20040087866

  Date filed: October 30, 2002

  Abstract: A split-night sleep diagnostic system is provided for diagnosing and treating **sleep apnea** in a single night. The diagnostic system includes a blower, a respiratory interface and a conduit connected between the blower and the respiratory interface. Also included is a valve disposed along the conduit. The valve includes an aperture formed in the conduit between the blower and the respiratory interface, and a valve member movable between a first position partially occluding the conduit so that air flows through the aperture and a second position blocking the aperture so that continuous positive airway pressure is provided to a patient. Both diagnosis and titration can be performed using a single system at a single location over the course of a single night.

  Excerpt(s): The present invention relates generally to a method and an apparatus for treating apnea and, more particularly, to a method and an apparatus for diagnosing and treating **sleep apnea** in a single night.... The term "apnea", as used herein, is meant to encompass any type of breathing disorder, for example, apnea (complete cessation of breathing), patency obstruction, partial obstruction, apnea that arises in patients with various cardiac, cerebrovascular and endocrine conditions unrelated to the state of the upper airway, or the like.... Sleep apnea arises during sleep when a patient undergoes repeated cessation of breathing. The cessation is caused by an obstruction of the throat air passage. Repeated cessation of breathing reduces blood oxygen and disturbs sleep. Reduction of blood oxygen can cause heart attacks and strokes, while sleep disturbances or fragmentation can produce excessive daytime sleepiness.

Web site: http://appft1.uspto.gov/netahtml/PTO/search-bool.html

- **Use of somatostatin receptor agonists in the treatment of human disorders of sleep hypoxia and oxygen deprivation**

  Inventor(s): Young, Charles W.; (New York, NY)

  Correspondence: FROMMER LAWRENCE & HAUG; 745 FIFTH AVENUE- 10TH FL.; NEW YORK; NY; 10151; US

  Patent Application Number: 20030083241

  Date filed: October 25, 2002

  Abstract: The invention relates to a method of treating diverse human disorders that may arise, in part, out of sleep hypoxia and oxygen deprivation occurring in the context of sleep apnea/hypopnea disturbances. The disorders that may be treated by the invention comprise gastroesophageal reflux disease (GERD), asthma-associated gastroesophageal reflux (GER), GER-associated asthma, asthma, cardiomyopathy, cardioarrhythmia, congestive heart failure, sudden infant death syndrome, and diverse neurologic conditions. The mode of treatment uses somatostatin receptor ligands (SstRLs), particularly somatostatin-receptor agonists. The invention concerns the method of treatment utilizing, and compositions comprising SstRLs and somatostatin receptor agonists, including agonists of the somatostatin receptor types 2 and 5, particularly, the type 2A receptor (SsR-2A), including octreotide and lanreotide.

  Excerpt(s): The invention relates to a method of using somatostatin receptor agonists to treat diverse human disorders of sleep hypoxia and oxygen deprivation, including but not limited to: 1) gastroesophageal reflux disease (GERD), asthma-associated gastroesophageal reflux (GER), GER-associated asthma, and asthma; 2) **obstructive sleep apnea** (OSA), and OSA-associated conditions, including GER, asthma, cardiomyopathy, cardioarrhythmia, congestive heart failure, median nerve compression neuropathy (carpal tunnel syndrome) and cognitive impairment; as well as sleep apnea-associated sudden infant death syndrome (SIDS), 3) **central sleep apnea** (CSA), as well as CSA-associated conditions, including GER, cardiomyopathy, cardioarrhythmia, congestive heart failure, and cognitive impairment; 4) mixed pattern sleep apneas, including but not limited to post-vascular occlusion **sleep apnea,** dementia-associated **sleep apnea,** amyotrophic lateral sclerosis-associated **sleep apnea,** myasthenia gravis-associated **sleep apnea,** and alcoholism-related **sleep apnea;** 5) excess calpain-activation disorders in tissues where the injured cell population expresses somatostatin receptors; including, but not limited to the central nervous system, peripheral nerves, heart, liver, kidney, and gastrointestinal tract.... Various documents are cited in this text. Citations in the text can be by way of a citation to a document in the reference list, e.g., by way of an author(s) and document year, whereby full citation in the text is to a document that may or may not also be listed in the reference list.... There is no admission that any of the various documents cited in this text are prior art as to the present invention. Any document having as an author or inventor person or persons named as an inventor herein is a document that is not by another as to the inventor of entity herein. All documents cited in this text ("herein cited documents") and all documents cited or referenced in herein cited documents are hereby incorporated herein by reference.

Web site: http://appft1.uspto.gov/netahtml/PTO/search-bool.html

- **Using activity-based rest disturbance as a metric of sleep apnea**

  Inventor(s): Florio, Joseph J.; (La Canada, CA)

  Correspondence: PACESETTER, INC.; 15900 VALLEY VIEW COURT; SYLMAR; CA; 91392-9221; US

  Patent Application Number: 20040002742

  Date filed: June 27, 2002

  Abstract: An implantable cardiac device is programmed to monitor short term activity changes that occur while a patient is at rest to produce a sleep disturbance metric that is useful in analyzing and/or treating **sleep apnea.** After the implantable cardiac device confirms that a patient is at rest, the device monitors an instantaneous signal from an activity sensor to detect variances from normal rest mode activity. When the variances exceed a preset threshold for a short time period (e.g., less than 30-40 sec.), the patient is presumed to be experiencing a form of sleep disturbance as opposed to conscious or wakeful activity. These short term events are recorded as sleep disturbance events. The sleep disturbance metric are reported to a physician as a diagnostic to help ascertain the severity of **sleep apnea** or to evaluate the effectiveness of pacing therapies being applied to treat **sleep apnea.**

Excerpt(s): The present invention generally relates to implantable cardiac devices, and particularly, to techniques for monitoring sleep disturbances as a metric for determining severity of **sleep apnea** and/or for evaluating pacing therapies for treating **sleep apnea.**.. Sleep apnea is a condition in which a person stops breathing for a short time while sleeping. **Sleep apnea** has multiple classifications based on the source of dysfunction. **Obstructive sleep apnea** results from mechanical blockage of the airway, for example, due to the weight of fatty neck tissue compressing the trachea. **Central sleep apnea** results from neurological dysfunction. Mixed **sleep apnea** has a combination of mechanical and neurological cause.... Symptoms of **sleep apnea** include snoring, breath holding during sleep, rapid awakening with gasping for air, morning headaches, depression, irritability, loss of memory, lack of energy, high risk of automobile and workplace accidents, and lack of high quality sleep and resulting daytime grogginess and sleepiness. **Sleep apnea** is rarely fatal but is linked to high blood pressure and increased probability of heart disease, stroke, and arrhythmias. Patients with coronary artery disease who have a blood oxygen level lowered by sleep-disordered breathing may be at risk of ventricular arrhythmia and nocturnal sudden death. Furthermore, sleep-disordered breathing may cause coronary artery disease and hypertension.

Web site: http://appft1.uspto.gov/netahtml/PTO/search-bool.html

- **Ventilation interface for sleep apnea therapy**

  Inventor(s): Wood, Thomas J.; (Waycross, GA)

  Correspondence: HARNESS, DICKEY & PIERCE, P.L.C.; P.O. BOX 8910; RESTON; VA; 20195; US

  Patent Application Number: 20040020493

  Date filed: July 2, 2003

  Abstract: The ventilation interface for **sleep apnea** therapy interfaces a ventilation device to the patient's airways. The ventilation interface includes a pair of nasal inserts made from flexible, resilient silicone which are oval shaped in cross-section and slightly tapered from a base proximal the ventilation supply to the distal tip end. A bead flange is disposed about the exterior of each insert at the distal end of the insert. A bleed port for release of exhaled air is defined through a conical vent projecting normally to the path of the incoming air flow, and continues through a nipple extending to the exterior of the air conduit. In one embodiment, a pair of nasal inserts are integral with a nasal cannula body, with bleed ports axially aligned with each insert. In another embodiment, each insert is independently connected to a separate, thin-walled, flexible supply line.

Excerpt(s): This is a continuation-in-part of application Ser. No. 09/524,371, filed Mar. 13, 2000.... The present invention relates to ventilation devices, and particularly to a ventilation device having a nasal inserts which are inserted into the nostrils and seal against the nostrils without the aid of harnesses, head straps, adhesive tape or other external devices, and having exhalation ports designed to eliminate whistling noises, the ventilation interface having particular utility in various modes of therapy for **obstructive sleep apnea**... Sleep apnea is a potentially lethal affliction in which breathing stops recurrently during sleep. **Sleep apnea** may be of the obstructive type (sometimes known as the pickwickian syndrome) in which the upper airway is blocked in spite of airflow drive; the central type with decreased respiratory drive; or a mixed type. Breathing may cease for periods long enough to cause or to exacerbate cardiac conditions, and may be accompanied by swallowing of the tongue. **Sleep apnea** frequently results in-fitful periods of both day and night sleeping with drowsiness and exhaustion, leaving the patient physically and mentally debilitated.

Web site: http://appft1.uspto.gov/netahtml/PTO/search-bool.html

- **Ventilatory assistance for treatment of cardiac failure and Cheyne-stokes breathing**

  Inventor(s): Berthon-Jones, Michael; (Leonay, AU)

  Correspondence: Gottlieb, Rackman & Reisman, P.C.; 270 Madison Avenue; New York; NY; 10016-0601; US

  Patent Application Number: 20030154979

  Date filed: February 26, 2003

  Abstract: Method and apparatus for the treatment of cardiac failure, Cheyne Stokes breathing or **central sleep apnea** are disclosed. A subject is provided with ventilatory support, for example positive pressure ventilatory support using a blower and mask. Respiratory airflow is determined. From the respiratory airflow are derived a measure of instantaneous ventilation (for example half the absolute value of the respiratory airflow) and a measure of longterm average ventilation (for example the instantaneous ventilation low pass filtered with a 100 second time constant). A target ventilation is taken as 95% of the longterm average ventilation. The instantaneous ventilation is fed as the input signal to a clipped integral controller, with the target ventilation as the reference signal. The output of the controller determines the degree of ventilatory support. Clipping is typically to between half and double the degree of support that would do all the respirator work. A third measure of ventilation, for example instantaneous ventilation low pass filtered with a time constant of 5 seconds, is calculated. Ventilatory support is in phase with the subject's respiratory airflow to the fuzzy extent that this ventilation is above target, and at a preset rate conversely.

Excerpt(s): The invention relates to methods and apparatus for the provision of positive pressure ventilatory assistance for patients with cardiac failure or Cheyne-Stokes breathing from any cause, including **central sleep apnea,** cardiac failure or stroke.... In this specification, respiratory airflow is intended to refer to the instantaneous flow of gas into or out of the lungs. The term "average" is intended to mean any measure of central tendency or the result of any low pass filtering operation. Ventilatory support is intended to mean any procedure which has a similar effect as the respiratory muscles, particularly the supply of breathable gas under varying positive pressure to the airway via a nosemask, face mask, endotracheal tube, tracheotomy tube, or the like, but also including other procedures such as negative pressure ventilation, cuirasse, iron lung, external chest compression, or rocking bed ventilation. According to common usage, ventilation can mean either a procedure, as in the expression "positive pressure ventilation", or a measure of average respiratory airflow over a period of time. Instantaneous ventilation is intended to mean the volume inspired over a short period of time less than several seconds. Equally it can be calculated at the volume expired over such a period, or it can be the average of the two. For example, measures of instantaneous ventilation would include half the average of the absolute value of the respiratory airflow, calculated over a time interval short compared with several seconds, or half the absolute value of the respiratory airflow, low pass filtered with a time constant short compared with several seconds. For technical reasons to be explained below in the best embodiment, instantaneous ventilation is taken as half the absolute value of the instantaneous respiratory airflow, is averaged over an arbitrarily short period of time. However, it is not intended that the invention is limited to calculating instantaneous ventilation in this way.... The term "varying A inversely with B" is intended in the broad sense of increasing A if B is decreasing, and decreasing A if B is increasing.

Web site: http://appft1.uspto.gov/netahtml/PTO/search-bool.html

Keeping Current

In order to stay informed about patents and patent applications dealing with sleep apnea, you can access the U.S. Patent Office archive via the Internet at the following Web address: **http://www.uspto.gov/patft/index.html**. You will see two broad options: (1) Issued Patent, and (2) Published Applications. To see a list of issued patents, perform the following steps: Under "Issued Patents," click "Quick Search." Then, type "sleep apnea" (or synonyms) into the "Term 1" box. After clicking on the search button, scroll down to see the various patents which have been granted to date on sleep apnea.

You can also use this procedure to view pending patent applications concerning sleep apnea. Simply go back to the following Web address: **http://www.uspto.gov/patft/index.html**. Select "Quick Search" under "Published Applications." Then proceed with the steps listed above.

Vocabulary Builder

Alertness: A state of readiness to detect and respond to certain specified small changes occurring at random intervals in the environment. [NIH]

Ameliorating: A changeable condition which prevents the consequence of a failure or accident from becoming as bad as it otherwise would. [NIH]

Discrimination: The act of qualitative and/or quantitative differentiation between two or more stimuli. [NIH]

EMG: Recording of electrical activity or currents in a muscle. [NIH]

Exhaustion: The feeling of weariness of mind and body. [NIH]

Extender: Any of several colloidal substances of high molecular weight, used as a blood or plasma substitute in transfusion for increasing the volume of the circulating blood. [NIH]

Gravis: Eruption of watery blisters on the skin among those handling animals and animal products. [NIH]

Involuntary: Reaction occurring without intention or volition. [NIH]

Ligands: A RNA simulation method developed by the MIT. [NIH]

Migration: The systematic movement of genes between populations of the same species, geographic race, or variety. [NIH]

Pacemakers: A center or a substance that controls the rhythm of a body process; the term usually refers to the cardiac pacemaker. [NIH]

Phenyl: Ingredient used in cold and flu remedies. [NIH]

Prone: Having the front portion of the body downwards. [NIH]

CHAPTER 5. BOOKS ON SLEEP APNEA

Overview

This chapter provides bibliographic book references relating to sleep apnea. You have many options to locate books on sleep apnea. The simplest method is to go to your local bookseller and inquire about titles that they have in stock or can special order for you. Some patients, however, feel uncomfortable approaching their local booksellers and prefer online sources (e.g. **www.amazon.com** and **www.bn.com**). In addition to online booksellers, excellent sources for book titles on sleep apnea include the Combined Health Information Database and the National Library of Medicine. Once you have found a title that interests you, visit your local public or medical library to see if it is available for loan.

Book Summaries: Federal Agencies

The Combined Health Information Database collects various book abstracts from a variety of healthcare institutions and federal agencies. To access these summaries, go directly to **http://chid.nih.gov/detail/detail.html**. You will need to use the "Detailed Search" option. To find book summaries, use the drop boxes at the bottom of the search page where "You may refine your search by." Select the dates and language you prefer. For the format option, select "Monograph/Book." Now type "sleep apnea" (or synonyms) into the "For these words:" box. You will only receive results on books. You should check back periodically with this database which is updated every 3 months. The following is a typical result when searching for books on sleep apnea:

- **Mayo Clinic on High Blood Pressure**

  Source: New York, NY: Kensington Publishing. 1999. 180 p.

Contact: Available from Mayo Clinic. 200 First Street, S.W., Rochester, MN 55905. (800) 291-1128 or (507) 284-2511. Fax (507) 284-0161. Website: www.mayo.edu. PRICE: $14.95 plus shipping and handling. ISBN: 1893005011.

Summary: This book focuses on what people who have high blood pressure can do to better manage their blood pressure and keep it at a safe level. The book begins with a chapter that explains the basics of blood pressure, how high blood pressure develops, and why it can be harmful. This is followed by a chapter that identifies unmodifiable and modifiable risk factors for high blood pressure. Unmodifiable risk factors include race, age, family history, and gender. Modifiable risk factors include obesity, inactivity, tobacco use, sodium sensitivity, low potassium, excessive alcohol consumption, stress, chronic illness, high cholesterol, diabetes, **sleep apnea,** and heart failure. Other topics addressed in this chapter include secondary high blood pressure and ways of preventing high blood pressure. The third chapter focuses on the diagnosis and treatment of high blood pressure. Topics include measuring blood pressure, receiving a diagnosis, getting a medical evaluation, and deciding on treatment with either medication or lifestyle changes. Subsequent chapters discuss determining a healthy weight, losing weight, becoming more physically active, and eating well using the Dietary Approaches to Stop Hypertension (DASH) plan. The following chapters detail the effects of sodium, tobacco, alcohol, caffeine, and stress on blood pressure. Another chapter focuses on the mode of action and side effects of various medications used in controlling high blood pressure, including diuretics, beta blockers, angiotensin-converting enzyme inhibitors, angiotensin II receptor blockers, calcium antagonists, alpha blockers, central acting agents, and direct vasodilators. Remaining chapters examine factors unique to women, management of high blood pressure among specific populations and groups, treatment of difficult-to-control high blood pressure, management of a hypertensive emergency, and home monitoring of blood pressure. The book also includes a week of menus based on the recommendations of the DASH eating plan. 17 figures. 2 tables.

- **Annual Review of Diabetes 2003**

  Source: Alexandria, VA: American Diabetes Association. 2003. 168 p.

  Contact: Available from American Diabetes Association. 1701 North Beauregard Street, Alexandria, VA 22311. (800) 232-3472. E-mail: AskADA@diabetes.org. Fax: (770) 442-9742. Website: www.diabetes.org. PRICE: $49.95 plus shipping and handling.

Summary: This issue of the Annual Review of Diabetes includes twenty research articles in three categories: epidemiology and pathogenesis, treatment, and complications. Specific topics include the rise of childhood type 1 diabetes in the 20th century; immunological markers in the diagnosis and prediction of autoimmune type 1a diabetes; adults with prediabetes; the energy homeostasis system and weight gain; the metabolic syndrome and incidence of type 2 diabetes; the peroxisome proliferator; the use of oral glucose tolerance tests in clinical practice; the economic costs of diabetes in the United States; diet and exercise among adults with type 2 diabetes; trends for achieving weight loss and increased physical activity; postprandial (after a meal) glucose control; strategies for the treatment of dyslipidemia; self-management education of adults with type 2 diabetes and its impact on glycemic control; common drug pathways and interactions; the interactions of prescribed medications and over-the-counter medications; obstructive **sleep apnea** in patients with diabetes; gestational diabetes and the incidence of type 2 diabetes; glucose monitoring in gestational diabetes; genetic studies of late diabetes complications; and eating disorders in adolescent girls and young adult women with type 1 diabetes. Each article concludes with a list of references.

- **Ear, Nose, and Throat Disorders Sourcebook**

  Source: Detroit, MI: Omnigraphics, Inc. 1998. 576 p.

  Contact: Available from Omnigraphics, Inc. Penobscot Building, Detroit, MI 48226. (800) 234-1340. Fax (800) 875-1340. PRICE: $78.00. ISBN: 0780802063.

  Summary: This reference book provides information about some of the most common disorders of the ears, nose, and throat. The text describes diseases and their accompanying symptoms, as well as treatment options and current research initiatives. The book's 67 chapters are arranged in six parts: introduction, disorders of the inner and outer ear, vestibular disorders, disorders of the nose and sinuses, disorders of the throat, and cancers related to the ears, nose, and throat. Specific disorders and topics include otitis externa, otitis media, allergy, perforated eardrum, cholesteatoma, otosclerosis, tinnitus, hyperacusis, ear surgery, dizziness, BPPV (benign paraoxysmal positional vertigo), labyrinthitis, Meniere's disease, perilymph fistula, sinusitis, rhinitis, antihistamines, nosebleeds, smell and taste problems, sore throats, hoarseness, swallowing disorders, salivary glands, snoring, **sleep apnea,** spasmodic dysphonia, laryngeal diseases and disorders, smoking cessation, head and neck cancer, cancer of the oral cavity and upper throat, esophageal cancer, and oropharyngeal cancer. Simple line drawings illustrate some of the anatomical concepts discussed. The book also includes a glossary of terms and an annotated directory of organizational resources with addresses, telephone numbers, e-mail addresses, and web site locations.

Book Summaries: Online Booksellers

Commercial Internet-based booksellers, such as Amazon.com and Barnes & Noble.com, offer summaries which have been supplied by each title's publisher. Some summaries also include customer reviews. Your local bookseller may have access to in-house and commercial databases that index all published books (e.g. Books in Print®). The following have been recently listed with online booksellers as relating to sleep apnea (sorted alphabetically by title; follow the hyperlink to view more details at Amazon.com):

- **30 Years Sleep Apnea Syndrome (Respiration)** by G. Barthlen, H. Matthys; ISBN: 3805565836; http://www.amazon.com/exec/obidos/ASIN/3805565836/icongroupinterna
- **GUILLEMINAULT SLEEP APNEA SYNDROMES** by C GUILLEMINAULT; ISBN: 0471608815; http://www.amazon.com/exec/obidos/ASIN/0471608815/icongroupinterna
- **Obstructive Sleep Apnea Syndrome: Clinical Research and Treatment** by Christian Guilleminault, Markku Partinen; ISBN: 0881675857; http://www.amazon.com/exec/obidos/ASIN/0881675857/icongroupinterna
- **Obstructive Sleep Apnea Syndrome: Diagnosis and Treatment (Continuing Education Program (American Academy of Otolaryngology--Head and Neck Surgery Foundation).)** by B. Tucker Woodson, et al; ISBN: 1567720501; http://www.amazon.com/exec/obidos/ASIN/1567720501/icongroupinterna
- **Sleep Apnea and Rhonchopathy: 3rd World Congress on Sleep Apnea and Phonchopathy, Tokyo, September 21-23, 1991** by Kiyoshi Togawa; ISBN: 380555611X; http://www.amazon.com/exec/obidos/ASIN/380555611X/icongroupinterna
- **Snoring and Obstructive Sleep Apnea Syndrome: A Controversial Issue** by J.-P. Guyot; ISBN: 3805571887; http://www.amazon.com/exec/obidos/ASIN/3805571887/icongroupinterna

- **Snoring Can Kill!!: Discover How Sleep Apnea Can Be Ruining Your Life** by Joseph L. Goldstein; ISBN: 0966893956; http://www.amazon.com/exec/obidos/ASIN/0966893956/icongroupinterna

Chapters on Sleep Apnea

Frequently, sleep apnea will be discussed within a book, perhaps within a specific chapter. In order to find chapters that are specifically dealing with sleep apnea, an excellent source of abstracts is the Combined Health Information Database. You will need to limit your search to book chapters and sleep apnea using the "Detailed Search" option. Go directly to the following hyperlink: **http://chid.nih.gov/detail/detail.html**. To find book chapters, use the drop boxes at the bottom of the search page where "You may refine your search by." Select the dates and language you prefer, and the format option "Book Chapter." By making these selections and typing in "sleep apnea" (or synonyms) into the "For these words:" box, you will only receive results on chapters in books. The following is a typical result when searching for book chapters on sleep apnea:

- **Respiratory Disorders**

  Source: in Scully, C. and Cawson, R.A. Medical Problems in Dentistry. 4th ed. Woburn, MA: Butterworth-Heinemann. 1998. p. 154-172.

  Contact: Available from Butterworth-Heinemann. 225 Wildwood Avenue, Woburn, MA 01801-2041. (800) 366-2665 or (781) 904-2500. Fax (800) 446-6520 or (781) 933-6333. E-mail: orders@bhusa.com. Website: www.bh.com. PRICE: $110.00. ISBN: 0723610568.

  Summary: Respiratory disorders are common and may significantly affect dental treatment, especially general anesthesia. Respiratory diseases are often also a contraindication to opioids, benzodiazepines and other respiratory depressants. This chapter on respiratory disorders is from a text that covers the general medical and surgical conditions relevant to the oral health care sciences. Topics include upper respiratory tract viral infections, sinusitis, lower respiratory tract infections, pulmonary tuberculosis, Legionnaire's disease (legionellosis), lung abscess, bronchiectasis, cystic fibrosis, chronic obstructive airways diseases, asthma, bronchogenic carcinoma (lung cancer), occupational lung disease, sarcoidosis, postoperative respiratory complications (including aspiration of gastric contents), obstructive **sleep apnea** syndrome, and respiratory distress syndromes (RDS). For each disease, the authors discuss general aspects, diagnosis and management issues, dental aspects, and patient care strategies. The chapter includes a summary of the points covered. 1 figure. 5 tables. 51 references.

- **Oral Surgery**

  Source: in Sutton, A.L. Dental Care and Oral Health Sourcebook. 2nd ed. Detroit, MI: Omnigraphics. 2003. p. 295-312.

  Contact: Available from Omnigraphics. 615 Griswold Street, Detroit, MI 48226. (313) 961-1340. Fax: (313) 961-1383. E-mail: progers@omnigraphics.com. www.omnigraphics.com. PRICE: $78.00; plus shipping and handling. ISBN: 780806344.

  Summary: The scope of oral and maxillofacial surgery encompasses the diagnosis, surgical and related management of diseases, injuries, and defects that involve both the functional and esthetic aspects of the oral and maxillofacial regions. This includes preventive, reconstructive, or emergency care for the teeth, mouth, jaws, and facial structures. After four years of postgraduate dental education, an oral and maxillofacial surgeon completes four or more years of intensive, postdoctoral, hospital-based surgical residency training. This chapter on oral surgery is from a book that provides information about dental care and oral health at all stages of life. The chapter offers four sections: a description of the oral and maxillofacial surgeon specialty; a description of oral and maxillofacial surgery; corrective jaw surgery; and nutrition after oral surgery. Specific topics include office surgery, dentoalveolar surgery, reconstructive surgery, dental implants, facial infections, facial trauma, facial pain, oral pathology, orofacial deformities, snoring and obstructive **sleep apnea,** cosmetic maxillofacial surgery, impacted teeth, unequal jaw growth, dentures, and nutritional strategies. The chapter includes nutritious, calorie-dense recipes for food ideas during the convalescence period after oral surgery.

- **How Vocal Abilities Can Be Limited by Anatomical Abnormalities and Bodily Injuries**

  Source: in Thurman, L. and Welch, G., eds. Bodymind and Voice: Foundations of Voice Education, Volumes 1-3. 2nd ed. Collegeville, MN: VoiceCare Network. 2000. p. 582-585.

  Contact: Available from National Center for Voice and Speech (NCVS). Book Sales, 334 Speech and Hearing Center, University of Iowa, Iowa City, IA 52242. Website: www.ncvs.org. PRICE: $75.00 plus shipping and handling. ISBN: 0874141230.

  Summary: This chapter on anatomical abnormalities and bodily injuries is from a multi-volume text that brings a biopsychosocial approach to the study of the voice. The authors use the phrase 'bodyminds' to describe the interrelationship of perception, memory, learning, behavior, and health, as they combine to affect all environmental interactions, adaptations, and learning. The books are written for teachers, voice professionals, people who use their voices on an avocational basis, and interested members of the general public. This chapter notes that malformations of auditory (hearing) and neural vocal anatomy can have genetic sources, and can lead to abnormalities of speaking or singing functions. Insufficient sensorimotor stimulation during late gestation and childhood can result in underdeveloped neural networks, suboptimum neural capabilities, or functional abnormalities that can affect vocal self expression. Bodily injuries of many types and in many different parts of the body also can impact upon voice and speech. Manifestations of injury may be subtle and short lived, or overt and permanent. The chapter covers morphologic voice disorders, including laryngeal webs, congenital anomalies of the vocal tract, obstructive **sleep apnea** syndrome (OSAS), swollen soft palate, short soft palate, cleft palate, and enlarged turbinates; and injury to vocal skeleton or soft tissues, including trauma to the anterior neck or cervical spine, laryngeal fracture, mandibular (lower jaw) fracture, trauma to the torso, iatrogenic (physician caused) trauma, recurrent laryngeal nerve injury, vocal fold mucosal scarring, intubation injury, and acquired laryngeal webs. 22 references.

- **Lungs and Pleura**

  Source: in Daugirdas, J.T. and Ing, T.S., eds. Handbook of Dialysis. 2nd ed. Boston, MA: Little, Brown and Company. 1994. p. 598-603.

  Contact: Available from Lippincott-Raven Publishers. 12107 Insurance Way, Hagerstown, MD 21740. (800) 777-2295. Fax (301) 824-7390. E-mail: lrorders@phl.lrpub.com. Website: http://www.lrpub.com. PRICE: $37.95. ISBN: 0316173835.

  Summary: This chapter on complications affecting the lungs and pleura is from a handbook that outlines all aspects of dialysis therapy, emphasizing the management of dialysis patients. Topics include pulmonary edema, pleural effusion, infection, dyspnea during dialysis, respiratory failure due to hyperkalemia, hypophosphatemia, or glucose load, dosages of pulmonary drugs in dialysis patients, and **sleep apnea** syndrome in dialysis patients. The author presents information in outline form, for easy reference. 17 references.

- **How Vocal Abilities Can Be Limited by Non-Infectious Diseases and Disorders of the Respiratory and Digestive Systems**

  Source: in Thurman, L. and Welch, G., eds. Bodymind and Voice: Foundations of Voice Education, Volumes 1-3. 2nd ed. Collegeville, MN: VoiceCare Network. 2000. p. 546-555.

  Contact: Available from National Center for Voice and Speech (NCVS). Book Sales, 334 Speech and Hearing Center, University of Iowa, Iowa City, IA 52242. Website: www.ncvs.org. PRICE: $75.00 plus shipping and handling. ISBN: 0874141230.

  Summary: This chapter on noninfectious diseases and disorders of the respiratory and digestive systems is from a multi-volume text that brings a biopsychosocial approach to the study of the voice. The authors use the phrase 'bodyminds' to describe the interrelationship of perception, memory, learning, behavior, and health, as they combine to affect all environmental interactions, adaptations, and learning. The books are written for teachers, voice professionals, people who use their voices on an avocational basis, and interested members of the general public. This chapter describes the effects of smoking and other pollutants, sinusitis and rhinitis, laryngitis, bronchitis and other pulmonary (lung) diseases, the effects of outdoor and indoor air pollution, normal and disordered nasal (nose) conditions, asthma, obstructive **sleep apnea,** emphysema, and gastroesophageal reflux disease (GERD, the return of stomach acid to the esophagus and larynx). GERD can result in hoarseness, lowering of the average speaking pitch range, increased effort when singing, and a 'tired voice.' Asthma can affect voice primarily by decreasing the ability of the respiratory system to inhale and then pressurize the lung air to create sufficient breathflow between the vocal folds. Asthma symptoms can be triggered by inhalation of allergens or pollutant particles of irritant chemicals, infection, cold air, vigorous exercise, acute neuropsychobiological distress, or even vigorous singing. 68 references.

- **Pediatric Phonatory Disorders**

  Source: in Andrews, M.L. Manual of Voice Treatment: Pediatrics Through Geriatrics. 2nd ed. San Diego, CA: Singular Publishing Group, Inc. 1999. p. 151-217.

  Contact: Available from Singular Publishing Group, Inc. 401 West 'A' Street, Suite 325, San Diego, CA 92101-7904. (800) 521-8545 or (619) 238-6777. Fax (800) 774-8398 or (619) 238-6789. E-mail: singpub@singpub.com. Website: www.singpub.com. PRICE: $55.00 plus shipping and handling. ISBN: 1565939880.

Summary: This chapter on pediatric phonatory disorders is from a resource book for clinicians and clinicians in training who are treating patients with voice disorders. The chapter offers five sections: preschool children, school age children, pediatric voice problems associated with other conditions (hearing impairment, cerebral palsy, craniofacial dysmorphology, nasal obstruction, obstructive **sleep apnea** syndrome, trauma, lesions), the voice at puberty, and the treatment of resonance disorders. The chapter discusses the physiologic systems relevant to voice production from a developmental perspective. To emphasize the importance of complete case history information, the relevance of the possible effects on voice of infant airway obstruction and medical and surgical treatments to alleviate it are reviewed. Other topics include the reasons for tracheotomy and possible complications and sequelae of this surgery; the common symptoms of vocal disruption in school age children; hyperfunctional and hypofunctional patterns associated with respiration, phonation, resonance, and psychodynamics; and the importance of explaining the effects of specific voice disorders in children to their parents, teachers, and allied health professionals. 9 figures. 3 tables.

- **Voice Surgery**

  Source: in Sataloff, R.T., ed. Professional Voice: The Science and Art of Clinical Care. 2nd ed. San Diego, CA: Singular Publishing Group, Inc. 1997. p. 603-645.

  Contact: Available from Singular Publishing Group, Inc. 401 West 'A' Street, Suite 325, San Diego, CA 92101-7904. (800) 521-8545 or (619) 238-6777. Fax (800) 774-8398 or (619) 238-6789. E-mail: singpub@singpub.com. Website: www.singpub.com. PRICE: $325.00 plus shipping and handling. ISBN: 1565937287.

  Summary: This chapter, from a book on the clinical care of the professional voice, reviews the current thinking regarding voice surgery. Most surgical procedures for voice disorders can be performed endoscopically, obviating the need for external incisions and minimizing the amount of tissue disruption. The author stresses that, when endoscopic visualization is not adequate because of patient anatomy, disease extent, or other factors, the surgeon should not compromise the results of treatment or risk patient injury by attempting to complete an endoscopic procedure. Topics include patient selection and consent, documentation (preoperative assessment), timing of voice surgery, indirect laryngoscopy, direct laryngoscopy, anesthesia (local and general), instrumentation, laryngeal microsurgery, contact endoscopy, vocal fold cysts, vocal fold polyps, varicosities and ectatic vessels and vocal fold hemorrhage, Reinke's edema, granulomas and vocal process ulcers, papillomas, ventricular fold cysts, epiglottic cysts, laryngoceles, miscellaneous masses, sulcus vocalis, laryngeal webs, bowed vocal folds, presbyphonia, vocal fold paralysis and framework dysfunction, Teflon injection, Gelfoam injection, collagen injection, autologous fat injection, removal of Teflon, thyroplasty, nomenclature, arytenoid adduction or rotation, nerve anastomosis, nerve muscle pedicle surgery, arytenoid reduction for arytenoid dislocation, arytenoidectomy, voice rest, and related surgery, including that for velopharyngeal insufficiency and obstructive **sleep apnea** syndrome in professional voice users. 31 figures. 1 table. 99 references.

- **Oral Cavity, Pharynx and Esophagus**

  Source: in Strome, M.; Kelly, J.H.; Fried, M.P., eds. Manual of Otolaryngology: Diagnosis and Therapy. 2nd ed. Boston, MA: Little, Brown and Company. 1992. p. 137-171.

  Contact: Available from Little, Brown and Company. 34 Beacon Street, Boston, MA 02108. (800) 759-0190. PRICE: $27.50 plus shipping and handling. ISBN: 0316819689.

  Summary: This chapter, from a reference manual detailing the essentials of otolaryngology and head and neck surgery, discusses the oral cavity, pharynx, and esophagus. Topics covered include oropharyngeal anatomy; physical examination of the pharynx; infectious pharyngitis, including acute bacterial pharyngotonsillitis, diptheria, infectious mononucleosis, Vincent's angina, candidiasis, syphilis, gonococcal pharyngitis, tuberculosis, viral pharyngitis, lingual tonsillitis, nasopharyngitis, and AIDS; noninfectious etiology, including pemphigus, retropharyngeal abscess, parapharyngeal abscess, and submandibular space abscess (Ludwig's angina); allergic edema; tissue hypertrophy, including adenotonsillar hypertrophy, and obstructive **sleep apnea;** congenital obstruction, including Pierre-Robin syndrome, Thornwald's bursa or nasopharyngeal cyst, and choanal atresia; cysts and neoplasms; dysphasia; and esophageal disorders. The manual summarizes the signs and symptoms, diagnosis, and treatment for each disease or disorder. 26 references.

General Home References

In addition to references for sleep apnea, you may want a general home medical guide that spans all aspects of home healthcare. The following list is a recent sample of such guides (sorted alphabetically by title; hyperlinks provide rankings, information, and reviews at Amazon.com):

- **100 Questions About Sleep and Sleep Disorders** by Sudhansu Chokroverty, M.D.; Paperback - 110 pages, 1st edition (February 15, 2001), Blackwell Science Inc; ISBN: 0865425833; **http://www.amazon.com/exec/obidos/ASIN/0865425833/icongroupinterna**
- **The Bible Cure for Sleep Disorders** by Don Colbert; Paperback - 96 pages (March 2001), Siloam Press; ISBN: 0884197484; **http://www.amazon.com/exec/obidos/ASIN/0884197484/icongroupinterna**
- **Sleep and Its Disorders : What You Should Know** by Robert G. Hooper, M.D., Melissa Mulera (Illustrator); Paperback - 176 pages (January 2001), Just Peachy Press; ISBN: 0970002645; **http://www.amazon.com/exec/obidos/ASIN/0970002645/icongroupinterna**
- **Sleep Disorders Sourcebook: Basic Consumer Health Information About Sleep and Its Disorders, Including Insomnia, Sleepwalking, Sleep Apmea, Restless)** by Jenifer Swanson (Editor); Library Binding - 600 pages (January 1999), Omnigraphics, Inc.; ISBN: 0780802349; **http://www.amazon.com/exec/obidos/ASIN/0780802349/icongroupinterna**
- **Sleeping Well: The Sourcebook for Sleep and Sleep Disorders (The Facts for Life)** by Michael J. Thorpy, M.D., Jan Yager; Paperback - 342 pages (October 2001), Checkmark Books; ISBN: 0816040907; **http://www.amazon.com/exec/obidos/ASIN/0816040907/icongroupinterna**

Vocabulary Builder

Abscess: A localized, circumscribed collection of pus. [NIH]

Adduction: The rotation of an eye toward the midline (nasally). [NIH]

Dysphonia: Difficulty or pain in speaking; impairment of the voice. [NIH]

Eardrum: A thin, tense membrane forming the greater part of the outer wall of the tympanic cavity and separating it from the external auditory meatus; it constitutes the boundary between the external and middle ear. [NIH]

Infections: The illnesses caused by an organism that usually does not cause disease in a person with a normal immune system. [NIH]

Microsurgery: Surgical procedures on the cellular level; a light microscope and miniaturized instruments are used. [NIH]

Networks: Pertaining to a nerve or to the nerves, a meshlike structure of interlocking fibers or strands. [NIH]

Palsy: Disease of the peripheral nervous system occurring usually after many years of increased lead absorption. [NIH]

Papilloma: A benign epithelial neoplasm which may arise from the skin, mucous membranes or glandular ducts. [NIH]

Paralysis: Loss or impairment of muscle function or sensation. [NIH]

Pedicle: Embryonic link between the optic vesicle or optic cup and the forebrain or diencephalon, which becomes the optic nerve. [NIH]

Perilymph: The fluid contained within the space separating the membranous from the osseous labyrinth of the ear. [NIH]

Pitch: The subjective awareness of the frequency or spectral distribution of a sound. [NIH]

Pleural: A circumscribed area of hyaline whorled fibrous tissue which appears on the surface of the parietal pleura, on the fibrous part of the diaphragm or on the pleura in the interlobar fissures. [NIH]

Potassium: It is essential to the ability of muscle cells to contract. [NIH]

Salivary: The duct that convey saliva to the mouth. [NIH]

Submandibular: Four to six lymph glands, located between the lower jaw and the submandibular salivary gland. [NIH]

Trauma: Any injury, wound, or shock, must frequently physical or structural shock, producing a disturbance. [NIH]

Ulcer: A localized necrotic lesion of the skin or a mucous surface. [NIH]

Vasodilators: Any nerve or agent which induces dilatation of the blood vessels. [NIH]

CHAPTER 6. PERIODICALS AND NEWS ON SLEEP APNEA

Overview

Keeping up on the news relating to sleep apnea can be challenging. Subscribing to targeted periodicals can be an effective way to stay abreast of recent developments on sleep apnea. Periodicals include newsletters, magazines, and academic journals.

In this chapter, we suggest a number of news sources and present various periodicals that cover sleep apnea beyond and including those which are published by patient associations mentioned earlier. We will first focus on news services, and then on periodicals. News services, press releases, and newsletters generally use more accessible language, so if you do chose to subscribe to one of the more technical periodicals, make sure that it uses language you can easily follow.

News Services and Press Releases

Well before articles show up in newsletters or the popular press, they may appear in the form of a press release or a public relations announcement. One of the simplest ways of tracking press releases on sleep apnea is to search the news wires. News wires are used by professional journalists, and have existed since the invention of the telegraph. Today, there are several major "wires" that are used by companies, universities, and other organizations to announce new medical breakthroughs. In the following sample of sources, we will briefly describe how to access each service. These services only post recent news intended for public viewing.

PR Newswire

Perhaps the broadest of the wires is PR Newswire Association, Inc. To access this archive, simply go to **http://www.prnewswire.com**. Below the search box, select the option "The last 30 days." In the search box, type "sleep apnea" or synonyms. The search results are shown by order of relevance. When reading these press releases, do not forget that the sponsor of the release may be a company or organization that is trying to sell a particular product or therapy. Their views, therefore, may be biased.

Reuters Health

The Reuters' Medical News and Health eLine databases can be very useful in exploring news archives relating to sleep apnea. While some of the listed articles are free to view, others can be purchased for a nominal fee. To access this archive, go to **http://www.reutershealth.com/en/index.html** and search by "sleep apnea" (or synonyms). The following was recently listed in this archive for sleep apnea:

- **Obstructive sleep apnea treatment improves cardiovascular outcomes**
  Source: Reuters Medical News
  Date: June 16, 2004
- **Treating sleep apnea could cut road deaths**
  Source: Reuters Health eLine
  Date: May 07, 2004
- **Most sleep apnea patients can go home after surgery**
  Source: Reuters Health eLine
  Date: April 30, 2004
- **No link found between SIDS and obstructive sleep apnea in parents**
  Source: Reuters Medical News
  Date: April 05, 2004
- **White coat hypertension common in sleep apnea patients**
  Source: Reuters Medical News
  Date: March 29, 2004
- **Treatment of sleep apnea offers many benefits for CHF patients**
  Source: Reuters Medical News
  Date: February 10, 2004
- **Intranasal steroids curb sleep apnea severity in patients with rhinitis**
  Source: Reuters Industry Breifing
  Date: January 16, 2004

- **Home oximetry fails to reliably detect obstructive sleep apnea in children**
  Source: Reuters Medical News
  Date: December 26, 2003
- **CORRECTION: Obstructive sleep apnea may impair insulin sensitivity in obesity**
  Source: Reuters Medical News
  Date: September 22, 2003
- **Children with obstructive sleep apnea show distinct pattern of airway motion**
  Source: Reuters Medical News
  Date: May 05, 2003
- **CPAP improves heart failure and sleep apnea in patients with both disorders**
  Source: Reuters Medical News
  Date: March 26, 2003
- **Viasys gets FDA clearance for new sleep apnea system**
  Source: Reuters Industry Breifing
  Date: January 28, 2003
- **Headaches common in sleep apnea patients**
  Source: Reuters Medical News
  Date: August 16, 2002
- **Viasys sleep apnea device gains FDA clearance**
  Source: Reuters Industry Breifing
  Date: May 28, 2002
- **Study links sleep apnea with risk of blood clots**
  Source: Reuters Health eLine
  Date: May 21, 2002
- **Favorable results of laser surgery for sleep apnea deteriorate with time**
  Source: Reuters Medical News
  Date: April 15, 2002
- **Dental appliances improves sleep apnea index without adverse effects**
  Source: Reuters Medical News
  Date: March 26, 2002
- **Atrial overdrive pacing reduces sleep apnea episodes in bradycardia patients**
  Source: Reuters Medical News
  Date: February 06, 2002

- **Obstructive sleep apnea linked to peripheral vasoconstriction**
  Source: Reuters Medical News
  Date: January 28, 2002
- **Size of upper airway explains lower prevalence of sleep apnea in women**
  Source: Reuters Medical News
  Date: November 27, 2001
- **CPAP improves cardiac function in sleep apnea patients**
  Source: Reuters Medical News
  Date: October 09, 2001
- **Cephalon's Provigil looks promising as adjunct in sleep apnea patients**
  Source: Reuters Industry Breifing
  Date: October 09, 2001
- **Short trial of CPAP for sleep apnea predicts long-term use**
  Source: Reuters Medical News
  Date: September 05, 2001
- **Treating sleep apnea reduces car crash risk**
  Source: Reuters Health eLine
  Date: June 19, 2001

The NIH

Within MEDLINEplus, the NIH has made an agreement with the New York Times Syndicate, the AP News Service, and Reuters to deliver news that can be browsed by the public. Search news releases at **http://www.nlm.nih.gov/medlineplus/alphanews_a.html.** MEDLINEplus allows you to browse across an alphabetical index. Or you can search by date at **http://www.nlm.nih.gov/medlineplus/newsbydate.html**. Often, news items are indexed by MEDLINEplus within their search engine.

Business Wire

Business Wire is similar to PR Newswire. To access this archive, simply go to **http://www.businesswire.com**. You can scan the news by industry category or company name.

Market Wire

Market Wire is more focused on technology than the other wires. To browse the latest press releases by topic, such as alternative medicine, biotechnology, fitness, healthcare, legal, nutrition, and pharmaceuticals, log on to Market Wire's Medical/Health channel at the following hyperlink **http://www.marketwire.com/mw/release_index?channel=MedicalHealth**. Market Wire's home page is **http://www.marketwire.com/mw/home**. From here, type "sleep apnea" (or synonyms) into the search box, and click on "Search News." As this service is technology oriented, you may wish to use it when searching for press releases covering diagnostic procedures or tests.

Search Engines

Free-to-view news can also be found in the news section of your favorite search engines (see the health news page at Yahoo: **http://dir.yahoo.com/Health/News_and_Media/,** or use this Web site's general news search page **http://news.yahoo.com/.** Type in "sleep apnea" (or synonyms). If you know the name of a company that is relevant to sleep apnea, you can go to any stock trading Web site (such as **www.etrade.com**) and search for the company name there. News items across various news sources are reported on indicated hyperlinks.

BBC

Covering news from a more European perspective, the British Broadcasting Corporation (BBC) allows the public free access to their news archive located at **http://www.bbc.co.uk/**. Search by "sleep apnea" (or synonyms).

Newsletters on Sleep Apnea

Given their focus on current and relevant developments, newsletters are often more useful to patients than academic articles. You can find newsletters using the Combined Health Information Database (CHID). You will need to use the "Detailed Search" option. To access CHID, go directly to the following hyperlink: **http://chid.nih.gov/detail/detail.html**. Your investigation must limit the search to "Newsletter" and "sleep apnea." Go to the bottom of the search page where "You may refine your search by." Select the dates and language that you prefer. For the format option, select "Newsletter." By making these selections and typing in "sleep apnea" or synonyms into the "For these words:" box, you will only receive results on newsletters. The following list was generated using the options described above:

- **Wake-Up Call: The Wellness Letter for Snoring and Apnea**

  Source: Washington, DC: American Sleep Apnea Association. 1994-.

  Contact: Available from American Sleep Apnea Association, 2025 Pennsylvania Avenue, NW, Suite 905, Washington, DC 20006. (202) 293-3650, (202) 293-3656 (Fax), asaa@nicom.com (Email), http://www.asaa@nicom.com (Website). Free with membership fee of $25.00 to persons living in the U.S.; membership fee is $50.00 for persons living outside the U.S.

  Summary: This newsletter is intended to keep snorers and sufferers of **sleep apnea** up to date on the treatment and management of these conditions. A typical issue includes articles on treatment and management, medical complications associated with the disorders (e.g., cardiovascular disease), risk factors for apnea, funding for research, patient advocacy, health policy, and public health campaigns; a question-and-answer column written by a sleep disorders specialist; and information on the activities of the AWAKE (Alert, Well and Keeping Energetic) Network, a nationwide network of mutual help and health awareness groups for individuals who suffer from sleep-disordered breathing.

Academic Periodicals covering Sleep Apnea

Academic periodicals can be a highly technical yet valuable source of information on sleep apnea. We have compiled the following list of periodicals known to publish articles relating to sleep apnea and which are currently indexed within the National Library of Medicine's PubMed database (follow hyperlinks to view more information, summaries, etc., for each). In addition to these sources, to keep current on articles written on sleep apnea published by any of the periodicals listed below, you can simply follow the hyperlink indicated or go to **www.ncbi.nlm.nih.gov/pubmed**. Type the periodical's name into the search box to find the latest studies published.

If you want complete details about the historical contents of a periodical, you can also visit **http://www.ncbi.nlm.nih.gov/entrez/jrbrowser.cgi**. Here, type in the name of the journal or its abbreviation, and you will receive an index of published articles. At **http://locatorplus.gov/** you can retrieve more indexing information on medical periodicals (e.g. the name of the publisher). Select the button "Search LOCATORplus." Then type in the name of the journal and select the advanced search option "Journal Title Search." The following is a sample of periodicals which publish articles on sleep apnea:

- **Aana Journal. (AANA J)**
  http://www.ncbi.nlm.nih.gov/entrez/jrbrowser.cgi?field=0®exp=Aana+Journal&dispmax=20&dispstart=0

- **Acta Anaesthesiologica Scandinavica. (Acta Anaesthesiol Scand)**
  http://www.ncbi.nlm.nih.gov/entrez/jrbrowser.cgi?field=0®exp=Acta+Anaesthesiologica+Scandinavica&dispmax=20&dispstart=0

- **Acta Neurologica Scandinavica. (Acta Neurol Scand)**
  http://www.ncbi.nlm.nih.gov/entrez/jrbrowser.cgi?field=0®exp=Acta+Neurologica+Scandinavica&dispmax=20&dispstart=0

- **Acta Odontologica Scandinavica. (Acta Odontol Scand)**
  http://www.ncbi.nlm.nih.gov/entrez/jrbrowser.cgi?field=0®exp=Acta+Odontologica+Scandinavica&dispmax=20&dispstart=0

- **Acta Oto-Laryngologica. (Acta Otolaryngol)**
  http://www.ncbi.nlm.nih.gov/entrez/jrbrowser.cgi?field=0®exp=Acta+Oto-Laryngologica&dispmax=20&dispstart=0

- **Ajr. American Journal of Roentgenology. (AJR Am J Roentgenol)**
  http://www.ncbi.nlm.nih.gov/entrez/jrbrowser.cgi?field=0®exp=Ajr.+American+Journal+of+Roentgenology&dispmax=20&dispstart=0

- **Allergy and Asthma Proceedings : the Official Journal of Regional and State Allergy Societies. (Allergy Asthma Proc)**
  http://www.ncbi.nlm.nih.gov/entrez/jrbrowser.cgi?field=0®exp=Allergy+and+Asthma+Proceedings+:+the+Official+Journal+of+Regional+and+State+Allergy+Societies&dispmax=20&dispstart=0

- **American Family Physician. (Am Fam Physician)**
  http://www.ncbi.nlm.nih.gov/entrez/jrbrowser.cgi?field=0®exp=American+Family+Physician&dispmax=20&dispstart=0

- **American Journal of Hypertension : Journal of the American Society of Hypertension. (Am J Hypertens)**
http://www.ncbi.nlm.nih.gov/entrez/jrbrowser.cgi?field=0®exp=American+Journal+of+Hypertension+:+Journal+of+the+American+Society+of+Hypertension&dispmax=20&dispstart=0

- **American Journal of Ophthalmology. (Am J Ophthalmol)**
http://www.ncbi.nlm.nih.gov/entrez/jrbrowser.cgi?field=0®exp=American+Journal+of+Ophthalmology&dispmax=20&dispstart=0

- **American Journal of Orthodontics and Dentofacial Orthopedics : Official Publication of the American Association of Orthodontists, Its Constituent Societies, and the American Board of Orthodontics. (Am J Orthod Dentofacial Orthop)**
http://www.ncbi.nlm.nih.gov/entrez/jrbrowser.cgi?field=0®exp=American+Journal+of+Orthodontics+and+Dentofacial+Orthopedics+:+Official+Publication+of+the+American+Association+of+Orthodontists,+Its+Constituent+Societies,+and+the+American+Board+of+Orthodon

  <Title>American Journal of Otolaryngology. (Am J Otolaryngol)
http://www.ncbi.nlm.nih.gov/entrez/jrbrowser.cgi?field=0®exp=American+Journal+of+Otolaryngology&dispmax=20&dispstart=0

- **American Journal of Physical Medicine & Rehabilitation / Association of Academic Physiatrists. (Am J Phys Med Rehabil)**
http://www.ncbi.nlm.nih.gov/entrez/jrbrowser.cgi?field=0®exp=American+Journal+of+Physical+Medicine+&+Rehabilitation+/+Association+of+Academic+Physiatrists&dispmax=20&dispstart=0

- **American Journal of Physiology. Heart and Circulatory Physiology. (Am J Physiol Heart Circ Physiol)**
http://www.ncbi.nlm.nih.gov/entrez/jrbrowser.cgi?field=0®exp=American+Journal+of+Physiology.+Heart+and+Circulatory+Physiology&dispmax=20&dispstart=0

- **American Journal of Respiratory and Critical Care Medicine. (Am J Respir Crit Care Med)**
http://www.ncbi.nlm.nih.gov/entrez/jrbrowser.cgi?field=0®exp=American+Journal+of+Respiratory+and+Critical+Care+Medicine&dispmax=20&dispstart=0

- **American Journal of Respiratory Medicine : Drugs, Devices, and Other Interventions. (Am J Respir Med)**
http://www.ncbi.nlm.nih.gov/entrez/jrbrowser.cgi?field=0®exp=American+Journal+of+Respiratory+Medicine+:+Drugs,+Devices,+and+Other+Interventions&dispmax=20&dispstart=0

- **American Journal of Rhinology. (Am J Rhinol)**
http://www.ncbi.nlm.nih.gov/entrez/jrbrowser.cgi?field=0®exp=American+Journal+of+Rhinology&dispmax=20&dispstart=0

- **Anesthesia and Analgesia. (Anesth Analg)**
http://www.ncbi.nlm.nih.gov/entrez/jrbrowser.cgi?field=0®exp=Anesthesia+and+Analgesia&dispmax=20&dispstart=0

- **Annals of Internal Medicine. (Ann Intern Med)**
http://www.ncbi.nlm.nih.gov/entrez/jrbrowser.cgi?field=0®exp=Annals+of+Internal+Medicine&dispmax=20&dispstart=0

- **Annals of Noninvasive Electrocardiology : the Official Journal of the International Society for Holter and Noninvasive Electrocardiology, Inc. (Ann Noninvasive Electrocardiol)**
http://www.ncbi.nlm.nih.gov/entrez/jrbrowser.cgi?field=0®exp=Annals+of+Noninvasive+Electrocardiology+:+the+Official+Journal+of+the+International+Society+for+Holter+and+Noninvasive+Electrocardiology,+Inc&dispmax=20&dispstart=0

- **Annals of Plastic Surgery. (Ann Plast Surg)**
http://www.ncbi.nlm.nih.gov/entrez/jrbrowser.cgi?field=0®exp=Annals+of+Plastic+Surgery&dispmax=20&dispstart=0

- **Archives of Internal Medicine. (Arch Intern Med)**
http://www.ncbi.nlm.nih.gov/entrez/jrbrowser.cgi?field=0®exp=Archives+of+Internal+Medicine&dispmax=20&dispstart=0

- **Archives of Otolaryngology--Head & Neck Surgery. (Arch Otolaryngol Head Neck Surg)**
http://www.ncbi.nlm.nih.gov/entrez/jrbrowser.cgi?field=0®exp=Archives+of+Otolaryngology--Head+&+Neck+Surgery&dispmax=20&dispstart=0

- **Archives of Pediatrics & Adolescent Medicine. (Arch Pediatr Adolesc Med)**
  http://www.ncbi.nlm.nih.gov/entrez/jrbrowser.cgi?field=0®exp=Archives+of+Pediatrics+&+Adolescent+Medicine&dispmax=20&dispstart=0

- **Biological Research for Nursing. (Biol Res Nurs)**
  http://www.ncbi.nlm.nih.gov/entrez/jrbrowser.cgi?field=0®exp=Biological+Research+for+Nursing&dispmax=20&dispstart=0

- **Blood Pressure Monitoring. (Blood Press Monit)**
  http://www.ncbi.nlm.nih.gov/entrez/jrbrowser.cgi?field=0®exp=Blood+Pressure+Monitoring&dispmax=20&dispstart=0

- **Brazilian Journal of Medical and Biological Research = Revista Brasileira De Pesquisas Medicas E Biologicas / Sociedade Brasileira De Biofisica. [et Al.. (Braz J Med Biol Res)**
  http://www.ncbi.nlm.nih.gov/entrez/jrbrowser.cgi?field=0®exp=Brazilian+Journal+of+Medical+and+Biological+Research+=+Revista+Brasileira+De+Pesquisas+Medicas+E+Biologicas+/+Sociedade+Brasileira+De+Biofisica+.+[et+Al.+&dispmax=20&dispstart=0

- **Canadian Journal of Anaesthesia = Journal Canadien D'anesthesie. (Can J Anaesth)**
  http://www.ncbi.nlm.nih.gov/entrez/jrbrowser.cgi?field=0®exp=Canadian+Journal+of+Anaesthesia+=+Journal+Canadien+D'anesthesie&dispmax=20&dispstart=0

- **Chinese Medical Journal. (Chin Med J (Engl))**
  http://www.ncbi.nlm.nih.gov/entrez/jrbrowser.cgi?field=0®exp=Chinese+Medical+Journal&dispmax=20&dispstart=0

- **Clinical Hemorheology and Microcirculation. (Clin Hemorheol Microcirc)**
  http://www.ncbi.nlm.nih.gov/entrez/jrbrowser.cgi?field=0®exp=Clinical+Hemorheology+and+Microcirculation&dispmax=20&dispstart=0

- **Clinics in Chest Medicine. (Clin Chest Med)**
  http://www.ncbi.nlm.nih.gov/entrez/jrbrowser.cgi?field=0®exp=Clinics+in+Chest+Medicine&dispmax=20&dispstart=0

- **Current Hypertension Reports. (Curr Hypertens Rep)**
http://www.ncbi.nlm.nih.gov/entrez/jrbrowser.cgi?field=0®exp=Current+Hypertension+Reports&dispmax=20&dispstart=0

- **Current Opinion in Pulmonary Medicine. (Curr Opin Pulm Med)**
http://www.ncbi.nlm.nih.gov/entrez/jrbrowser.cgi?field=0®exp=Current+Opinion+in+Pulmonary+Medicine&dispmax=20&dispstart=0

- **Early Human Development. (Early Hum Dev)**
http://www.ncbi.nlm.nih.gov/entrez/jrbrowser.cgi?field=0®exp=Early+Human+Development&dispmax=20&dispstart=0

- **Endocrinology and Metabolism Clinics of North America. (Endocrinol Metab Clin North Am)**
http://www.ncbi.nlm.nih.gov/entrez/jrbrowser.cgi?field=0®exp=Endocrinology+and+Metabolism+Clinics+of+North+America&dispmax=20&dispstart=0

- **European Journal of Clinical Investigation. (Eur J Clin Invest)**
http://www.ncbi.nlm.nih.gov/entrez/jrbrowser.cgi?field=0®exp=European+Journal+of+Clinical+Investigation&dispmax=20&dispstart=0

- **European Surgical Research. Europaische Chirurgische Forschung. Recherches Chirurgicales Europeennes. (Eur Surg Res)**
http://www.ncbi.nlm.nih.gov/entrez/jrbrowser.cgi?field=0®exp=European+Surgical+Research.+Europaische+Chirurgische+Forschung.+Recherches+Chirurgicales+Europeennes&dispmax=20&dispstart=0

- **Federal Register. (Fed Regist)**
http://www.ncbi.nlm.nih.gov/entrez/jrbrowser.cgi?field=0®exp=Federal+Register&dispmax=20&dispstart=0

- **Geriatric Nursing (New York, N... (Geriatr Nurs)**
http://www.ncbi.nlm.nih.gov/entrez/jrbrowser.cgi?field=0®exp=Geriatric+Nursing+(New+York,+N.+.+&dispmax=20&dispstart=0

- **Harvard Health Letter / from Harvard Medical School. (Harv Health Lett)**
http://www.ncbi.nlm.nih.gov/entrez/jrbrowser.cgi?field=0®exp=Harvard+Health+Letter+/+from+Harvard+Medical+School&dispmax=20&dispstart=0

- **Ieee Transactions on Bio-Medical Engineering. (IEEE Trans Biomed Eng)**
  http://www.ncbi.nlm.nih.gov/entrez/jrbrowser.cgi?field=0®exp=Ieee+Transactions+on+Bio-Medical+Engineering&dispmax=20&dispstart=0

- **International Journal of Pediatric Otorhinolaryngology. (Int J Pediatr Otorhinolaryngol)**
  http://www.ncbi.nlm.nih.gov/entrez/jrbrowser.cgi?field=0®exp=International+Journal+of+Pediatric+Otorhinolaryngology&dispmax=20&dispstart=0

- **International Journal of Psychiatry in Medicine. (Int J Psychiatry Med)**
  http://www.ncbi.nlm.nih.gov/entrez/jrbrowser.cgi?field=0®exp=International+Journal+of+Psychiatry+in+Medicine&dispmax=20&dispstart=0

- **Jama : the Journal of the American Medical Association. (JAMA)**
  http://www.ncbi.nlm.nih.gov/entrez/jrbrowser.cgi?field=0®exp=Jama+:+the+Journal+of+the+American+Medical+Association&dispmax=20&dispstart=0

- **Journal of Applied Physiology (Bethesda, Md. : 1985). (J Appl Physiol)**
  http://www.ncbi.nlm.nih.gov/entrez/jrbrowser.cgi?field=0®exp=Journal+of+Applied+Physiology+(Bethesda,+Md.+:+1985)&dispmax=20&dispstart=0

- **Journal of Clinical Ultrasound : Jcu. (J Clin Ultrasound)**
  http://www.ncbi.nlm.nih.gov/entrez/jrbrowser.cgi?field=0®exp=Journal+of+Clinical+Ultrasound+:+Jcu&dispmax=20&dispstart=0

- **Journal of Hypertension. (J Hypertens)**
  http://www.ncbi.nlm.nih.gov/entrez/jrbrowser.cgi?field=0®exp=Journal+of+Hypertension&dispmax=20&dispstart=0

- **Journal of Oral and Maxillofacial Surgery : Official Journal of the American Association of Oral and Maxillofacial Surgeons. (J Oral Maxillofac Surg)**
  http://www.ncbi.nlm.nih.gov/entrez/jrbrowser.cgi?field=0®exp=Journal+of+Oral+and+Maxillofacial+Surgery+:+Official+Journal+of+the+American+Association+of+Oral+and+Maxillofacial+Surgeons&dispmax=2

0&dispstart=0

- **Journal of Pediatric Hematology/Oncology : Official Journal of the American Society of Pediatric Hematology/Oncology. (J Pediatr Hematol Oncol)**
http://www.ncbi.nlm.nih.gov/entrez/jrbrowser.cgi?field=0®exp=Journal+of+Pediatric+Hematology/Oncology+:+Official+Journal+of+the+American+Society+of+Pediatric+Hematology/Oncology&dispmax=20&dispstart=0

- **Journal of Psychosomatic Research. (J Psychosom Res)**
http://www.ncbi.nlm.nih.gov/entrez/jrbrowser.cgi?field=0®exp=Journal+of+Psychosomatic+Research&dispmax=20&dispstart=0

- **Journal of Sleep Research. (J Sleep Res)**
http://www.ncbi.nlm.nih.gov/entrez/jrbrowser.cgi?field=0®exp=Journal+of+Sleep+Research&dispmax=20&dispstart=0

- **Journal of the International Neuropsychological Society : Jins. (J Int Neuropsychol Soc)**
http://www.ncbi.nlm.nih.gov/entrez/jrbrowser.cgi?field=0®exp=Journal+of+the+International+Neuropsychological+Society+:+Jins&dispmax=20&dispstart=0

- **Magnetic Resonance Imaging. (Magn Reson Imaging)**
http://www.ncbi.nlm.nih.gov/entrez/jrbrowser.cgi?field=0®exp=Magnetic+Resonance+Imaging&dispmax=20&dispstart=0

- **Mayo Clinic Proceedings. (Mayo Clin Proc)**
http://www.ncbi.nlm.nih.gov/entrez/jrbrowser.cgi?field=0®exp=Mayo+Clinic+Proceedings&dispmax=20&dispstart=0

- **Methods of Information in Medicine. (Methods Inf Med)**
http://www.ncbi.nlm.nih.gov/entrez/jrbrowser.cgi?field=0®exp=Methods+of+Information+in+Medicine&dispmax=20&dispstart=0

- **Neuropsychopharmacology : Official Publication of the American College of Neuropsychopharmacology. (Neuropsychopharmacology)**
http://www.ncbi.nlm.nih.gov/entrez/jrbrowser.cgi?field=0®exp=Neuropsychopharmacology+:+Official+Publication+of+the+American+College+of+Neuropsychopharmacology&dispmax=20&dispstart=0

- **Obesity Research. (Obes Res)**
http://www.ncbi.nlm.nih.gov/entrez/jrbrowser.cgi?field=0®exp=Obesity+Research&dispmax=20&dispstart=0

- **Obesity Surgery : the Official Journal of the American Society for Bariatric Surgery and of the Obesity Surgery Society of Australia and New Zealand. (Obes Surg)**
http://www.ncbi.nlm.nih.gov/entrez/jrbrowser.cgi?field=0®exp=Obesity+Surgery+:+the+Official+Journal+of+the+American+Society+for+Bariatric+Surgery+and+of+the+Obesity+Surgery+Society+of+Australia+and+New+Zealand&dispmax=20&dispstart=0

- **Otolaryngology and Head and Neck Surgery. (Otolaryngol Head Neck Surg)**
http://www.ncbi.nlm.nih.gov/entrez/jrbrowser.cgi?field=0®exp=Otolaryngology+and+Head+and+Neck+Surgery&dispmax=20&dispstart=0

- **Pediatric Pulmonology. (Pediatr Pulmonol)**
http://www.ncbi.nlm.nih.gov/entrez/jrbrowser.cgi?field=0®exp=Pediatric+Pulmonology&dispmax=20&dispstart=0

- **Plastic and Reconstructive Surgery. (Plast Reconstr Surg)**
http://www.ncbi.nlm.nih.gov/entrez/jrbrowser.cgi?field=0®exp=Plastic+and+Reconstructive+Surgery&dispmax=20&dispstart=0

- **Postgraduate Medicine. (Postgrad Med)**
http://www.ncbi.nlm.nih.gov/entrez/jrbrowser.cgi?field=0®exp=Postgraduate+Medicine&dispmax=20&dispstart=0

- **Psychiatry and Clinical Neurosciences. (Psychiatry Clin Neurosci)**
http://www.ncbi.nlm.nih.gov/entrez/jrbrowser.cgi?field=0®exp=Psychiatry+and+Clinical+Neurosciences&dispmax=20&dispstart=0

- **Respiration Physiology. (Respir Physiol)**
http://www.ncbi.nlm.nih.gov/entrez/jrbrowser.cgi?field=0®exp=Respiration+Physiology&dispmax=20&dispstart=0

- **Respiration; International Review of Thoracic Diseases. (Respiration)**
http://www.ncbi.nlm.nih.gov/entrez/jrbrowser.cgi?field=0®exp=Respiration;+International+Review+of+Thoracic+Diseases&dispmax=20&di

spstart=0

- **Respiratory Medicine. (Respir Med)**
http://www.ncbi.nlm.nih.gov/entrez/jrbrowser.cgi?field=0®exp=Respiratory+Medicine&dispmax=20&dispstart=0

- **Respiratory Physiology & Neurobiology. (Respir Physiol Neurobiol)**
http://www.ncbi.nlm.nih.gov/entrez/jrbrowser.cgi?field=0®exp=Respiratory+Physiology+&+Neurobiology&dispmax=20&dispstart=0

- **Sleep & Breathing = Schlaf & Atmung. (Sleep Breath)**
http://www.ncbi.nlm.nih.gov/entrez/jrbrowser.cgi?field=0®exp=Sleep+&+Breathing+=+Schlaf+&+Atmung&dispmax=20&dispstart=0

- **Sleep Medicine Reviews. (Sleep Med Rev)**
http://www.ncbi.nlm.nih.gov/entrez/jrbrowser.cgi?field=0®exp=Sleep+Medicine+Reviews&dispmax=20&dispstart=0

- **Sleep Medicine. (Sleep Med)**
http://www.ncbi.nlm.nih.gov/entrez/jrbrowser.cgi?field=0®exp=Sleep+Medicine&dispmax=20&dispstart=0

- **Spinal Cord : the Official Journal of the International Medical Society of Paraplegia. (Spinal Cord)**
http://www.ncbi.nlm.nih.gov/entrez/jrbrowser.cgi?field=0®exp=Spinal+Cord+:+the+Official+Journal+of+the+International+Medical+Society+of+Paraplegia&dispmax=20&dispstart=0

- **The American Journal of Cardiology. (Am J Cardiol)**
http://www.ncbi.nlm.nih.gov/entrez/jrbrowser.cgi?field=0®exp=The+American+Journal+of+Cardiology&dispmax=20&dispstart=0

- **The American Journal of Gastroenterology. (Am J Gastroenterol)**
http://www.ncbi.nlm.nih.gov/entrez/jrbrowser.cgi?field=0®exp=The+American+Journal+of+Gastroenterology&dispmax=20&dispstart=0

- **The American Journal of Medicine. (Am J Med)**
http://www.ncbi.nlm.nih.gov/entrez/jrbrowser.cgi?field=0®exp=The+American+Journal+of+Medicine&dispmax=20&dispstart=0

- **The American Journal of Psychiatry. (Am J Psychiatry)**
http://www.ncbi.nlm.nih.gov/entrez/jrbrowser.cgi?field=0®exp=Th

e+American+Journal+of+Psychiatry&dispmax=20&dispstart=0

- **The Annals of Otology, Rhinology, and Laryngology. (Ann Otol Rhinol Laryngol)**
  http://www.ncbi.nlm.nih.gov/entrez/jrbrowser.cgi?field=0®exp=The+Annals+of+Otology,+Rhinology,+and+Laryngology&dispmax=20&dispstart=0

- **The Cleft Palate-Craniofacial Journal : Official Publication of the American Cleft Palate-Craniofacial Association. (Cleft Palate Craniofac J)**
  http://www.ncbi.nlm.nih.gov/entrez/jrbrowser.cgi?field=0®exp=The+Cleft+Palate-Craniofacial+Journal+:+Official+Publication+of+the+American+Cleft+Palate-Craniofacial+Association&dispmax=20&dispstart=0

- **The Journal of Arthroplasty. (J Arthroplasty)**
  http://www.ncbi.nlm.nih.gov/entrez/jrbrowser.cgi?field=0®exp=The+Journal+of+Arthroplasty&dispmax=20&dispstart=0

- **The Journal of Asthma : Official Journal of the Association for the Care of Asthma. (J Asthma)**
  http://www.ncbi.nlm.nih.gov/entrez/jrbrowser.cgi?field=0®exp=The+Journal+of+Asthma+:+Official+Journal+of+the+Association+for+the+Care+of+Asthma&dispmax=20&dispstart=0

- **The Journal of Clinical Endocrinology and Metabolism. (J Clin Endocrinol Metab)**
  http://www.ncbi.nlm.nih.gov/entrez/jrbrowser.cgi?field=0®exp=The+Journal+of+Clinical+Endocrinology+and+Metabolism&dispmax=20&dispstart=0

- **The Journal of Family Practice. (J Fam Pract)**
  http://www.ncbi.nlm.nih.gov/entrez/jrbrowser.cgi?field=0®exp=The+Journal+of+Family+Practice&dispmax=20&dispstart=0

- **The Journal of Otolaryngology. (J Otolaryngol)**
  http://www.ncbi.nlm.nih.gov/entrez/jrbrowser.cgi?field=0®exp=The+Journal+of+Otolaryngology&dispmax=20&dispstart=0

- **The Journal of Pediatrics. (J Pediatr)**
  http://www.ncbi.nlm.nih.gov/entrez/jrbrowser.cgi?field=0®exp=The+Journal+of+Pediatrics&dispmax=20&dispstart=0

- **The Journal of the American Dental Association. (J Am Dent Assoc)**
  http://www.ncbi.nlm.nih.gov/entrez/jrbrowser.cgi?field=0®exp=The+Journal+of+the+American+Dental+Association&dispmax=20&dispstart=0

- **The Laryngoscope. (Laryngoscope)**
  http://www.ncbi.nlm.nih.gov/entrez/jrbrowser.cgi?field=0®exp=The+Laryngoscope&dispmax=20&dispstart=0

- **The Medical Clinics of North America. (Med Clin North Am)**
  http://www.ncbi.nlm.nih.gov/entrez/jrbrowser.cgi?field=0®exp=The+Medical+Clinics+of+North+America&dispmax=20&dispstart=0

- **The New England Journal of Medicine. (N Engl J Med)**
  http://www.ncbi.nlm.nih.gov/entrez/jrbrowser.cgi?field=0®exp=The+New+England+Journal+of+Medicine&dispmax=20&dispstart=0

CHAPTER 7. PHYSICIAN GUIDELINES AND DATABASES

Overview

Doctors and medical researchers rely on a number of information sources to help patients with their conditions. Many will subscribe to journals or newsletters published by their professional associations or refer to specialized textbooks or clinical guides published for the medical profession. In this chapter, we focus on databases and Internet-based guidelines created or written for this professional audience.

NIH Guidelines

For the more common diseases, The National Institutes of Health publish guidelines that are frequently consulted by physicians. Publications are typically written by one or more of the various NIH Institutes. For physician guidelines, commonly referred to as "clinical" or "professional" guidelines, you can visit the following Institutes:

- Office of the Director (OD); guidelines consolidated across agencies available at **http://www.nih.gov/health/consumer/conkey.htm**
- National Institute of General Medical Sciences (NIGMS); fact sheets available at **http://www.nigms.nih.gov/news/facts/**
- National Library of Medicine (NLM); extensive encyclopedia (A.D.A.M., Inc.) with guidelines: **http://www.nlm.nih.gov/medlineplus/healthtopics.html**
- National Heart, Lung, and Blood Institute (NHLBI); guidelines available at **http://www.nhlbi.nih.gov/guidelines/index.htm**

The NHLBI, in particular, suggests the following publications to physicians:

Sleep Disorders

- Restless Legs Syndrome: Detection and Management in Primary Care: **http://www.nhlbi.nih.gov/health/prof/sleep/rls_gde.htm**
- Sleep Apnea: Is Your Patient at Risk?: **http://www.nhlbi.nih.gov/health/prof/sleep/slpaprsk.htm**
- Insomnia: Assessment and Management in Primary Care: **http://www.nhlbi.nih.gov/health/prof/sleep/insom_pc.htm**
- Problem Sleepiness in Your Patient: **http://www.nhlbi.nih.gov/health/prof/sleep/pslp_pat.htm**
- Working Group Report on Problem Sleepiness: **http://www.nhlbi.nih.gov/health/prof/sleep/pslp_wg.htm**
- National Center on Sleep Disorders Pamphlet: **http://www.nhlbi.nih.gov/health/prof/sleep/sleep.txt**

Sleep in Youth

- Awake At the Wheel Materials: **http://www.nhlbi.nih.gov/health/public/sleep/aaw/awake.htm**
- Educating Youth About Sleep and Drowsy Driving: **http://www.nhlbi.nih.gov/health/prof/sleep/dwydrv_y.htm**
- Drowsy Driving and Automobile Crashes: **http://www.nhlbi.nih.gov/health/prof/sleep/drsy_drv.htm**

Additional Resources

- National Center on Sleep Disorders Research Web Site: **http://www.nhlbi.nih.gov/about/ncsdr/index.htm**
- Trans-NIH Sleep Research Coordinating Committee Annual Report: **http://www.nhlbi.nih.gov/health/prof/sleep/sleep00.htm**
- Sleep Disorders Research Advisory Board (SDRAB): **http://www.nhlbi.nih.gov/meetings/sdrab/index.htm**
- National Sleep Disorders Research Plan: **http://www.nhlbi.nih.gov/health/prof/sleep/reschpln.htm**
- List of Publications: **http://www.nhlbi.nih.gov/health/pubs/index.htm**
- Information Center: **http://www.nhlbi.nih.gov/health/infoctr/index.htm**

- Sleep Information for Patients/Public: **http://www.nhlbi.nih.gov/health/public/sleep/index.htm**

NIH Databases

In addition to the various Institutes of Health that publish professional guidelines, the NIH has designed a number of databases for professionals.[23] Physician-oriented resources provide a wide variety of information related to the biomedical and health sciences, both past and present. The format of these resources varies. Searchable databases, bibliographic citations, full text articles (when available), archival collections, and images are all available. The following are referenced by the National Library of Medicine:[24]

- **Bioethics:** Access to published literature on the ethical, legal and public policy issues surrounding healthcare and biomedical research. This information is provided in conjunction with the Kennedy Institute of Ethics located at Georgetown University, Washington, D.C.: **http://www.nlm.nih.gov/databases/databases_bioethics.html**
- **HIV/AIDS Resources:** Describes various links and databases dedicated to HIV/AIDS research: **http://www.nlm.nih.gov/pubs/factsheets/aidsinfs.html**
- **NLM Online Exhibitions:** Describes "Exhibitions in the History of Medicine": **http://www.nlm.nih.gov/exhibition/exhibition.html**. Additional resources for historical scholarship in medicine: **http://www.nlm.nih.gov/hmd/hmd.html**
- **Biotechnology Information:** Access to public databases. The National Center for Biotechnology Information conducts research in computational biology, develops software tools for analyzing genome data, and disseminates biomedical information for the better understanding of molecular processes affecting human health and disease: **http://www.ncbi.nlm.nih.gov/**
- **Population Information:** The National Library of Medicine provides access to worldwide coverage of population, family planning, and related health issues, including family planning technology and programs, fertility, and population law and policy: **http://www.nlm.nih.gov/databases/databases_population.html**

---

[23] Remember, for the general public, the National Library of Medicine recommends the databases referenced in MEDLINE*plus* (**http://medlineplus.gov/** or **http://www.nlm.nih.gov/medlineplus/databases.html**).

[24] See **http://www.nlm.nih.gov/databases/databases.html**.

- **Cancer Information:** Access to caner-oriented databases: **http://www.nlm.nih.gov/databases/databases_cancer.html**
- **Profiles in Science:** Offering the archival collections of prominent twentieth-century biomedical scientists to the public through modern digital technology: **http://www.profiles.nlm.nih.gov/**
- **Chemical Information:** Provides links to various chemical databases and references: **http://sis.nlm.nih.gov/Chem/ChemMain.html**
- **Clinical Alerts:** Reports the release of findings from the NIH-funded clinical trials where such release could significantly affect morbidity and mortality: **http://www.nlm.nih.gov/databases/alerts/clinical_alerts.html**
- **Space Life Sciences:** Provides links and information to space-based research (including NASA): **http://www.nlm.nih.gov/databases/databases_space.html**
- **MEDLINE:** Bibliographic database covering the fields of medicine, nursing, dentistry, veterinary medicine, the healthcare system, and the pre-clinical sciences: **http://www.nlm.nih.gov/databases/databases_medline.html**
- **Toxicology and Environmental Health Information (TOXNET):** Databases covering toxicology and environmental health: **http://sis.nlm.nih.gov/Tox/ToxMain.html**
- **Visible Human Interface:** Anatomically detailed, three-dimensional representations of normal male and female human bodies: **http://www.nlm.nih.gov/research/visible/visible_human.html**

While all of the above references may be of interest to physicians who study and treat sleep apnea, the following are particularly noteworthy.

The NLM Gateway[25]

The NLM (National Library of Medicine) Gateway is a Web-based system that lets users search simultaneously in multiple retrieval systems at the U.S. National Library of Medicine (NLM). It allows users of NLM services to initiate searches from one Web interface, providing "one-stop searching" for many of NLM's information resources or databases.[26] One target audience for the Gateway is the Internet user who is new to NLM's online resources and

---

[25] Adapted from NLM: **http://gateway.nlm.nih.gov/gw/Cmd?Overview.x.**

[26] The NLM Gateway is currently being developed by the Lister Hill National Center for Biomedical Communications (LHNCBC) at the National Library of Medicine (NLM) of the National Institutes of Health (NIH).

does not know what information is available or how best to search for it. This audience may include physicians and other healthcare providers, researchers, librarians, students, and, increasingly, patients, their families, and the public.[27] To use the NLM Gateway, simply go to the search site at **http://gateway.nlm.nih.gov/gw/Cmd**. Type "sleep apnea" (or synonyms) into the search box and click "Search." The results will be presented in a tabular form, indicating the number of references in each database category.

Results Summary

Category	Items Found
Journal Articles	12115
Books / Periodicals / Audio Visual	170
Consumer Health	819
Meeting Abstracts	13
Other Collections	45
Total	13162

HSTAT[28]

HSTAT is a free, Web-based resource that provides access to full-text documents used in healthcare decision-making.[29] HSTAT's audience includes healthcare providers, health service researchers, policy makers, insurance companies, consumers, and the information professionals who serve these groups. HSTAT provides access to a wide variety of publications, including clinical practice guidelines, quick-reference guides for clinicians, consumer health brochures, evidence reports and technology assessments from the Agency for Healthcare Research and Quality (AHRQ), as well as AHRQ's Put Prevention Into Practice.[30] Simply search by "sleep apnea" (or synonyms) at the following Web site: **http://text.nlm.nih.gov**.

---

[27] Other users may find the Gateway useful for an overall search of NLM's information resources. Some searchers may locate what they need immediately, while others will utilize the Gateway as an adjunct tool to other NLM search services such as PubMed® and MEDLINEplus®. The Gateway connects users with multiple NLM retrieval systems while also providing a search interface for its own collections. These collections include various types of information that do not logically belong in PubMed, LOCATORplus, or other established NLM retrieval systems (e.g., meeting announcements and pre-1966 journal citations). The Gateway will provide access to the information found in an increasing number of NLM retrieval systems in several phases.

[28] Adapted from HSTAT: **http://www.nlm.nih.gov/pubs/factsheets/hstat.html**.

[29] The HSTAT URL is **http://hstat.nlm.nih.gov/**.

[30] Other important documents in HSTAT include: the National Institutes of Health (NIH) Consensus Conference Reports and Technology Assessment Reports; the HIV/AIDS

Coffee Break: Tutorials for Biologists[31]

Some patients may wish to have access to a general healthcare site that takes a scientific view of the news and covers recent breakthroughs in biology that may one day assist physicians in developing treatments. To this end, we recommend "Coffee Break," a collection of short reports on recent biological discoveries. Each report incorporates interactive tutorials that demonstrate how bioinformatics tools are used as a part of the research process. Currently, all Coffee Breaks are written by NCBI staff.[32] Each report is about 400 words and is usually based on a discovery reported in one or more articles from recently published, peer-reviewed literature.[33] This site has new articles every few weeks, so it can be considered an online magazine of sorts,

---

Treatment Information Service (ATIS) resource documents; the Substance Abuse and Mental Health Services Administration's Center for Substance Abuse Treatment (SAMHSA/CSAT) Treatment Improvement Protocols (TIP) and Center for Substance Abuse Prevention (SAMHSA/CSAP) Prevention Enhancement Protocols System (PEPS); the Public Health Service (PHS) Preventive Services Task Force's *Guide to Clinical Preventive Services*; the independent, nonfederal Task Force on Community Services *Guide to Community Preventive Services*; and the Health Technology Advisory Committee (HTAC) of the Minnesota Health Care Commission (MHCC) health technology evaluations.

[31] Adapted from **http://www.ncbi.nlm.nih.gov/Coffeebreak/Archive/FAQ.html**.

[32] The figure that accompanies each article is frequently supplied by an expert external to NCBI, in which case the source of the figure is cited. The result is an interactive tutorial that tells a biological story.

[33] After a brief introduction that sets the work described into a broader context, the report focuses on how a molecular understanding can provide explanations of observed biology and lead to therapies for diseases. Each vignette is accompanied by a figure and hypertext links that lead to a series of pages that interactively show how NCBI tools and resources are used in the research process.

and intended for general background information. You can access Coffee Break at **http://www.ncbi.nlm.nih.gov/Coffeebreak/**.

Other Commercial Databases

In addition to resources maintained by official agencies, other databases exist that are commercial ventures addressing medical professionals. Here are some examples that may interest you:

- **CliniWeb International:** Index and table of contents to selected clinical information on the Internet; see **http://www.ohsu.edu/cliniweb/**.
- **Medical World Search:** Searches full text from thousands of selected medical sites on the Internet; see **http://www.mwsearch.com/**.

CHAPTER 8. DISSERTATIONS ON SLEEP APNEA

Overview

University researchers are active in studying almost all known diseases. The result of research is often published in the form of Doctoral or Master's dissertations. You should understand, therefore, that applied diagnostic procedures and/or therapies can take many years to develop after the thesis that proposed the new technique or approach was written.

In this chapter, we will give you a bibliography on recent dissertations relating to sleep apnea. You can read about these in more detail using the Internet or your local medical library. We will also provide you with information on how to use the Internet to stay current on dissertations.

Dissertations on Sleep Apnea

ProQuest Digital Dissertations is the largest archive of academic dissertations available. From this archive, we have compiled the following list covering dissertations devoted to sleep apnea. You will see that the information provided includes the dissertation's title, its author, and the author's institution. To read more about the following, simply use the Internet address indicated. The following covers recent dissertations dealing with sleep apnea:

- **A comparison between a telemedicine and traditional management model of care with nasal continuous positive airway pressure use among individuals with obstructive sleep apnea syndrome** by Taylor,

Yvonne Lynette; DrPH from The George Washington University, 2003, 185 pages
http://wwwlib.umi.com/dissertations/fullcit/3100979

- **Cognitive and behavioral effects of obstructive sleep apnea in toddlers with Down syndrome** by Gaither, Rebecca Ann; PhD from Illinois Institute of Technology, 2003, 49 pages
http://wwwlib.umi.com/dissertations/fullcit/3087837
- **Subjective and objective treatment outcomes of maxillomandibular advancement for the treatment of obstructive sleep apnea syndrome** by Robertson, Chad Gregory; MSc from Dalhousie University (Canada), 2003, 82 pages
http://wwwlib.umi.com/dissertations/fullcit/MQ79520

Keeping Current

As previously mentioned, an effective way to stay current on dissertations dedicated to sleep apnea is to use the database called *ProQuest Digital Dissertations* via the Internet, located at the following Web address: **http://wwwlib.umi.com/dissertations.** The site allows you to freely access the last two years of citations and abstracts. Ask your medical librarian if the library has full and unlimited access to this database. From the library, you should be able to do more complete searches than with the limited 2-year access available to the general public.

PART III. APPENDICES

ABOUT PART III

Part III is a collection of appendices on general medical topics which may be of interest to patients with sleep apnea and related conditions.

Appendix A. Researching Your Medications

Overview

There are a number of sources available on new or existing medications which could be prescribed to patients with sleep apnea. While a number of hard copy or CD-Rom resources are available to patients and physicians for research purposes, a more flexible method is to use Internet-based databases. In this chapter, we will begin with a general overview of medications. We will then proceed to outline official recommendations on how you should view your medications. You may also want to research medications that you are currently taking for other conditions as they may interact with medications for sleep apnea. Research can give you information on the side effects, interactions, and limitations of prescription drugs used in the treatment of sleep apnea. Broadly speaking, there are two sources of information on approved medications: public sources and private sources. We will emphasize free-to-use public sources.

Your Medications: The Basics[34]

The Agency for Health Care Research and Quality has published extremely useful guidelines on how you can best participate in the medication aspects of sleep apnea. Taking medicines is not always as simple as swallowing a pill. It can involve many steps and decisions each day. The AHCRQ recommends that patients with sleep apnea take part in treatment decisions. Do not be afraid to ask questions and talk about your concerns. By taking a moment to ask questions early, you may avoid problems later. Here are some points to cover each time a new medicine is prescribed:

---

[34] This section is adapted from AHCRQ: **http://www.ahcpr.gov/consumer/ncpiebro.htm**.

- Ask about all parts of your treatment, including diet changes, exercise, and medicines.
- Ask about the risks and benefits of each medicine or other treatment you might receive.
- Ask how often you or your doctor will check for side effects from a given medication.

Do not hesitate to ask what is important to you about your medicines. You may want a medicine with the fewest side effects, or the fewest doses to take each day. You may care most about cost, or how the medicine might affect how you live or work. Or, you may want the medicine your doctor believes will work the best. Telling your doctor will help him or her select the best treatment for you.

Do not be afraid to "bother" your doctor with your concerns and questions about medications for sleep apnea. You can also talk to a nurse or a pharmacist. They can help you better understand your treatment plan. Feel free to bring a friend or family member with you when you visit your doctor. Talking over your options with someone you trust can help you make better choices, especially if you are not feeling well. Specifically, ask your doctor the following:

- The name of the medicine and what it is supposed to do.
- How and when to take the medicine, how much to take, and for how long.
- What food, drinks, other medicines, or activities you should avoid while taking the medicine.
- What side effects the medicine may have, and what to do if they occur.
- If you can get a refill, and how often.
- About any terms or directions you do not understand.
- What to do if you miss a dose.
- If there is written information you can take home (most pharmacies have information sheets on your prescription medicines; some even offer large-print or Spanish versions).

Do not forget to tell your doctor about all the medicines you are currently taking (not just those for sleep apnea). This includes prescription medicines and the medicines that you buy over the counter. Then your doctor can avoid giving you a new medicine that may not work well with the medications you take now. When talking to your doctor, you may wish to prepare a list of medicines you currently take, the reason you take them, and how you take them. Be sure to include the following information for each:

- Name of medicine
- Reason taken
- Dosage
- Time(s) of day

Also include any over-the-counter medicines, such as:

- Laxatives
- Diet pills
- Vitamins
- Cold medicine
- Aspirin or other pain, headache, or fever medicine
- Cough medicine
- Allergy relief medicine
- Antacids
- Sleeping pills
- Others (include names)

Learning More about Your Medications

Because of historical investments by various organizations and the emergence of the Internet, it has become rather simple to learn about the medications your doctor has recommended for sleep apnea. One such source is the United States Pharmacopeia. In 1820, eleven physicians met in Washington, D.C. to establish the first compendium of standard drugs for the United States. They called this compendium the "U.S. Pharmacopeia (USP)." Today, the USP is a non-profit organization consisting of 800 volunteer scientists, eleven elected officials, and 400 representatives of state associations and colleges of medicine and pharmacy. The USP is located in Rockville, Maryland, and its home page is located at **www.usp.org**. The USP currently provides standards for over 3,700 medications. The resulting USP DI® Advice for the Patient® can be accessed through the National Library of Medicine of the National Institutes of Health. The database is partially derived from lists of federally approved medications in the Food and Drug Administration's (FDA) Drug Approvals database.[35]

While the FDA database is rather large and difficult to navigate, the Phamacopeia is both user-friendly and free to use. It covers more than 9,000 prescription and over-the-counter medications. To access this database, simply type the following hyperlink into your Web browser: **http://www.nlm.nih.gov/medlineplus/druginformation.html**. To view examples of a given medication (brand names, category, description, preparation, proper use, precautions, side effects, etc.), simply follow the hyperlinks indicated within the United States Pharmacopeia (USP).

Commercial Databases

In addition to the medications listed in the USP above, a number of commercial sites are available by subscription to physicians and their institutions. You may be able to access these sources from your local medical library or your doctor's office.

Reuters Health Drug Database

The Reuters Health Drug Database can be searched by keyword at the hyperlink: **http://www.reutershealth.com/frame2/drug.html**.

Mosby's GenRx

Mosby's GenRx database (also available on CD-Rom and book format) covers 45,000 drug products including generics and international brands. It provides prescribing information, drug interactions, and patient information. Information can be obtained at the following hyperlink: **http://www.genrx.com/Mosby/PhyGenRx/group.html**.

PDR*health*

The PDR*health* database is a free-to-use, drug information search engine that has been written for the public in layman's terms. It contains FDA-approved drug information adapted from the Physicians' Desk Reference (PDR)

[35] Though cumbersome, the FDA database can be freely browsed at the following site: **www.fda.gov/cder/da/da.htm**.

database. PDR*health* can be searched by brand name, generic name, or indication. It features multiple drug interactions reports. Search PDR*health* at **http://www.pdrhealth.com/drug_info/index.html**.

Other Web Sites

A number of additional Web sites discuss drug information. As an example, you may like to look at **www.drugs.com** which reproduces the information in the Pharmacopeia as well as commercial information. You may also want to consider the Web site of the Medical Letter, Inc. which allows users to download articles on various drugs and therapeutics for a nominal fee: **http://www.medletter.com/**.

Contraindications and Interactions (Hidden Dangers)

Some of the medications mentioned in the previous discussions can be problematic for patients with sleep apnea--not because they are used in the treatment process, but because of contraindications, or side effects. Medications with contraindications are those that could react with drugs used to treat sleep apnea or potentially create deleterious side effects in patients with sleep apnea. You should ask your physician about any contraindications, especially as these might apply to other medications that you may be taking for common ailments.

Drug-drug interactions occur when two or more drugs react with each other. This drug-drug interaction may cause you to experience an unexpected side effect. Drug interactions may make your medications less effective, cause unexpected side effects, or increase the action of a particular drug. Some drug interactions can even be harmful to you.

Be sure to read the label every time you use a nonprescription or prescription drug, and take the time to learn about drug interactions. These precautions may be critical to your health. You can reduce the risk of potentially harmful drug interactions and side effects with a little bit of knowledge and common sense.

Drug labels contain important information about ingredients, uses, warnings, and directions which you should take the time to read and understand. Labels also include warnings about possible drug interactions. Further, drug labels may change as new information becomes available. This is why it's especially important to read the label every time you use a medication. When your doctor prescribes a new drug, discuss all over-the-counter and prescription medications, dietary supplements, vitamins, botanicals, minerals and herbals you take as well as the foods you eat. Ask your pharmacist for the package insert for each prescription drug you take. The package insert provides more information about potential drug interactions.

A Final Warning

At some point, you may hear of alternative medications from friends, relatives, or in the news media. Advertisements may suggest that certain alternative drugs can produce positive results for patients with sleep apnea. Exercise caution--some of these drugs may have fraudulent claims, and others may actually hurt you. The Food and Drug Administration (FDA) is the official U.S. agency charged with discovering which medications are likely to improve the health of patients with sleep apnea. The FDA warns patients to watch out for[36]:

- Secret formulas (real scientists share what they know)
- Amazing breakthroughs or miracle cures (real breakthroughs don't happen very often; when they do, real scientists do not call them amazing or miracles)
- Quick, painless, or guaranteed cures
- If it sounds too good to be true, it probably isn't true.

If you have any questions about any kind of medical treatment, the FDA may have an office near you. Look for their number in the blue pages of the phone book. You can also contact the FDA through its toll-free number, 1-888-INFO-FDA (1-888-463-6332), or on the World Wide Web at **www.fda.gov**.

General References

In addition to the resources provided earlier in this chapter, the following general references describe medications (sorted alphabetically by title; hyperlinks provide rankings, information and reviews at Amazon.com):

- **Complete Guide to Prescription and Nonprescription Drugs 2001 (Complete Guide to Prescription and Nonprescription Drugs, 2001)** by H. Winter Griffith, Paperback 16th edition (2001), Medical Surveillance;

---

[36] This section has been adapted from **http://www.fda.gov/opacom/lowlit/medfraud.html**.

ISBN: 0942447417;
http://www.amazon.com/exec/obidos/ASIN/039952634X/icongroupinterna

- **The Essential Guide to Prescription Drugs, 2001** by James J. Rybacki, James W. Long; Paperback - 1274 pages (2001), Harper Resource; ISBN: 0060958162;
http://www.amazon.com/exec/obidos/ASIN/0060958162/icongroupinterna
- **Handbook of Commonly Prescribed Drugs** by G. John Digregorio, Edward J. Barbieri; Paperback 16th edition (2001), Medical Surveillance; ISBN: 0942447417;
http://www.amazon.com/exec/obidos/ASIN/0942447417/icongroupinterna
- **Johns Hopkins Complete Home Encyclopedia of Drugs 2nd ed.** by Simeon Margolis (Ed.), Johns Hopkins; Hardcover - 835 pages (2000), Rebus; ISBN: 0929661583;
http://www.amazon.com/exec/obidos/ASIN/0929661583/icongroupinterna
- **Medical Pocket Reference: Drugs 2002** by Springhouse Paperback 1st edition (2001), Lippincott Williams & Wilkins Publishers; ISBN: 1582550964;
http://www.amazon.com/exec/obidos/ASIN/1582550964/icongroupinterna
- **PDR** by Medical Economics Staff, Medical Economics Staff Hardcover - 3506 pages 55th edition (2000), Medical Economics Company; ISBN: 1563633752;
http://www.amazon.com/exec/obidos/ASIN/1563633752/icongroupinterna
- **Pharmacy Simplified: A Glossary of Terms** by James Grogan; Paperback - 432 pages, 1st edition (2001), Delmar Publishers; ISBN: 0766828581;
http://www.amazon.com/exec/obidos/ASIN/0766828581/icongroupinterna
- **Physician Federal Desk Reference** by Christine B. Fraizer; Paperback 2nd edition (2001), Medicode Inc; ISBN: 1563373971;
http://www.amazon.com/exec/obidos/ASIN/1563373971/icongroupinterna
- **Physician's Desk Reference Supplements** Paperback - 300 pages, 53 edition (1999), ISBN: 1563632950;
http://www.amazon.com/exec/obidos/ASIN/1563632950/icongroupinterna

Vocabulary Builder

The following vocabulary builder gives definitions of words used in this chapter that have not been defined in previous chapters:

Contraindications: Any factor or sign that it is unwise to pursue a certain kind of action or treatment, e. g. giving a general anesthetic to a person with pneumonia. [NIH]

APPENDIX B. RESEARCHING NUTRITION

Overview

Since the time of Hippocrates, doctors have understood the importance of diet and nutrition to patients' health and well-being. Since then, they have accumulated an impressive archive of studies and knowledge dedicated to this subject. Based on their experience, doctors and healthcare providers may recommend particular dietary supplements to patients with sleep apnea. Any dietary recommendation is based on a patient's age, body mass, gender, lifestyle, eating habits, food preferences, and health condition. It is therefore likely that different patients with sleep apnea may be given different recommendations. Some recommendations may be directly related to sleep apnea, while others may be more related to the patient's general health. These recommendations, themselves, may differ from what official sources recommend for the average person.

In this chapter we will begin by briefly reviewing the essentials of diet and nutrition that will broadly frame more detailed discussions of sleep apnea. We will then show you how to find studies dedicated specifically to nutrition and sleep apnea.

Food and Nutrition: General Principles

What Are Essential Foods?

Food is generally viewed by official sources as consisting of six basic elements: (1) fluids, (2) carbohydrates, (3) protein, (4) fats, (5) vitamins, and (6) minerals. Consuming a combination of these elements is considered to be a healthy diet:

- **Fluids** are essential to human life as 80-percent of the body is composed of water. Water is lost via urination, sweating, diarrhea, vomiting, diuretics (drugs that increase urination), caffeine, and physical exertion.
- **Carbohydrates** are the main source for human energy (thermoregulation) and the bulk of typical diets. They are mostly classified as being either simple or complex. Simple carbohydrates include sugars which are often consumed in the form of cookies, candies, or cakes. Complex carbohydrates consist of starches and dietary fibers. Starches are consumed in the form of pastas, breads, potatoes, rice, and other foods. Soluble fibers can be eaten in the form of certain vegetables, fruits, oats, and legumes. Insoluble fibers include brown rice, whole grains, certain fruits, wheat bran and legumes.
- **Proteins** are eaten to build and repair human tissues. Some foods that are high in protein are also high in fat and calories. Food sources for protein include nuts, meat, fish, cheese, and other dairy products.
- **Fats** are consumed for both energy and the absorption of certain vitamins. There are many types of fats, with many general publications recommending the intake of unsaturated fats or those low in cholesterol.

Vitamins and minerals are fundamental to human health, growth, and, in some cases, disease prevention. Most are consumed in your diet (exceptions being vitamins K and D which are produced by intestinal bacteria and sunlight on the skin, respectively). Each vitamin and mineral plays a different role in health. The following outlines essential vitamins:

- **Vitamin A** is important to the health of your eyes, hair, bones, and skin; sources of vitamin A include foods such as eggs, carrots, and cantaloupe.
- **Vitamin B^1**, also known as thiamine, is important for your nervous system and energy production; food sources for thiamine include meat, peas, fortified cereals, bread, and whole grains.
- **Vitamin B^2**, also known as riboflavin, is important for your nervous system and muscles, but is also involved in the release of proteins from nutrients; food sources for riboflavin include dairy products, leafy vegetables, meat, and eggs.
- **Vitamin B^3**, also known as niacin, is important for healthy skin and helps the body use energy; food sources for niacin include peas, peanuts, fish, and whole grains
- **Vitamin B^6**, also known as pyridoxine, is important for the regulation of cells in the nervous system and is vital for blood formation; food sources for pyridoxine include bananas, whole grains, meat, and fish.

- **Vitamin B^{12}** is vital for a healthy nervous system and for the growth of red blood cells in bone marrow; food sources for vitamin B^{12} include yeast, milk, fish, eggs, and meat.
- **Vitamin C** allows the body's immune system to fight various diseases, strengthens body tissue, and improves the body's use of iron; food sources for vitamin C include a wide variety of fruits and vegetables.
- **Vitamin D** helps the body absorb calcium which strengthens bones and teeth; food sources for vitamin D include oily fish and dairy products.
- **Vitamin E** can help protect certain organs and tissues from various degenerative diseases; food sources for vitamin E include margarine, vegetables, eggs, and fish.
- **Vitamin K** is essential for bone formation and blood clotting; common food sources for vitamin K include leafy green vegetables.
- **Folic Acid** maintains healthy cells and blood and, when taken by a pregnant woman, can prevent her fetus from developing neural tube defects; food sources for folic acid include nuts, fortified breads, leafy green vegetables, and whole grains.

It should be noted that it is possible to overdose on certain vitamins which become toxic if consumed in excess (e.g. vitamin A, D, E and K).

Like vitamins, minerals are chemicals that are required by the body to remain in good health. Because the human body does not manufacture these chemicals internally, we obtain them from food and other dietary sources. The more important minerals include:

- **Calcium** is needed for healthy bones, teeth, and muscles, but also helps the nervous system function; food sources for calcium include dry beans, peas, eggs, and dairy products.
- **Chromium** is helpful in regulating sugar levels in blood; food sources for chromium include egg yolks, raw sugar, cheese, nuts, beets, whole grains, and meat.
- **Fluoride** is used by the body to help prevent tooth decay and to reinforce bone strength; sources of fluoride include drinking water and certain brands of toothpaste.
- **Iodine** helps regulate the body's use of energy by synthesizing into the hormone thyroxine; food sources include leafy green vegetables, nuts, egg yolks, and red meat.

- **Iron** helps maintain muscles and the formation of red blood cells and certain proteins; food sources for iron include meat, dairy products, eggs, and leafy green vegetables.
- **Magnesium** is important for the production of DNA, as well as for healthy teeth, bones, muscles, and nerves; food sources for magnesium include dried fruit, dark green vegetables, nuts, and seafood.
- **Phosphorous** is used by the body to work with calcium to form bones and teeth; food sources for phosphorous include eggs, meat, cereals, and dairy products.
- **Selenium** primarily helps maintain normal heart and liver functions; food sources for selenium include wholegrain cereals, fish, meat, and dairy products.
- **Zinc** helps wounds heal, the formation of sperm, and encourage rapid growth and energy; food sources include dried beans, shellfish, eggs, and nuts.

The United States government periodically publishes recommended diets and consumption levels of the various elements of food. Again, your doctor may encourage deviations from the average official recommendation based on your specific condition. To learn more about basic dietary guidelines, visit the Web site: **http://www.health.gov/dietaryguidelines/**. Based on these guidelines, many foods are required to list the nutrition levels on the food's packaging. Labeling Requirements are listed at the following site maintained by the Food and Drug Administration: **http://www.cfsan.fda.gov/~dms/lab-cons.html**. When interpreting these requirements, the government recommends that consumers become familiar with the following abbreviations before reading FDA literature:[37]

- **DVs (Daily Values):** A new dietary reference term that will appear on the food label. It is made up of two sets of references, DRVs and RDIs.
- **DRVs (Daily Reference Values):** A set of dietary references that applies to fat, saturated fat, cholesterol, carbohydrate, protein, fiber, sodium, and potassium.
- **RDIs (Reference Daily Intakes):** A set of dietary references based on the Recommended Dietary Allowances for essential vitamins and minerals and, in selected groups, protein. The name "RDI" replaces the term "U.S. RDA."

[37] Adapted from the FDA: **http://www.fda.gov/fdac/special/foodlabel/dvs.html**.

- **RDAs (Recommended Dietary Allowances):** A set of estimated nutrient allowances established by the National Academy of Sciences. It is updated periodically to reflect current scientific knowledge.

What Are Dietary Supplements?[38]

Dietary supplements are widely available through many commercial sources, including health food stores, grocery stores, pharmacies, and by mail. Dietary supplements are provided in many forms including tablets, capsules, powders, gel-tabs, extracts, and liquids. Historically in the United States, the most prevalent type of dietary supplement was a multivitamin/mineral tablet or capsule that was available in pharmacies, either by prescription or "over the counter." Supplements containing strictly herbal preparations were less widely available. Currently in the United States, a wide array of supplement products are available, including vitamin, mineral, other nutrients, and botanical supplements as well as ingredients and extracts of animal and plant origin.

The Office of Dietary Supplements (ODS) of the National Institutes of Health is the official agency of the United States which has the expressed goal of acquiring "new knowledge to help prevent, detect, diagnose, and treat disease and disability, from the rarest genetic disorder to the common cold."[39] According to the ODS, dietary supplements can have an important impact on the prevention and management of disease and on the maintenance of health.[40] The ODS notes that considerable research on the effects of dietary supplements has been conducted in Asia and Europe where the use of plant products, in particular, has a long tradition. However, the overwhelming majority of supplements have not been studied scientifically. To explore the role of dietary supplements in the improvement of health care, the ODS plans, organizes, and supports conferences, workshops, and

---

[38] This discussion has been adapted from the NIH: **http://ods.od.nih.gov/showpage.aspx?pageid=46**.

[39] Contact: The Office of Dietary Supplements, National Institutes of Health, Building 31, Room 1B29, 31 Center Drive, MSC 2086, Bethesda, Maryland 20892-2086, Tel: (301) 435-2920, Fax: (301) 480-1845, E-mail: ods@nih.gov.

[40] Adapted from **http://ods.od.nih.gov/showpage.aspx?pageid=2**. The Dietary Supplement Health and Education Act defines dietary supplements as "a product (other than tobacco) intended to supplement the diet that bears or contains one or more of the following dietary ingredients: a vitamin, mineral, amino acid, herb or other botanical; or a dietary substance for use to supplement the diet by increasing the total dietary intake; or a concentrate, metabolite, constituent, extract, or combination of any ingredient described above; and intended for ingestion in the form of a capsule, powder, softgel, or gelcap, and not represented as a conventional food or as a sole item of a meal or the diet."

symposia on scientific topics related to dietary supplements. The ODS often works in conjunction with other NIH Institutes and Centers, other government agencies, professional organizations, and public advocacy groups.

To learn more about official information on dietary supplements, visit the ODS site at **http://dietary-supplements.info.nih.gov/**. Or contact:

The Office of Dietary Supplements
National Institutes of Health
Building 31, Room 1B29
31 Center Drive, MSC 2086
Bethesda, Maryland 20892-2086
Tel: (301) 435-2920
Fax: (301) 480-1845
E-mail: ods@nih.gov

Finding Studies on Sleep Apnea

The NIH maintains an office dedicated to patient nutrition and diet. The National Institutes of Health's Office of Dietary Supplements (ODS) offers a searchable bibliographic database called the IBIDS (International Bibliographic Information on Dietary Supplements). The IBIDS contains over 460,000 scientific citations and summaries about dietary supplements and nutrition as well as references to published international, scientific literature on dietary supplements such as vitamins, minerals, and botanicals.[41] IBIDS is available to the public free of charge through the ODS Internet page: **http://ods.od.nih.gov/databases/ibids.html**.

After entering the search area, you have three choices: (1) IBIDS Consumer Database, (2) Full IBIDS Database, or (3) Peer Reviewed Citations Only. We recommend that you start with the Consumer Database. While you may not find references for the topics that are of most interest to you, check back periodically as this database is frequently updated. More studies can be found by searching the Full IBIDS Database. Healthcare professionals and researchers generally use the third option, which lists peer-reviewed citations. In all cases, we suggest that you take advantage of the "Advanced

---

[41] Adapted from **http://ods.od.nih.gov**. IBIDS is produced by the Office of Dietary Supplements (ODS) at the National Institutes of Health to assist the public, healthcare providers, educators, and researchers in locating credible, scientific information on dietary supplements. IBIDS was developed and will be maintained through an interagency partnership with the Food and Nutrition Information Center of the National Agricultural Library, U.S. Department of Agriculture.

Search" option that allows you to retrieve up to 100 fully explained references in a comprehensive format. Type "sleep apnea" (or synonyms) into the search box. To narrow the search, you can also select the "Title" field.

The following information is typical of that found when using the "Full IBIDS Database" when searching using "sleep apnea" (or a synonym):

- **Clonidine and sleep apnea syndrome interaction: antagonism with yohimbine.**
  Author(s): Department of Emergency Medicine, Western Pennsylvania Hospital, Pittsburgh 15224, USA.
  Source: Roberge, R J Kimball, E T Rossi, J Warren, J J-Emerg-Med. 1998 Sep-October; 16(5): 727-30 0736-4679

- **Cure of sleep apnea syndrome after long-term nasal continuous positive airway pressure therapy and weight loss.**
  Author(s): Unite d'Explorations Electrophysiologiques du Systeme Nerveux, Cliniques Universitaires St. Luc, Brussels, Belgium.
  Source: Aubert Tulkens, G Culee, C Rodenstein, D O Sleepage 1989 June; 12(3): 216-22 0161-8105

- **Effect of autonomic blockade on heart rate and blood pressure in sleep apnea syndrome.**
  Author(s): Laboratoire du Sommeil, INSERM CJF 89 09, Hopital A. Beclere, Clamart, France.
  Source: Januel, B Laude, D Elghozi, J L Escourrou, P Blood-Press. 1995 July; 4(4): 226-31 0803-7051

- **Hormone replacement therapy may alleviate sleep apnea in menopausal women: a pilot study.**
  Author(s): Division of Reproductive Medicine and Infertility, Women and Infants Hospital, Brown University School of Medicine, Providence, RI 02905, USA.
  Source: Keefe, D L Watson, R Naftolin, F Menopause. 1999 Fall; 6(3): 196-200 1072-3714

- **Impact of obstructive sleep apnea and sleepiness on metabolic and cardivascular risk factors in the Swedish Obese Subjects (SOS) study.**
  Source: Grunstein, R.R. Stenlof, K. Sjostrom, L. Int-j-obes-relat-metab-disord. Avenel, NJ : The Macmillan Press Ltd. June 1995. volume 19 (6) page 410-418.

- **Influence of chronic barbiturate administration on sleep apnea after hypersomnia presentation: case study.**
  Author(s): Department of Psychiatry, University of Western Ontario. jatinder.Takhar@lhsc.on.ca

Source: Takhar, J Bishop, J J-Psychiatry-Neurosci. 2000 September; 25(4): 321-4 1180-4882

- **Is sleep apnea a predisposing factor for tobacco use?**
  Author(s): Department of Applied and Engineering Statistics, George Mason University, Fairfax VA, USA.
  Source: Schrand, J R Med-Hypotheses. 1996 December; 47(6): 443-8 0306-9877

- **Localization of site of obstruction in snorers and patients with obstructive sleep apnea syndrome: a comparison of fiberoptic nasopharyngoscopy and pressure measurements.**
  Author(s): Department of Otorhinolaryngology, Ullevaal University Hospital, Oslo, Norway.
  Source: Skatvedt, O Acta-Otolaryngol. 1993 March; 113(2): 206-9 0001-6489

- **MRI findings in the hypopharynx and the larynx of a patient with acromegaly associated with severe obstructive sleep apnea syndrome.**
  Author(s): 3rd Department of Internal Medicine, Miyazaki Medical College, Kiyotake, Japan.
  Source: Hidaka, H Katakami, H Miyazono, Y Matsukura, S Endocr-J. 1999 March; 46 Suppl: S105-8 0918-8959

- **Multiple cardiovascular risk factors in obstructive sleep apnea syndrome patients and an attempt at lifestyle modification using telemedicine-based education.**
  Author(s): The Third Department of Internal Medicine and Institute of Physical Fitness Sports Medicine, Aichi Medical University, Japan.
  Source: Oki, Y Shiomi, T Sasanabe, R Maekawa, M Hirota, I Usui, K Hasegawa, R Kobayashi, T Psychiatry-Clin-Neurosci. 1999 April; 53(2): 311-3 1323-1316

- **Nonsurgical management of the obstructive sleep apnea patient.**
  Author(s): Department of Oral and Maxillofacial Surgery, Baylor College of Dentistry, TX, USA.
  Source: Thornton, W K Roberts, D H J-Oral-Maxillofac-Surg. 1996 September; 54(9): 1103-8 0278-2391

- **Obstructive sleep apnea and obesity.**
  Author(s): Baylor College of Medicine, Houston, Texas.
  Source: Wittels, E H Thompson, S Otolaryngol-Clin-North-Am. 1990 August; 23(4): 751-60 0030-6665

- **The effect of sleep apnea on plasma and urinary catecholamines.**
  Author(s): Department of Psychiatry, University of California, San Diego, La Jolla 92093-0804, USA.

Source: Dimsdale, J E Coy, T Ziegler, M G Ancoli Israel, S Clausen, J Sleepage 1995 June; 18(5): 377-81 0161-8105

- **Treatment of obstructive sleep apnea syndrome with a Kampo-formula, San'o-shashin-to: a case report.**
  Author(s): Department of Neuropsychiatry, Faculty of Medicine, Toyama Medical and Pharmaceutical University, Japan.
  Source: Hisanaga, A Saitoh, O Fukuda, H Kurokawa, K Okabe, A Tachibana, H Hagino, H Mita, T Yamashita, I Tsutsumi, M Kurachi, M Itoh, T Psychiatry-Clin-Neurosci. 1999 April; 53(2): 303-5 1323-1316

Federal Resources on Nutrition

In addition to the IBIDS, the United States Department of Health and Human Services (HHS) and the United States Department of Agriculture (USDA) provide many sources of information on general nutrition and health. Recommended resources include:

- healthfinder®, HHS's gateway to health information, including diet and nutrition: **http://www.healthfinder.gov/scripts/SearchContext.asp?topic=238&page=0**
- The United States Department of Agriculture's Web site dedicated to nutrition information: **www.nutrition.gov**
- The Food and Drug Administration's Web site for federal food safety information: **www.foodsafety.gov**
- The National Action Plan on Overweight and Obesity sponsored by the United States Surgeon General: **http://www.surgeongeneral.gov/topics/obesity/**
- The Center for Food Safety and Applied Nutrition has an Internet site sponsored by the Food and Drug Administration and the Department of Health and Human Services: **http://vm.cfsan.fda.gov/**
- Center for Nutrition Policy and Promotion sponsored by the United States Department of Agriculture: **http://www.usda.gov/cnpp/**
- Food and Nutrition Information Center, National Agricultural Library sponsored by the United States Department of Agriculture: **http://www.nal.usda.gov/fnic/**
- Food and Nutrition Service sponsored by the United States Department of Agriculture: **http://www.fns.usda.gov/fns/**

Additional Web Resources

A number of additional Web sites offer encyclopedic information covering food and nutrition. The following is a representative sample:

- AOL: **http://search.aol.com/cat.adp?id=174&layer=&from=subcats**
- Family Village: **http://www.familyvillage.wisc.edu/med_nutrition.html**
- Google: **http://directory.google.com/Top/Health/Nutrition/**
- Open Directory Project: **http://dmoz.org/Health/Nutrition/**
- Yahoo.com: **http://dir.yahoo.com/Health/Nutrition/**
- WebMD®Health: **http://my.webmd.com/nutrition**
- WholeHealthMD.com: **http://www.wholehealthmd.com/reflib/0,1529,,00.html**

Vocabulary Builder

The following vocabulary builder defines words used in the references in this chapter that have not been defined in previous chapters:

Antagonism: Interference with, or inhibition of, the growth of a living organism by another living organism, due either to creation of unfavorable conditions (e. g. exhaustion of food supplies) or to production of a specific antibiotic substance (e. g. penicillin). [NIH]

APPENDIX C. FINDING MEDICAL LIBRARIES

Overview

At a medical library you can find medical texts and reference books, consumer health publications, specialty newspapers and magazines, as well as medical journals. In this Appendix, we show you how to quickly find a medical library in your area.

Preparation

Before going to the library, highlight the references mentioned in this sourcebook that you find interesting. Focus on those items that are not available via the Internet, and ask the reference librarian for help with your search. He or she may know of additional resources that could be helpful to you. Most importantly, your local public library and medical libraries have Interlibrary Loan programs with the National Library of Medicine (NLM), one of the largest medical collections in the world. According to the NLM, most of the literature in the general and historical collections of the National Library of Medicine is available on interlibrary loan to any library. NLM's interlibrary loan services are only available to libraries. If you would like to access NLM medical literature, then visit a library in your area that can request the publications for you.[42]

[42] Adapted from the NLM: **http://www.nlm.nih.gov/psd/cas/interlibrary.html**.

Finding a Local Medical Library

The quickest method to locate medical libraries is to use the Internet-based directory published by the National Network of Libraries of Medicine (NN/LM). This network includes 4626 members and affiliates that provide many services to librarians, health professionals, and the public. To find a library in your area, simply visit **http://nnlm.gov/members/adv.html** or call 1-800-338-7657.

Medical Libraries in the U.S. and Canada

In addition to the NN/LM, the National Library of Medicine (NLM) lists a number of libraries with reference facilities that are open to the public. The following is the NLM's list and includes hyperlinks to each library's Web site. These Web pages can provide information on hours of operation and other restrictions. The list below is a small sample of libraries recommended by the National Library of Medicine (sorted alphabetically by name of the U.S. state or Canadian province where the library is located)[43]:

- **Alabama:** Health InfoNet of Jefferson County (Jefferson County Library Cooperative, Lister Hill Library of the Health Sciences), **http://www.uab.edu/infonet/**
- **Alabama:** Richard M. Scrushy Library (American Sports Medicine Institute)
- **Arizona:** Samaritan Regional Medical Center: The Learning Center (Samaritan Health System, Phoenix, Arizona), **http://www.samaritan.edu/library/bannerlibs.htm**
- **California:** Kris Kelly Health Information Center (St. Joseph Health System, Humboldt), **http://www.humboldt1.com/~kkhic/index.html**
- **California:** Community Health Library of Los Gatos, **http://www.healthlib.org/orgresources.html**
- **California:** Consumer Health Program and Services (CHIPS) (County of Los Angeles Public Library, Los Angeles County Harbor-UCLA Medical Center Library) - Carson, CA, **http://www.colapublib.org/services/chips.html**
- **California:** Gateway Health Library (Sutter Gould Medical Foundation)
- **California:** Health Library (Stanford University Medical Center), **http://www-med.stanford.edu/healthlibrary/**

[43] Abstracted from **http://www.nlm.nih.gov/medlineplus/libraries.html**.

- **California:** Patient Education Resource Center - Health Information and Resources (University of California, San Francisco), **http://sfghdean.ucsf.edu/barnett/PERC/default.asp**
- **California:** Redwood Health Library (Petaluma Health Care District), **http://www.phcd.org/rdwdlib.html**
- **California:** Los Gatos PlaneTree Health Library, **http://planetreesanjose.org/**
- **California:** Sutter Resource Library (Sutter Hospitals Foundation, Sacramento), **http://suttermedicalcenter.org/library/**
- **California:** Health Sciences Libraries (University of California, Davis), **http://www.lib.ucdavis.edu/healthsci/**
- **California:** ValleyCare Health Library & Ryan Comer Cancer Resource Center (ValleyCare Health System, Pleasanton), **http://gaelnet.stmarys-ca.edu/other.libs/gbal/east/vchl.html**
- **California:** Washington Community Health Resource Library (Fremont), **http://www.healthlibrary.org/**
- **Colorado:** William V. Gervasini Memorial Library (Exempla Healthcare), **http://www.saintjosephdenver.org/yourhealth/libraries/**
- **Connecticut:** Hartford Hospital Health Science Libraries (Hartford Hospital), **http://www.harthosp.org/library/**
- **Connecticut:** Healthnet: Connecticut Consumer Health Information Center (University of Connecticut Health Center, Lyman Maynard Stowe Library), **http://library.uchc.edu/departm/hnet/**
- **Connecticut:** Waterbury Hospital Health Center Library (Waterbury Hospital, Waterbury), **http://www.waterburyhospital.com/library/consumer.shtml**
- **Delaware:** Consumer Health Library (Christiana Care Health System, Eugene du Pont Preventive Medicine & Rehabilitation Institute, Wilmington), **http://www.christianacare.org/health_guide/health_guide_pmri_health_info.cfm**
- **Delaware:** Lewis B. Flinn Library (Delaware Academy of Medicine, Wilmington), **http://www.delamed.org/chls.html**
- **Georgia:** Family Resource Library (Medical College of Georgia, Augusta), **http://cmc.mcg.edu/kids_families/fam_resources/fam_res_lib/frl.htm**
- **Georgia:** Health Resource Center (Medical Center of Central Georgia, Macon), **http://www.mccg.org/hrc/hrchome.asp**

- **Hawaii:** Hawaii Medical Library: Consumer Health Information Service (Hawaii Medical Library, Honolulu), **http://hml.org/CHIS/**
- **Idaho:** DeArmond Consumer Health Library (Kootenai Medical Center, Coeur d'Alene), **http://www.nicon.org/DeArmond/index.htm**
- **Illinois:** Health Learning Center of Northwestern Memorial Hospital (Chicago), **http://www.nmh.org/health_info/hlc.html**
- **Illinois:** Medical Library (OSF Saint Francis Medical Center, Peoria), **http://www.osfsaintfrancis.org/general/library/**
- **Kentucky:** Medical Library - Services for Patients, Families, Students & the Public (Central Baptist Hospital, Lexington), **http://www.centralbap.com/education/community/library.cfm**
- **Kentucky:** University of Kentucky - Health Information Library (Chandler Medical Center, Lexington), **http://www.mc.uky.edu/PatientEd/**
- **Louisiana:** Alton Ochsner Medical Foundation Library (Alton Ochsner Medical Foundation, New Orleans), **http://www.ochsner.org/library/**
- **Louisiana:** Louisiana State University Health Sciences Center Medical Library-Shreveport, **http://lib-sh.lsuhsc.edu/**
- **Maine:** Franklin Memorial Hospital Medical Library (Franklin Memorial Hospital, Farmington), **http://www.fchn.org/fmh/lib.htm**
- **Maine:** Gerrish-True Health Sciences Library (Central Maine Medical Center, Lewiston), **http://www.cmmc.org/library/library.html**
- **Maine:** Hadley Parrot Health Science Library (Eastern Maine Healthcare, Bangor), **http://www.emh.org/hll/hpl/guide.htm**
- **Maine:** Maine Medical Center Library (Maine Medical Center, Portland), **http://www.mmc.org/library/**
- **Maine:** Parkview Hospital (Brunswick), **http://www.parkviewhospital.org/**
- **Maine:** Southern Maine Medical Center Health Sciences Library (Southern Maine Medical Center, Biddeford), **http://www.smmc.org/services/service.php3?choice=10**
- **Maine:** Stephens Memorial Hospital's Health Information Library (Western Maine Health, Norway), **http://www.wmhcc.org/Library/**
- **Manitoba, Canada:** Consumer & Patient Health Information Service (University of Manitoba Libraries), **http://www.umanitoba.ca/libraries/units/health/reference/chis.html**

- **Manitoba, Canada:** J.W. Crane Memorial Library (Deer Lodge Centre, Winnipeg), **http://www.deerlodge.mb.ca/crane_library/about.asp**
- **Maryland:** Health Information Center at the Wheaton Regional Library (Montgomery County, Dept. of Public Libraries, Wheaton Regional Library), **http://www.mont.lib.md.us/healthinfo/hic.asp**
- **Massachusetts:** Baystate Medical Center Library (Baystate Health System), **http://www.baystatehealth.com/1024/**
- **Massachusetts:** Boston University Medical Center Alumni Medical Library (Boston University Medical Center), **http://med-libwww.bu.edu/library/lib.html**
- **Massachusetts:** Lowell General Hospital Health Sciences Library (Lowell General Hospital, Lowell), **http://www.lowellgeneral.org/library/HomePageLinks/WWW.htm**
- **Massachusetts:** Paul E. Woodard Health Sciences Library (New England Baptist Hospital, Boston), **http://www.nebh.org/health_lib.asp**
- **Massachusetts:** St. Luke's Hospital Health Sciences Library (St. Luke's Hospital, Southcoast Health System, New Bedford), **http://www.southcoast.org/library/**
- **Massachusetts:** Treadwell Library Consumer Health Reference Center (Massachusetts General Hospital), **http://www.mgh.harvard.edu/library/chrcindex.html**
- **Massachusetts:** UMass HealthNet (University of Massachusetts Medical School, Worchester), **http://healthnet.umassmed.edu/**
- **Michigan:** Botsford General Hospital Library - Consumer Health (Botsford General Hospital, Library & Internet Services), **http://www.botsfordlibrary.org/consumer.htm**
- **Michigan:** Helen DeRoy Medical Library (Providence Hospital and Medical Centers), **http://www.providence-hospital.org/library/**
- **Michigan:** Marquette General Hospital - Consumer Health Library (Marquette General Hospital, Health Information Center), **http://www.mgh.org/center.html**
- **Michigan:** Patient Education Resouce Center - University of Michigan Cancer Center (University of Michigan Comprehensive Cancer Center, Ann Arbor), **http://www.cancer.med.umich.edu/learn/leares.htm**
- **Michigan:** Sladen Library & Center for Health Information Resources - Consumer Health Information (Detroit), **http://www.henryford.com/body.cfm?id=39330**

- **Montana:** Center for Health Information (St. Patrick Hospital and Health Sciences Center, Missoula)
- **National:** Consumer Health Library Directory (Medical Library Association, Consumer and Patient Health Information Section), **http://caphis.mlanet.org/directory/index.html**
- **National:** National Network of Libraries of Medicine (National Library of Medicine) - provides library services for health professionals in the United States who do not have access to a medical library, **http://nnlm.gov/**
- **National:** NN/LM List of Libraries Serving the Public (National Network of Libraries of Medicine), **http://nnlm.gov/members/**
- **Nevada:** Health Science Library, West Charleston Library (Las Vegas-Clark County Library District, Las Vegas), **http://www.lvccld.org/special_collections/medical/index.htm**
- **New Hampshire:** Dartmouth Biomedical Libraries (Dartmouth College Library, Hanover), **http://www.dartmouth.edu/~biomed/resources.htmld/conshealth.htmld**
- **New Jersey:** Consumer Health Library (Rahway Hospital, Rahway), **http://www.rahwayhospital.com/library.htm**
- **New Jersey:** Dr. Walter Phillips Health Sciences Library (Englewood Hospital and Medical Center, Englewood), **http://www.englewoodhospital.com/links/index.htm**
- **New Jersey:** Meland Foundation (Englewood Hospital and Medical Center, Englewood), **http://www.geocities.com/ResearchTriangle/9360/**
- **New York:** Choices in Health Information (New York Public Library) - NLM Consumer Pilot Project participant, **http://www.nypl.org/branch/health/links.html**
- **New York:** Health Information Center (Upstate Medical University, State University of New York, Syracuse), **http://www.upstate.edu/library/hic/**
- **New York:** Health Sciences Library (Long Island Jewish Medical Center, New Hyde Park), **http://www.lij.edu/library/library.html**
- **New York:** ViaHealth Medical Library (Rochester General Hospital), **http://www.nyam.org/library/**
- **Ohio:** Consumer Health Library (Akron General Medical Center, Medical & Consumer Health Library), **http://www.akrongeneral.org/hwlibrary.htm**

- **Oklahoma:** The Health Information Center at Saint Francis Hospital (Saint Francis Health System, Tulsa), **http://www.sfh-tulsa.com/services/healthinfo.asp**
- **Oregon:** Planetree Health Resource Center (Mid-Columbia Medical Center, The Dalles), **http://www.mcmc.net/phrc/**
- **Pennsylvania:** Community Health Information Library (Milton S. Hershey Medical Center, Hershey), **http://www.hmc.psu.edu/commhealth/**
- **Pennsylvania:** Community Health Resource Library (Geisinger Medical Center, Danville), **http://www.geisinger.edu/education/commlib.shtml**
- **Pennsylvania:** HealthInfo Library (Moses Taylor Hospital, Scranton), **http://www.mth.org/healthwellness.html**
- **Pennsylvania:** Hopwood Library (University of Pittsburgh, Health Sciences Library System, Pittsburgh), **http://www.hsls.pitt.edu/guides/chi/hopwood/index_html**
- **Pennsylvania:** Koop Community Health Information Center (College of Physicians of Philadelphia), **http://www.collphyphil.org/kooppg1.shtml**
- **Pennsylvania:** Learning Resources Center - Medical Library (Susquehanna Health System, Williamsport), **http://www.shscares.org/services/lrc/index.asp**
- **Pennsylvania:** Medical Library (UPMC Health System, Pittsburgh), **http://www.upmc.edu/passavant/library.htm**
- **Quebec, Canada:** Medical Library (Montreal General Hospital), **http://www.mghlib.mcgill.ca/**
- **South Dakota:** Rapid City Regional Hospital Medical Library (Rapid City Regional Hospital), **http://www.rcrh.org/Services/Library/Default.asp**
- **Texas:** Houston HealthWays (Houston Academy of Medicine-Texas Medical Center Library), **http://hhw.library.tmc.edu/**
- **Washington:** Community Health Library (Kittitas Valley Community Hospital), **http://www.kvch.com/**
- **Washington:** Southwest Washington Medical Center Library (Southwest Washington Medical Center, Vancouver), **http://www.swmedicalcenter.com/body.cfm?id=72**

Appendix D. NIH Consensus Statement on the Treatment of Sleep Disorders of Older People

Overview

NIH Consensus Development Conferences are convened to evaluate available scientific information and resolve safety and efficacy issues related to biomedical technology. The resultant NIH Consensus Statements are intended to advance understanding of the technology or issue in question and to be useful to health professionals and the public.[44] Each NIH consensus statement is the product of an independent, non-Federal panel of experts and is based on the panel's assessment of medical knowledge available at the time the statement was written. Therefore, a consensus statement provides a "snapshot in time" of the state of knowledge of the conference topic.

The NIH makes the following caveat: "When reading or downloading NIH consensus statements, keep in mind that new knowledge is inevitably accumulating through medical research. Nevertheless, each NIH consensus statement is retained on this website in its original form as a record of the NIH Consensus Development Program."[45] The following concensus statement was posted on the NIH site and not indicated as "out of date" in March 2002. It was originally published, however, in March 1990.[46]

---

[44] This paragraph is adapted from the NIH: **http://odp.od.nih.gov/consensus/cons/cons.htm**.

[45] Adapted from the NIH: **http://odp.od.nih.gov/consensus/cons/consdate.htm.**

[46] **The Treatment of Sleep Disorders of Older People**. NIH Consensus Statement Online 1990 Mar 26-28 [cited 2002 February 21];8(3):1-22. **http://consensus.nih.gov/cons/078/078_statement.htm**

Abstract

The National Institutes of Health Consensus Development Conference on the Treatment of Sleep Disorders of Older People brought together clinical specialists in pulmonology, psychiatry, and psychology, geriatrics, internal medicine, other health care providers, and the public to address the cause, diagnosis, assessment, and specific treatments of sleep disorders of older people. Following 1 1/2 days of presentations by experts and discussion by the audience, a consensus panel weighed the scientific evidence and prepared a consensus statement.

Among their findings, the panel concluded that although sleep patterns change during the aging process most older people with sleep disturbances suffer from any of a variety of medical and psychosocial disorders. The panel recommended that the diagnostic evaluation of sleep disorders begin with a careful clinical evaluation performed by an informed primary care physician. When necessary, referrals should be made to individuals or centers with specialized skills and tools for therapy. The panel recognized two types of disorders for which treatment may be beneficial: obstructive sleep apnea and insomnia. The mainstay for treatment for sleep apnea is the use of nasal continuous positive airway pressure. A thorough medical evaluation is essential prior to initiating treatment for insomnia, as its causes may be of psychiatric, pharmacological, or medical origin. The panel recommended that hypnotic medications not be the mainstay of treatment for insomnia as they may have habit forming potential if overused.

The full text of the consensus panel's statement follows.

What Is the Treatment of Sleep Disorders of Older People?

The increase in the number of people over 65 and the rise in the proportion of older people represent a marked change in the demographic patterns in this country that will have profound social, economic, medical, and personal consequences. Individuals over 65 constituted 4 percent of the American population in 1900 and nearly 10 percent in 1972. By the year 2000, it is estimated that they will comprise over 13 percent of the population and by 2050 will represent more than 21 percent of Americans.

A large proportion of older people are at risk for disturbances of sleep that may be caused by many factors such as retirement and changes in social patterns, death of spouse and close friends, increased use of medications, concurrent diseases and changes in circadian rhythms. While changes in sleep patterns have been viewed as part of the normal aging process, new information indicates that many of these disturbances may be related to pathological processes that are associated with aging.

Although the exact numbers are not yet known, it has been estimated that disturbances of sleep afflict more than half of the people 65 and older who live at home and about two-thirds of those who live in long-term care facilities. Problems in sleep and daytime wakefulness disrupt not only the lives of older persons but also those of their families and caregivers. People over 65 years of age now constitute almost 13 percent of the American population but consume over 30 percent of all dispensed prescription drugs, as well as an unknown percentage of over-the-counter medicines. A large proportion of these drugs are sedatives and hypnotic agents, the safety and efficacy of which have not been established for older people. Nor has it been established to what extent drugs contribute to or alleviate problems of sleep. It is necessary to understand the causes of these disorders and to develop better treatment strategies, including non-pharmacological methods.

In addition to affecting the quality of life, troubled sleep has been implicated with excess mortality. Controversy also exists concerning the causes, diagnosis, assessment, and specific treatments of sleep disorders in older people.

In an effort to assess the current state of knowledge and determine what changes in sleep are clinically important, how sleep disorders are best diagnosed and treated, and how the public can establish good sleep practices, the National Institute on Aging, the Office of Medical Applications of Research, the National Institute of Neurological Disorders and Stroke, and the National Heart, Lung, and Blood Institute of the National Institutes of Health and the National Institute of Mental Health, convened this conference. Following 1-1/2 days of presentations by experts in the relevant fields, a consensus panel consisting of representatives from neurology, psychiatry, internal medicine, geriatric medicine, pulmonology, otolaryngology--head and neck surgery, epidemiology, biostatistics, pharmacology, and the public considered evidence and formulated a consensus statement responding to these key questions:

- What are the changes in sleep and wakefulness as functions of aging and of diseases of older people? What are the diagnostic criteria that establish clinical abnormalities? Which are clinically and epidemiologically important?

- What are the indications for a diagnostic evaluation? What sequence of assessment methods should be used to determine if the diagnostic criteria are met?
- What are the indications for the treatment of sleep disorders?
- What are the common medical practices and lay treatment practices and their health implications?
- What should the medical profession and general public know about good sleep hygiene and treatment of sleep disorders, and what should be done to increase awareness?
- What are the directions for future research?

Sleep and Wakefulness of Older People

Sleep is a distinctive and essential component of human behavior. Nearly a third of the life of a normal adult is spent sleeping. Sleep is divided into rapid eye movement (REM) and non-REM sleep. REM sleep is characterized by a low amplitude pattern in the EEG, an associated loss of muscle tone, and the presence of rapid eye movements. Non-REM sleep is characterized by sleep spindles and slow wave activity in the EEG. Sleep is differentially distributed into the dark portion of the daily cycle of light and dark. This regulation of sleep reflects basic brain mechanisms that provide the circadian organization of both behavioral and physiological processes.

During aging there are typical changes in the pattern of sleep. The amount of time spent in deeper levels of sleep diminishes. There is an associated increase in awakenings during sleep and in the total amount of time spent awake during the night. In part, these changes appear to represent a loss of effective circadian regulation of sleep.

In carefully screened, medically healthy, older subjects, there are relatively few individuals who have symptoms related to these changes in sleep and in the distribution of sleep and waking behaviors. Many older individuals, however, suffer from a variety of medical and psychosocial problems and these are very often associated with disturbances of sleep. These include psychiatric illnesses, particularly depression; Alzheimer's disease and other neurodegenerative diseases; cardiovascular disease; upper airway incompetence; pulmonary disease; arthritis; pain syndromes; prostatic disease; endocrinopathies; and other illnesses.

The diagnostic categories that establish clinical abnormalities of sleep arise from two sets of data. The first is derived from evaluation of the patient's history, which is classified into syndromes as have been described in the International Classification of Sleep Disorders. None of the disorders are specific for older people, but nearly all occur in this population. The second set comes from electrophysiological studies. Both provide valuable information, but each has its own limitations.

There is little agreement among workers in the field about what is clinically normal and what is clinically abnormal, except in extreme cases (for example, high values of indices of sleep disordered breathing). Also, measurements are not obtained in a standardized way. Much needs to be learned, and an important first step is to decide upon a standardized approach to data collection. The new classification scheme is an important first step in the standardization process.

In the assessment of the behavioral aspects of sleep, standardization is needed before epidemiological subpopulations can be defined and surveyed. The validity (including face validity) and reliability of standardized instruments and settings must be determined before sensitivity, specificity, and prevalence are assessed. Additional considerations are cost and ease of measurement. With standardized, agreed-upon instruments intra- and intersubject variability can be measured and linked with other clinical observations.

Standardized approaches to data collection for both the clinician and the researcher are particularly important in the measurement of variations over time. In many situations clinical action is based on an inference that the patient's condition has changed. If this judgment is guided by a psychometric instrument, then the reliability of the estimated change, in the presence of intrasubject variability, must be established.

The rapid and thorough evaluation of new and existing technology will aid in the development of standardized approaches to data collection. The evaluation begins with the specification of the clinical need. Comparisons with competing technology must be made as objectively as possible, and the ideal research design for accomplishing this is the randomized double-blind clinical trial.

It is difficult to answer questions about changes in sleep and wakefulness as functions of aging or of disease in older people because basic epidemiologic descriptive studies have not yet been carried out. Studies of the distribution of sleeping patterns and "disorders" need to be conducted in the "community" utilizing a representative sampling scheme so that the relationship of sleep patterns to possibly pertinent cultural, demographic, and other variables can be explored.

There is a need for epidemiological studies of sleep disorders: international and cross-cultural comparisons and case-control studies may confirm and generate etiological hypotheses. The natural history of certain sleep disorders is not well described: Do they spontaneously remit? What is the relationship to cardiovascular disease and life expectancy? Cohort studies may help advance our understanding of the natural history of these disorders.

Similarly, it is difficult to determine which diagnostic criteria are important in establishing clinical abnormalities. The field of sleep disorder research has largely approached this problem by attempting to separate "normal" from "abnormal" or "diseased." However, population distributions of the phenomena employed as diagnostic criteria (e.g., periodic movements in sleep or apneic episodes) are not well described. Current threshold values are usually not validated; and test characteristics (sensitivity, specificity, predictive values) are largely unavailable. Furthermore, inter- and intraobserver variation in test interpretation has been rarely studied.

While the severe forms of clinical entities, such as sleep apnea, are generally accepted and criteria agreed upon, mild and moderate forms are not well distinguished. Study of the distribution of these phenomena in populations, linking them to clinical outcomes, is lacking. For example, persons with a mild degree of periodic movements in sleep or apnea may be asymptomatic and not suffer any appreciable morbidity. It will be difficult to establish diagnostic criteria if the frequency of these events is not linked to natural history studies and eventual health outcomes and functional impairment.

Diagnostic Evaluation

Diagnostic evaluation begins with the recognition of a potential disorder by patient history or physician suspicion. Screening questions should include: 1) patient satisfaction with his or her sleep; 2) intrusion of sleep or fatigue into daily activities; and 3) complaint by bed partner or other observers of unusual behavior during sleep. A positive response to these questions should trigger a more detailed history of the onset, severity, duration, and pattern of the complaint, and lead to a differential diagnosis.

Three major types of sleep complaints are excessive sleepiness (hypersomnia), difficulty in initiating or maintaining sleep (insomnia), and strange or unusual behavior during sleep (parasomnias).

A careful medical history is needed to determine the presence and severity of concomitant disease. The history of snoring, breathing pauses, or periodic movements during sleep is sometimes better described by the bed partner or other observers. Prescribed medications, especially sedatives, alcohol use, and self medication can have a significant effect on sleep and may impair cardiopulmonary mechanisms during sleep. Psychiatric history and evaluation identify anxiety, depression, or major life events which are known to affect sleep habits or hygiene. In some cases the use of a patient sleep log to evaluate sleep/wakefulness patterns will serve to identify rhythmic or circadian disturbances or to document the magnitude of sleep intrusion into daily activities. Appropriate physical examination will depend upon the nature of the complaint and history elicited from the patient. For example, heavy snoring may necessitate a detailed examination of the nose and throat. Appropriate laboratory tests may be similarly indicated.

Given additional training and education, primary care physicians should be capable of initial assessment and management of the majority of sleep disorders presenting in the older population. When necessary, referrals should be made to individuals or a center with recognized skills in the indications for and application of more specialized tools, such as polysomnography or multiple sleep latency tests for diagnosis and recommendations for therapy.

Polysomnography is indicated when a sleep related breathing disorder is suspected and may be useful for certain behavior or movement disorders during sleep. Polysomnography followed by a multiple sleep latency test is useful for establishing the diagnosis of narcolepsy and for quantitating daytime sleepiness. At present, there are insufficient data to assess the value of polysomnography in the routine evaluation of insomnia, depression, or dementia.

Limited monitoring on an ambulatory basis may be useful to assess efficacy of therapy for sleep apnea. Technologic advances, standardization of variables, and cost-effectiveness need to be addressed before incorporating ambulatory monitors into epidemiologic studies or the clinical practice of sleep disorders medicine.

Treatment of Sleep Disorders

The goals of therapy of sleep disorders can be classified as:

- Reducing morbidity;
- Reducing excess mortality; and
- Improving quality of life for patient and family.

Sleep disorders have been classified extensively. The major focus of this conference could, however, be summarized as dealing with two primary types of complaints or disorders, for which there is evidence to suggest that treatment is beneficial. These consist of:

- The hypersomnias, primarily represented by obstructive sleep apnea; and
- The insomnia complaints, which can be due to a variety of psychiatric and medical disorders.

Indications for Treatment of Obstructive Sleep Apnea

Obstructive sleep apnea is a potentially reversible cause of daytime hypersomnia, which may be associated with comorbid conditions and even excess mortality. Effective treatment is available for many patients. Development of better and more effective treatment strategies should, however, be encouraged. Treatment is recommended for more severe degrees of this disorder. Objective indices of severity elicited by polysomnography should include a high index of respiratory disturbances per hour, repetitive episodes of hypoxemia, and an abnormally shortened sleep latency. Strict guidelines for therapy have not been adequately validated to dictate thresholds for distinguishing less severely affected patients. At the present time, considerable reliance is made on clinical judgment to initiate a therapeutic trial or regimen.

Indications for Treatment of Insomnia Complaints

Complaints of insomnia are very common in the older patient. Insomnia is a symptomatic expression of a constellation of medical conditions that are not entirely related one to another. Insomnia may be of psychiatric (e.g., depression, anxiety), physiological (e.g., central apnea, limb movement), pharmacological (e.g., prescribed or unprescribed drugs or alcohol), or of medical origin. It may coexist with other sleep disorders (such as apnea), but this may be merely coincidental.

Since insomnia has many causes, the indications for treatment are dependent on the etiology. A thorough medical evaluation is essential prior to initiating treatment. Indications for therapy will be driven by the underlying cause and severity of symptoms.

Attention was given to periodic movements in sleep which appear to be very common in the older patient. Certain pharmacological treatments appear to be effective in patients who find this condition distressing. There is, however, insufficient evidence at this time to indicate whether or not the disease state or its treatment affect morbidity in the older patient. Moreover, the long-term benefits and risks of treatment of periodic movements in sleep are unknown, and, therefore, further investigations are recommended.

Insomnia may also be related to circadian rhythm disorders. Amplitude and phase relationships are often altered in the older person. These changes may produce a variety of somatic complaints and sleep disturbances. Such alterations occur during shift work, transmeridian travel, or changes in daily routine or sleep patterns (earlier arousal and earlier bedtime tendency), or they may occur spontaneously.

Therapy should be directed toward appropriate control of the environment and adequate counseling of the patient and the employer. It may include appropriately timed bright light exposure.

Insomnia resulting from medical or psychiatric causes should be managed primarily by appropriate treatment of the underlying condition.

Common Medical Practices

Insomnia

Although hypnotic medication is frequently prescribed by physicians for insomnia and secured either across the counter or "extralegally," hypnotic medication should not be the mainstay of management for most of the causes of disturbed sleep.

Since a large proportion of individuals with chronic insomnia have psychiatric complaints, particularly depression, but also anxiety, panic states, alcoholism, and others, treatment should be directed toward the underlying disorder. In the case of depression the tricyclic antidepressants are frequently useful in the absence of contraindications. One can take advantage of the sedative effect of some of these agents in addition to their more specific effect on the depression. Some agents may actually cause sleeplessness and should be used in the morning.

Other diseases and conditions which cause or contribute to insomnia, such as congestive heart failure, hyperthyroidism, pulmonary disease, esophageal reflux, and arthritis, should be treated specifically with the reminder that medications such as steroids and theophylline may cause sleep disturbance, as can the timing of administration of diuretics.

Pharmacologic therapy may be helpful if it is determined that periodic movements in sleep are contributing to insomnia and require treatment. The long-term benefits of treatment have yet to be determined.

Other general measures such as sleep hygiene can be used as adjuncts to treatment of the specific causes of insomnia and tried when the cause is not clear or is unspecified. Sleep hygiene measures include regularization of bedtime (generally later rather than earlier); the use of the bedroom primarily for sleeping and sexual activity; exercise; avoidance of alcohol and caffeine; reduced evening fluid intake; and in the case of esophageal reflux, elevation of the head of the bed.

Short-term intermittent use of hypnotics and sedative tricyclics may be useful for temporary problems such as bereavement, dislocation, and situational anxiety. There are no studies that demonstrate their long term effectiveness. Given the changes in drug metabolism associated with increasing age, all medication should be used with caution, especially those with long half-lives. Older people should avoid over-the-counter sleep medication due to their anticholinergic effects and questionable efficacy. L-Tryptophan (another commonly used over-the-counter sleep-inducing agent) has been associated with eosinophilic myalgia syndrome and has been withdrawn from the market.

The role of pharmacological, behavioral, and phototherapeutic management of disorders of circadian rhythm regulation is currently under investigation.

Hypersomnia

When treatment is indicated for hypersomnia due to obstructive sleep apnea, certain general measures, if successfully initiated, may suffice. These include weight loss; avoidance of alcohol, sedatives and hypnotics; the avoidance of the supine sleeping position; and management of nasal and nasopharyngeal disease.

The mainstay of treatment is the use of nasal continuous positive airway pressure (CPAP), which is frequently successful. It and other devices (including tongue retaining and jaw advancing appliances and cervical collars) need further study.

Where other measures, including nasal CPAP, fail or are unacceptable, surgical procedures may become an appropriate alternative treatment. Uvulopalatopharyngoplasty has been reported to be successful. There is evidence that the procedure may have better success when tailored to a demonstrated site of obstruction. Tracheostomy may be required if other procedures are unacceptable or fail.

In all therapeutic interventions there should be long-term outcome assessment.

Good Sleep Hygiene and Treatment

The answer to this question involves defining the target audience, determining what information should be conveyed, and deciding how best to transmit the information.

Physicians and medical students, nurses, social workers and counselors, rehabilitation and respiratory therapists, discharge planners, and pharmacists and other allied health professionals are the groups to be approached first. We anticipate particular interest from providers of services to the older people including area agencies on aging, senior centers, and nursing homes.

Other special groups that are affected by sleep disorder issues include employers, pharmaceutical companies, members of the legal profession, and developers of technology. Funders of research, both public and private, must be involved in this developing field. Education also must be directed toward decision makers at local, state and national levels, including regulatory and legislative groups. There are also key decision makers in the private sector such as those in the insurance industry and health care systems.

Educational efforts must include the very groups we wish to help: the older persons, their families, and caregivers.

The information to be conveyed will differ in content, style, and depth depending on the audience--professionals, patients, and media. A particular educational emphasis is desirable for new physicians and researchers, even while it is recognized that there are many unanswered questions. Nevertheless there are general concepts that could be useful for all groups. The content should include concepts of sleep physiology and pathophysiology, and assessment and differential diagnosis.

Discussion of treatment approaches including technological devices, drugs, and lifestyle should address disadvantages as well as advantages. For audiences unfamiliar with the issue of sleep and the older person, the magnitude of the personal and societal toll in accidents, health, and unhappiness must be conveyed. Other key points include proper use of medications, preventive health measures, and good sleep hygiene practices. Individuals may satisfactorily cope with insomnia, and it may be transient. On the other hand, persistent insomnia may reflect major disease, and competent clinical consultation may be desirable.

Imagination and sustained effort are at the heart of the many educational efforts. For health professionals one goal is to include information on sleep in the curriculum of schools--not an easy task. More standard educational efforts include appropriate lay and professional publications, professional conferences, and continuing education. Lay or advocacy groups can contribute to the total educational effort, as well as benefit from it. Reaching the public can be facilitated by utilizing existing networks, for example, state and area agencies on aging, coordinated through the Administration on Aging. There are opportunities for communicating information in newsletters published by churches, hospitals, and senior centers. There is particular need to involve citizen groups who direct their efforts toward the older person. All media groups should be encouraged to discuss these issues.

The Public Health Service must take a more active role in educating and disseminating information to the public. Without such effort, this consensus report may not receive the wide dissemination it deserves.

Future Research

The conference presentations emphasized the problem of sleep disorders in older age due to the demographic shift in the American population to an increasing proportion in the over-65 age group, and to the public awareness of the interest of the medical community in diagnosis and treatment of these disorders.

The study of sleep and sleep disorders has advanced rapidly in the past 30 years. This advance has been most prominent in studies of normal sleep throughout the life span. However, the classification, diagnostic criteria, understanding of the basic mechanisms, natural history, and the efficacy of treatment in sleep disorders are still in early stages so that further research in all these areas is necessary. This is particularly true for the older population in whom these conditions may be more frequent and disruptive.

It is always difficult to define classification and diagnostic criteria in a relatively new area where clinical descriptions and observations predominate and where the interpretation of objective measures, even with existing and new technology, is hampered. Certainly, large studies of control populations with proper sampling methods are necessary. This is particularly the situation in older populations where controls without confounding disease are more difficult to obtain.

It is often necessary in alleviating illness to press forward with clinical descriptions and treatment even without knowledge of the basic mechanisms. However, it is only with elucidation of these mechanisms that rational approaches to therapy can be effected. The study of these disorders in older patients, who often have other diseases, affords some unusual opportunities. For example, how does the dopamine depletion in Parkinson's disease patients affect sleep architecture and cardiopulmonary adaptation? Also, older patients may take one or more drugs for other conditions, and this may afford an opportunity for clinical observations.

There have been extensive studies of sleep mechanisms in experimental animals. Efforts should be made to identify appropriate animal models for sleep disorders. Now it is possible to study old animals, including primates, and these studies should provide insight into the basic mechanisms of sleep changes in aging. The new interest in disordered circadian rhythms as a clinical observation opens up new areas of research.

Modern research techniques used in selected human cases might help identify biological markers for some of these disorders. Opportunities for clinical and pathological correlation should be encouraged. The application or development of new research techniques should provide added understanding of the neurobiology of sleep and its disorders.

The natural history of many sleep disorders has not been well described. Longitudinal studies into older age would clarify the progress of these disorders and their effect on morbidity and mortality. This is also necessary if one is to judge the efficacy of various treatment modalities. Important questions that can only be answered by long-term studies are whether some of the variations noted in the older population are the result of aging or of concomitant disease; whether these variations need to be tested further; and whether these variations are responsible for other medical conditions. This latter point needs clarification because of the questions regarding sleep apnea with oxygen desaturation and various forms of dementia.

An important area of study is the disruption of normal circadian rhythms by transmeridian time shifts, dislocation such as moving to a nursing home, and shift work. These may result in sleep disturbances with attendant problems with family, driving, and recreation.

It is obvious from the data presented that extensive studies need to be done to settle the question of benefits of treatment in these disorders. Carefully controlled studies of well defined clinical groups will be necessary to establish the benefit of various therapies. It is equally important in clinical trials to look at the efficacy of different means of sleep hygiene practices, not only for therapy but for prevention.

Added knowledge about the effectiveness of treatment should spur studies of cost effectiveness of diagnostic methods and therapies.

In all the areas mentioned there are many opportunities for basic and clinical research. The enhanced interest in the older population should provide both challenges and opportunities for investigators.

Conclusions and Recommendations

There is a need for epidemiologic investigations of sleep disorders: case control, cohort, and cross-cultural studies should be initiated. The information developed in these studies will aid in the understanding of the natural history, etiology, and prevention of sleep disorders.

- Evaluation of sleep disorders begins with careful clinical evaluation performed by an informed primary care physician.
- Standardization of clinical measures and assessment of the specificity and sensitivity of diagnostic procedures is essential.
- Advanced skills and diagnostic tools are available and should be applied in appropriate patients.
- The objective of sleep disorder therapy is to reduce morbidity and mortality and improve the quality of life.
- Obstructive sleep apnea is a potentially severe and treatable cause of daytime hypersomnia.
- Restoration of airway competence is the objective in the treatment of severe sleep apnea.
- Insomnia is a complaint with multiple causes and requires different treatments.
- Hypnotic medications should not be the mainstay of treatment of insomnia, are overused and have habit forming potential.
- The value of good sleep hygiene should not be underestimated in the prevention and treatment of insomnia.
- Widespread knowledge about sleep and its disorders is lacking, and education at all levels is needed.
- The Public Health Service must take an active role in educating the public.
- Powerful new techniques, such as brain imaging, molecular biological tools, and neurochemical analyses, should be used in human studies and animal models to explore the basic mechanisms of sleep and sleep disorders.
- Sleep disorders in older people offer unique opportunities to study integrative neurologic, psychiatric, and cardiopulmonary functions.
- Current and new therapies and technologies must be evaluated by randomized controlled clinical trials.
- The Health Care Financing Administration should review current reimbursement policies, and continue to explore clinical data set requirements as these reimbursement policies for sleep disorders evolve.

Appendix E. More on Problem Sleepiness

Overview[47]

Everyone feels sleepy at times. However, when sleepiness interferes with daily routines and activities, or reduces the ability to function, it is called "problem sleepiness." A person can be sleepy without realizing it. For example, a person may not feel sleepy during activities such as talking and listening to music at a party, but the same person can fall asleep while driving home afterward.

The following appendix is reproduced and adapted from the National Heart, Lung, and Blood Institute publication dedicated to problem sleepiness.

What Causes Problem Sleepiness?

You may have problem sleepiness if you:

- Consistently do not get enough sleep
- Get poor quality sleep
- Fall asleep while driving
- Struggle to stay awake when inactive such as when watching television or reading
- Have difficulty paying attention or concentrating at work, school, or home
- Have performance problems at work or school

[47] Adapted from the National Heart, Lung, and Blood Institute: **http://www.nhlbi.nih.gov/health/public/sleep/pslp_fs.pdf**.

- Are often told by others that you are sleepy
- Have difficulty remembering
- Have slowed responses
- Have difficulty controlling your emotions
- Must take naps on most days

Sleepiness can be due to the body's natural daily sleep-wake cycles, inadequate sleep, sleep disorders, or certain drugs.

Sleep-Wake Cycle

Each day there are two periods when the body experiences a natural tendency toward sleepiness: during the late night hours (generally between midnight and 7 a.m.) and again during the midafternoon (generally between 1 p.m. and 4 p.m.). If people are awake during these times, they have a higher risk of falling asleep unintentionally, especially if they haven't been getting enough sleep.

Inadequate Sleep

The amount of sleep needed each night varies among people. Each person needs a particular amount of sleep in order to be fully alert throughout the day. Research has shown that when healthy adults are allowed to sleep unrestricted, the average time slept is 8 to 8.5 hours. Some people need more than that to avoid problem sleepiness; others need less.

If a person does not get enough sleep, even on one night, a "sleep debt" begins to build and increases until enough sleep is obtained. Problem sleepiness occurs as the debt accumulates. Many people do not get enough sleep during the work week and then sleep longer on the weekends or days off to reduce their sleep debt. If too much sleep has been lost, sleeping in on the weekend may not completely reverse the effects of not getting enough sleep during the week.

Sleep Disorders

Sleep disorders such as sleep apnea, narcolepsy, restless legs syndrome, and insomnia can cause problem sleepiness. *Sleep apnea* is a serious disorder in which a person's breathing is interrupted during sleep, causing the individual to awaken many times during the night and experience problem sleepiness during the day. People with *narcolepsy* have excessive sleepiness during the day, even after sleeping enough at night. They may fall asleep at inappropriate times and places. *Restless legs syndrome (RLS)* causes a person to experience unpleasant sensations in the legs, often described as creeping, crawling, pulling, or painful. These sensations frequently occur in the evening, making it difficult for people with RLS to fall asleep, leading to problem sleepiness during the day. *Insomnia* is the perception of poor-quality sleep due to difficulty falling asleep, waking up during the night with difficulty returning to sleep, waking up too early in the morning, or unrefreshing sleep. Any of these sleep disorders can cause problem sleepiness.

Medical Conditions/Drugs

Certain medical conditions and drugs, including prescription medications, can also disrupt sleep and cause problem sleepiness. Examples include:

- Chronic illnesses such as asthma, congestive heart failure, rheumatoid arthritis, or any other chronically painful disorder.
- Some medications to treat high blood pressure, some heart medications, and asthma medications such as theophylline.
- Alcohol—Although some people use alcohol to help themselves fall asleep, it causes sleep disruption during the night, which can lead to problem sleepiness during the day. Alcohol is also a sedating drug that can, even in small amounts, make a sleepy person much more sleepy and at greater risk for car crashes and performance problems.
- Caffeine—Whether consumed in coffee, tea, soft drinks, or medications, caffeine makes it harder for many people to fall asleep and stay asleep. Caffeine stays in the body for about 3 to 7 hours, so even when taken earlier in the day it can cause problems with sleep at night.
- Nicotine from cigarettes or a skin patch is a stimulant and makes it harder to fall asleep and stay asleep.

Problem Sleepiness and Adolescents

Many U.S. high school and college students have signs of problem sleepiness, such as:

- Difficulty getting up for school

- Falling asleep at school
- Struggling to stay awake while doing homework

The need for sleep may be 9 hours or more per night as a person goes through adolescence. At the same time, many teens begin to show a preference for a later bed time, which may be due to a biological change. Teens tend to stay up later but have to get up early for school, resulting in their getting much less sleep than they need.

Many factors contribute to problem sleepiness in teens and young adults, but the main causes are not getting enough sleep and irregular sleep schedules. Some of the factors that influence adolescent sleep include:

- Social activities with peers that lead to later bedtimes
- Homework to be done in the evenings
- Early wake-up times due to early school start times
- Parents being less involved in setting and enforcing bedtimes
- Employment, sports, or other extracurricular activities that decrease the time available for sleep

Teens and young adults who do not get enough sleep are at risk for problems such as:

- Automobile crashes
- Poor performance in school and poor grades
- Depressed moods
- Problems with peer and adult relationships

Many adolescents have part-time jobs in addition to their classes and other activities. High school students who work more than 20 hours per week have more problem sleepiness and may use more caffeine, nicotine, and alcohol than those who work less than 20 hours per week or not at all.

Shift Work And Problem Sleepiness

About 20 million Americans (20 to 25 percent of workers) perform shift work. Most shift workers get less sleep over 24 hours than day workers. Sleep loss is greatest for night shift workers, those who work early morning shifts, and female shift workers with children at home. About 60 to 70 percent of shift workers have difficulty sleeping and/or problem sleepiness.

The human sleep-wake system is designed to prepare the body and mind for sleep at night and wakefulness during the day. These natural rhythms make it difficult to sleep during daylight hours and to stay awake during the night hours, even in people who are well rested. It is possible that the human body never completely adjusts to nighttime activity and daytime sleep, even in those who work permanent night shifts.

In addition to the sleep-wake system, environmental factors can influence sleepiness in shift workers. Because our society is strongly day-oriented, shift workers who try to sleep during the day are often interrupted by noise, light, telephones, family members, and other distractions. In contrast, the nighttime sleep of day workers is largely protected by social customs that keep noises and interruptions to a minimum.

Problem sleepiness in shift workers may result in:

- Increased risk for automobile crashes, especially while driving home after the night shift
- Decreased quality of life
- Decreased productivity (night work performance may be slower and less accurate than day performance)
- Increased risk of accidents and injuries at work

What Can Help?

Sleep—There Is No Substitute!

Many people simply do not allow enough time for sleep on a regular basis. A first step may be to evaluate daily activities and sleep-wake patterns to determine how much sleep is obtained. If you are consistently getting less than 8 hours of sleep per night, more sleep may be needed. A good approach is to gradually move to an earlier bedtime. For example, if an extra hour of sleep is needed, try going to bed 15 minutes earlier each night for four nights and then keep the last bedtime. This method will increase the amount of time in bed without causing a sudden change in schedule. However, if work or family schedules do not permit the earlier bedtime, a 30- to 60-minute daily nap may help.

Medications/Drugs

In general, medications do not help problem sleepiness, and some make it worse. *Caffeine* can reduce sleepiness and increase alertness, but only temporarily. It can also cause problem sleepiness to become worse by interrupting sleep.

While *alcohol* may shorten the time it takes to fall asleep, it can disrupt sleep later in the night, and therefore add to the problem sleepiness.

Medications may be prescribed for patients in certain situations. For example, the short-term use of sleeping pills has been shown to be helpful in patients diagnosed with acute insomnia. Long-term use of sleep medication is recommended only for the treatment of specific sleep disorders.

If You're Sleepy—Don't Drive!

A person who is sleepy and drives is at high risk for an automobile crash. Planning ahead may help reduce that risk. For example, the following tips may help when planning a long distance car trip:

- Get a good night's sleep before leaving
- Avoid driving between midnight and 7 a.m.
- Change drivers often to allow for rest periods
- Schedule frequent breaks

If you are a shift worker, the following may help:

- Decreasing the amount of night work
- Increasing the total amount of sleep by adding naps and lengthening the amount of time allotted for sleep
- Increasing the intensity of light at work
- Having a predictable schedule of night shifts
- Eliminating sound and light in the bedroom during daytime sleep
- Using caffeine (only during the first part of the shift) to promote alertness at night
- Possibly using prescription sleeping pills to help daytime sleep on an occasional basis (check with your doctor)

If you think you are getting enough sleep, but still feel sleepy during the day, check with your doctor to be sure your sleepiness is not due to a sleep disorder.

ONLINE GLOSSARIES

The Internet provides access to a number of free-to-use medical dictionaries and glossaries. The National Library of Medicine has compiled the following list of online dictionaries:

- ADAM Medical Encyclopedia (A.D.A.M., Inc.), comprehensive medical reference: **http://www.nlm.nih.gov/medlineplus/encyclopedia.html**
- MedicineNet.com Medical Dictionary (MedicineNet, Inc.): **http://www.medterms.com/Script/Main/hp.asp**
- Merriam-Webster Medical Dictionary (Inteli-Health, Inc.): **http://www.intelihealth.com/IH/**
- Multilingual Glossary of Technical and Popular Medical Terms in Eight European Languages (European Commission) - Danish, Dutch, English, French, German, Italian, Portuguese, and Spanish: **http://allserv.rug.ac.be/~rvdstich/eugloss/welcome.html**
- On-line Medical Dictionary (CancerWEB): **http://www.graylab.ac.uk/omd/**
- Technology Glossary (National Library of Medicine) - Health Care Technology: **http://www.nlm.nih.gov/nichsr/ta101/ta10108.htm**
- Terms and Definitions (Office of Rare Diseases): **http://rarediseases.info.nih.gov/ord/glossary_a-e.html**

Beyond these, MEDLINEplus contains a very user-friendly encyclopedia covering every aspect of medicine (licensed from A.D.A.M., Inc.). The ADAM Medical Encyclopedia can be accessed via the following Web site address: **http://www.nlm.nih.gov/medlineplus/encyclopedia.html**. ADAM is also available on commercial Web sites such as Web MD (**http://my.webmd.com/adam/asset/adam_disease_articles/a_to_z/a**) and drkoop.com (**http://www.drkoop.com/**). Topics of interest can be researched by using keywords before continuing elsewhere, as these basic definitions and concepts will be useful in more advanced areas of research. You may choose to print various pages specifically relating to sleep apnea and keep them on file. The NIH, in particular, suggests that patients with sleep apnea visit the following Web sites in the ADAM Medical Encyclopedia:

- **Basic Guidelines for Sleep Apnea**

  Central sleep apnea
  Web site:
  http://www.nlm.nih.gov/medlineplus/ency/article/003997.htm

Obstructive sleep apnea
Web site:
http://www.nlm.nih.gov/medlineplus/ency/article/000811.htm

- **Signs & Symptoms for Sleep Apnea**

Apnea
Web site:
http://www.nlm.nih.gov/medlineplus/ency/article/003069.htm

Blood pressure, high
Web site:
http://www.nlm.nih.gov/medlineplus/ency/article/003082.htm

Breath cessation
Web site:
http://www.nlm.nih.gov/medlineplus/ency/article/003069.htm

Cessation of breathing
Web site:
http://www.nlm.nih.gov/medlineplus/ency/article/003069.htm

Confusion
Web site:
http://www.nlm.nih.gov/medlineplus/ency/article/003205.htm

Consciousness, decreased
Web site:
http://www.nlm.nih.gov/medlineplus/ency/article/003202.htm

Decreased consciousness
Web site:
http://www.nlm.nih.gov/medlineplus/ency/article/003202.htm

Drowsiness
Web site:
http://www.nlm.nih.gov/medlineplus/ency/article/003208.htm

Edema
Web site:
http://www.nlm.nih.gov/medlineplus/ency/article/003103.htm

Hallucinations
Web site:
http://www.nlm.nih.gov/medlineplus/ency/article/003258.htm

Headaches
Web site:
http://www.nlm.nih.gov/medlineplus/ency/article/003024.htm

Hypoxia
Web site:
http://www.nlm.nih.gov/medlineplus/ency/article/003215.htm

Lethargy
Web site:
http://www.nlm.nih.gov/medlineplus/ency/article/003088.htm

Memory loss
Web site:
http://www.nlm.nih.gov/medlineplus/ency/article/003257.htm

No breathing
Web site:
http://www.nlm.nih.gov/medlineplus/ency/article/003069.htm

Obese
Web site:
http://www.nlm.nih.gov/medlineplus/ency/article/003101.htm

Sleepiness
Web site:
http://www.nlm.nih.gov/medlineplus/ency/article/003208.htm

Snoring
Web site:
http://www.nlm.nih.gov/medlineplus/ency/article/003207.htm

Somnolence
Web site:
http://www.nlm.nih.gov/medlineplus/ency/article/003208.htm

Swelling, overall
Web site:
http://www.nlm.nih.gov/medlineplus/ency/article/003103.htm

Weight gain
Web site:
http://www.nlm.nih.gov/medlineplus/ency/article/003084.htm

- **Diagnostics and Tests for Sleep Apnea**

Arterial blood gases
Web site:
http://www.nlm.nih.gov/medlineplus/ency/article/003855.htm

ECG
Web site:
http://www.nlm.nih.gov/medlineplus/ency/article/003868.htm

Sleep studies
Web site:
http://www.nlm.nih.gov/medlineplus/ency/article/003932.htm

- **Surgery and Procedures for Sleep Apnea**

Adenoidectomy
Web site:
http://www.nlm.nih.gov/medlineplus/ency/article/003011.htm

Tonsillectomy
Web site:
http://www.nlm.nih.gov/medlineplus/ency/article/003013.htm

Tracheostomy
Web site:
http://www.nlm.nih.gov/medlineplus/ency/article/002955.htm

- **Background Topics for Sleep Apnea**

Alcohol use
Web site:
http://www.nlm.nih.gov/medlineplus/ency/article/001944.htm

Incidence
Web site:
http://www.nlm.nih.gov/medlineplus/ency/article/002387.htm

Intentional weight loss
Web site:
http://www.nlm.nih.gov/medlineplus/ency/article/001940.htm

Labored breathing
Web site:
http://www.nlm.nih.gov/medlineplus/ency/article/000007.htm

Nasal CPAP
Web site:
http://www.nlm.nih.gov/medlineplus/ency/article/001916.htm

Obstructed airway
Web site:
http://www.nlm.nih.gov/medlineplus/ency/article/000036.htm

Physical examination
Web site:
http://www.nlm.nih.gov/medlineplus/ency/article/002274.htm

Weight management
Web site:
http://www.nlm.nih.gov/medlineplus/ency/article/001943.htm

Weight reduction
Web site:
http://www.nlm.nih.gov/medlineplus/ency/article/001940.htm

Online Dictionary Directories

The following are additional online directories compiled by the National Library of Medicine, including a number of specialized medical dictionaries and glossaries:

- Medical Dictionaries: Medical & Biological (World Health Organization): **http://www.who.int/hlt/virtuallibrary/English/diction.htm#Medical**
- MEL-Michigan Electronic Library List of Online Health and Medical Dictionaries (Michigan Electronic Library): **http://mel.lib.mi.us/health/health-dictionaries.html**
- Patient Education: Glossaries (DMOZ Open Directory Project): **http://dmoz.org/Health/Education/Patient_Education/Glossaries/**

- Web of Online Dictionaries (Bucknell University): **http://www.yourdictionary.com/diction5.html#medicine**

SLEEP APNEA GLOSSARY

The following is a complete glossary of terms used in this sourcebook. The definitions are derived from official public sources including the National Institutes of Health [NIH] and the European Union [EU]. After this glossary, we list a number of additional hardbound and electronic glossaries and dictionaries that you may wish to consult.

Abscess: A localized, circumscribed collection of pus. [NIH]

Adduction: The rotation of an eye toward the midline (nasally). [NIH]

Adenoma: A benign tumor originating from, or having the appearance of, glandular epithelium; of endocrine or exocrine origin. [NIH]

Adjustment: The dynamic process wherein the thoughts, feelings, behavior, and biophysiological mechanisms of the individual continually change to adjust to the environment. [NIH]

Airway: A device for securing unobstructed passage of air into and out of the lungs during general anesthesia. [NIH]

Alertness: A state of readiness to detect and respond to certain specified small changes occurring at random intervals in the environment. [NIH]

Ameliorating: A changeable condition which prevents the consequence of a failure or accident from becoming as bad as it otherwise would. [NIH]

Antagonism: Interference with, or inhibition of, the growth of a living organism by another living organism, due either to creation of unfavorable conditions (e. g. exhaustion of food supplies) or to production of a specific antibiotic substance (e. g. penicillin). [NIH]

Apnea: Cessation of breathing. [NIH]

Attenuated: Strain with weakened or reduced virulence. [NIH]

Attenuation: Reduction of transmitted sound energy or its electrical equivalent. [NIH]

Axonal: Condition associated with metabolic derangement of the entire neuron and is manifest by degeneration of the distal portion of the nerve fiber. [NIH]

Berger: A binocular loupe with the lenses mounted at the anterior end of a light-excluding chamber fitting over the eyes and held in place by an elastic headband. [NIH]

Bioengineering: The application of engineering principles to the solution of biological problems, for example, remote-handling devices, life-support systems, controls, and displays. [NIH]

Biophysics: The science of physical phenomena and processes in living organisms. [NIH]

Brachial: All the nerves from the arm are ripped from the spinal cord. [NIH]

Catecholamine: A group of chemical substances manufactured by the adrenal medulla and secreted during physiological stress. [NIH]

CDNA: Synthetic DNA reverse transcribed from a specific RNA through the action of the enzyme reverse transcriptase. DNA synthesized by reverse transcriptase using RNA as a template. [NIH]

Circadian: Repeated more or less daily, i. e. on a 23- to 25-hour cycle. [NIH]

Clamp: A u-shaped steel rod used with a pin or wire for skeletal traction in the treatment of certain fractures. [NIH]

Cofactor: A substance, microorganism or environmental factor that activates or enhances the action of another entity such as a disease-causing agent. [NIH]

Competency: The capacity of the bacterium to take up DNA from its surroundings. [NIH]

Confounder: A factor of confusion which blurs a specific connection between a disease and a probable causal factor which is being studied. [NIH]

Consultation: A deliberation between two or more physicians concerning the diagnosis and the proper method of treatment in a case. [NIH]

Continuum: An area over which the vegetation or animal population is of constantly changing composition so that homogeneous, separate communities cannot be distinguished. [NIH]

Contraindications: Any factor or sign that it is unwise to pursue a certain kind of action or treatment, e. g. giving a general anesthetic to a person with pneumonia. [NIH]

Cortisol: A steroid hormone secreted by the adrenal cortex as part of the body's response to stress. [NIH]

Cytokine: Small but highly potent protein that modulates the activity of many cell types, including T and B cells. [NIH]

Deletion: A genetic rearrangement through loss of segments of DNA (chromosomes), bringing sequences, which are normally separated, into close proximity. [NIH]

Density: The logarithm to the base 10 of the opacity of an exposed and processed film. [NIH]

Discrete: Made up of separate parts or characterized by lesions which do not become blended; not running together; separate. [NIH]

Discrimination: The act of qualitative and/or quantitative differentiation between two or more stimuli. [NIH]

Dysphonia: Difficulty or pain in speaking; impairment of the voice. [NIH]

Eardrum: A thin, tense membrane forming the greater part of the outer wall of the tympanic cavity and separating it from the external auditory meatus; it constitutes the boundary between the external and middle ear. [NIH]

EEG: A graphic recording of the changes in electrical potential associated with the activity of the cerebral cortex made with the electroencephalogram. [NIH]

Electrode: Component of the pacing system which is at the distal end of the lead. It is the interface with living cardiac tissue across which the stimulus is transmitted. [NIH]

EMG: Recording of electrical activity or currents in a muscle. [NIH]

Empirical: A treatment based on an assumed diagnosis, prior to receiving confirmatory laboratory test results. [NIH]

Eosinophilic: A condition found primarily in grinding workers caused by a reaction of the pulmonary tissue, in particular the eosinophilic cells, to dust that has entered the lung. [NIH]

Estrogen: One of the two female sex hormones. [NIH]

Evoke: The electric response recorded from the cerebral cortex after stimulation of a peripheral sense organ. [NIH]

Excitatory: When cortical neurons are excited, their output increases and each new input they receive while they are still excited raises their output markedly. [NIH]

Exhaustion: The feeling of weariness of mind and body. [NIH]

Expiratory: The volume of air which leaves the breathing organs in each expiration. [NIH]

Extender: Any of several colloidal substances of high molecular weight, used as a blood or plasma substitute in transfusion for increasing the volume of the circulating blood. [NIH]

Extraocular: External to or outside of the eye. [NIH]

Fat: Total lipids including phospholipids. [NIH]

Fatigue: The feeling of weariness of mind and body. [NIH]

Fold: A plication or doubling of various parts of the body. [NIH]

Forearm: The part between the elbow and the wrist. [NIH]

Generator: Any system incorporating a fixed parent radionuclide from which is produced a daughter radionuclide which is to be removed by elution or by any other method and used in a radiopharmaceutical. [NIH]

Genetics: The biological science that deals with the phenomena and mechanisms of heredity. [NIH]

Gestational: Psychosis attributable to or occurring during pregnancy. [NIH]

Glossectomy: Amputation of the tongue. [NIH]

Gravis: Eruption of watery blisters on the skin among those handling animals and animal products. [NIH]

Heterogeneity: The property of one or more samples or populations which implies that they are not identical in respect of some or all of their parameters, e. g. heterogeneity of variance. [NIH]

Impairment: In the context of health experience, an impairment is any loss or abnormality of psychological, physiological, or anatomical structure or function. [NIH]

Incisor: Anything adapted for cutting; any one of the four front teeth in each jaw. [NIH]

Infancy: The period of complete dependency prior to the acquisition of competence in walking, talking, and self-feeding. [NIH]

Infections: The illnesses caused by an organism that usually does not cause disease in a person with a normal immune system. [NIH]

Initiation: Mutation induced by a chemical reactive substance causing cell changes; being a step in a carcinogenic process. [NIH]

Insight: The capacity to understand one's own motives, to be aware of one's own psychodynamics, to appreciate the meaning of symbolic behavior. [NIH]

Involuntary: Reaction occurring without intention or volition. [NIH]

Lag: The time elapsing between application of a stimulus and the resulting reaction. [NIH]

Latency: The period of apparent inactivity between the time when a stimulus is presented and the moment a response occurs. [NIH]

Ligands: A RNA simulation method developed by the MIT. [NIH]

Linkage: The tendency of two or more genes in the same chromosome to remain together from one generation to the next more frequently than expected according to the law of independent assortment. [NIH]

Loop: A wire usually of platinum bent at one end into a small loop (usually 4 mm inside diameter) and used in transferring microorganisms. [NIH]

Microsurgery: Surgical procedures on the cellular level; a light microscope and miniaturized instruments are used. [NIH]

Migration: The systematic movement of genes between populations of the same species, geographic race, or variety. [NIH]

Modification: A change in an organism, or in a process in an organism, that is acquired from its own activity or environment. [NIH]

Monitor: An apparatus which automatically records such physiological signs as respiration, pulse, and blood pressure in an anesthetized patient or one undergoing surgical or other procedures. [NIH]

Morphological: Relating to the configuration or the structure of live organs. [NIH]

MRNA: The RNA molecule that conveys from the DNA the information that is to be translated into the structure of a particular polypeptide molecule. [NIH]

Narcolepsy: A condition of unknown cause characterized by a periodic uncontrollable tendency to fall asleep. [NIH]

Nerve: A cordlike structure of nervous tissue that connects parts of the nervous system with other tissues of the body and conveys nervous impulses to, or away from, these tissues. [NIH]

Networks: Pertaining to a nerve or to the nerves, a meshlike structure of interlocking fibers or strands. [NIH]

Nuclei: A body of specialized protoplasm found in nearly all cells and containing the chromosomes. [NIH]

Nucleus: A body of specialized protoplasm found in nearly all cells and containing the chromosomes. [NIH]

Otology: The branch of medicine which deals with the diagnosis and treatment of the disorders and diseases of the ear. [NIH]

Outpatient: A patient who is not an inmate of a hospital but receives diagnosis or treatment in a clinic or dispensary connected with the hospital. [NIH]

Pacemakers: A center or a substance that controls the rhythm of a body process; the term usually refers to the cardiac pacemaker. [NIH]

Palsy: Disease of the peripheral nervous system occurring usually after many years of increased lead absorption. [NIH]

Papilloma: A benign epithelial neoplasm which may arise from the skin, mucous membranes or glandular ducts. [NIH]

Paralysis: Loss or impairment of muscle function or sensation. [NIH]

Patch: A piece of material used to cover or protect a wound, an injured part, etc.: a patch over the eye. [NIH]

Pathologies: The study of abnormality, especially the study of diseases. [NIH]

Pediatrics: The branch of medical science concerned with children and their diseases. [NIH]

Pedicle: Embryonic link between the optic vesicle or optic cup and the forebrain or diencephalon, which becomes the optic nerve. [NIH]

Perilymph: The fluid contained within the space separating the membranous from the osseous labyrinth of the ear. [NIH]

Phenotypes: An organism as observed, i. e. as judged by its visually perceptible characters resulting from the interaction of its genotype with the environment. [NIH]

Phenyl: Ingredient used in cold and flu remedies. [NIH]

Pitch: The subjective awareness of the frequency or spectral distribution of a sound. [NIH]

Plasticity: In an individual or a population, the capacity for adaptation: a) through gene changes (genetic plasticity) or b) through internal physiological modifications in response to changes of environment (physiological plasticity). [NIH]

Pleural: A circumscribed area of hyaline whorled fibrous tissue which appears on the surface of the parietal pleura, on the fibrous part of the diaphragm or on the pleura in the interlobar fissures. [NIH]

Polymorphism: The occurrence together of two or more distinct forms in the same population. [NIH]

Pontine: A brain region involved in the detection and processing of taste. [NIH]

Postsynaptic: Nerve potential generated by an inhibitory hyperpolarizing stimulation. [NIH]

Potassium: It is essential to the ability of muscle cells to contract. [NIH]

Potentiate: A degree of synergism which causes the exposure of the organism to a harmful substance to worsen a disease already contracted. [NIH]

Potentiation: An overall effect of two drugs taken together which is greater than the sum of the effects of each drug taken alone. [NIH]

Probe: An instrument used in exploring cavities, or in the detection and dilatation of strictures, or in demonstrating the potency of channels; an elongated instrument for exploring or sounding body cavities. [NIH]

Prone: Having the front portion of the body downwards. [NIH]

Protocol: The detailed plan for a clinical trial that states the trial's rationale, purpose, drug or vaccine dosages, length of study, routes of administration, who may participate, and other aspects of trial design. [NIH]

Race: A population within a species which exhibits general similarities within itself, but is both discontinuous and distinct from other populations of that species, though not sufficiently so as to achieve the status of a taxon. [NIH]

Reliability: Used technically, in a statistical sense, of consistency of a test with itself, i. e. the extent to which we can assume that it will yield the same result if repeated a second time. [NIH]

Reticular: Coarse-fibered, netlike dermis layer. [NIH]

Retractor: An instrument designed for pulling aside tissues to improve exposure at operation; an instrument for drawing back the edge of a wound. [NIH]

Salivary: The duct that convey saliva to the mouth. [NIH]

Schizophrenia: A mental disorder characterized by a special type of disintegration of the personality. [NIH]

Secretory: Secreting; relating to or influencing secretion or the secretions. [NIH]

Segmental: Describing or pertaining to a structure which is repeated in similar form in successive segments of an organism, or which is undergoing segmentation. [NIH]

Segregation: The separation in meiotic cell division of homologous chromosome pairs and their contained allelomorphic gene pairs. [NIH]

Sensor: A device designed to respond to physical stimuli such as temperature, light, magnetism or movement and transmit resulting impulses for interpretation, recording, movement, or operating control. [NIH]

Specialist: In medicine, one who concentrates on 1 special branch of medical science. [NIH]

Specificity: Degree of selectivity shown by an antibody with respect to the number and types of antigens with which the antibody combines, as well as with respect to the rates and the extents of these reactions. [NIH]

Spectrometer: An apparatus for determining spectra; measures quantities such as wavelengths and relative amplitudes of components. [NIH]

Sperm: The fecundating fluid of the male. [NIH]

Splint: A rigid appliance used for the immobilization of a part or for the correction of deformity. [NIH]

Stimulus: That which can elicit or evoke action (response) in a muscle, nerve, gland or other excitable issue, or cause an augmenting action upon any function or metabolic process. [NIH]

Stromal: Large, veil-like cell in the bone marrow. [NIH]

Submandibular: Four to six lymph glands, located between the lower jaw and the submandibular salivary gland. [NIH]

Superoxide: Derivative of molecular oxygen that can damage cells. [NIH]

Supine: Having the front portion of the body upwards. [NIH]

Synapse: The region where the processes of two neurons come into close contiguity, and the nervous impulse passes from one to the other; the fibers of the two are intermeshed, but, according to the general view, there is no direct contiguity. [NIH]

Synchrony: The normal physiologic sequencing of atrial and ventricular activation and contraction. [NIH]

TATA: One sequence thought to be important for the transcription initiation in eukaryotes was found in most of the yeast genes. It is an AT-rich region with the canonical sequence TATA/AATA usually located 25-32 bp upstream from the transcription initiation site. [NIH]

Temporal: One of the two irregular bones forming part of the lateral surfaces and base of the skull, and containing the organs of hearing. [NIH]

Therapeutics: The branch of medicine which is concerned with the treatment of diseases, palliative or curative. [NIH]

Threshold: For a specified sensory modality (e. g. light, sound, vibration), the lowest level (absolute threshold) or smallest difference (difference threshold, difference limen) or intensity of the stimulus discernible in prescribed conditions of stimulation. [NIH]

Tractus: A part of some structure, usually that part along which something passes. [NIH]

Translation: The process whereby the genetic information present in the linear sequence of ribonucleotides in mRNA is converted into a corresponding sequence of amino acids in a protein. It occurs on the ribosome and is unidirectional. [NIH]

Translational: The cleavage of signal sequence that directs the passage of the protein through a cell or organelle membrane. [NIH]

Transmitter: A chemical substance which effects the passage of nerve impulses from one cell to the other at the synapse. [NIH]

Trauma: Any injury, wound, or shock, must frequently physical or structural shock, producing a disturbance. [NIH]

Tubercle: A rounded elevation on a bone or other structure. [NIH]

Ubiquitin: A highly conserved 76 amino acid-protein found in all eukaryotic cells. [NIH]

Ulcer: A localized necrotic lesion of the skin or a mucous surface. [NIH]

Uvula: Uvula palatinae; specifically, the tongue-like process which projects from the middle of the posterior edge of the soft palate. [NIH]

Vasodilators: Any nerve or agent which induces dilatation of the blood vessels. [NIH]

Vitro: Descriptive of an event or enzyme reaction under experimental investigation occurring outside a living organism. Parts of an organism or microorganism are used together with artificial substrates and/or conditions. [NIH]

Windpipe: A rigid tube, 10 cm long, extending from the cricoid cartilage to the upper border of the fifth thoracic vertebra. [NIH]

General Dictionaries and Glossaries

While the above glossary is essentially complete, the dictionaries listed here cover virtually all aspects of medicine, from basic words and phrases to more advanced terms (sorted alphabetically by title; hyperlinks provide rankings, information and reviews at Amazon.com):

- **Dictionary of Medical Acronymns & Abbreviations** by Stanley Jablonski (Editor), Paperback, 4th edition (2001), Lippincott Williams & Wilkins Publishers, ISBN: 1560534605, **http://www.amazon.com/exec/obidos/ASIN/1560534605/icongroupinterna**
- **Dictionary of Medical Terms : For the Nonmedical Person (Dictionary of Medical Terms for the Nonmedical Person, Ed 4)** by Mikel A. Rothenberg, M.D, et al, Paperback - 544 pages, 4th edition (2000), Barrons Educational Series, ISBN: 0764112015, **http://www.amazon.com/exec/obidos/ASIN/0764112015/icongroupinterna**
- **A Dictionary of the History of Medicine** by A. Sebastian, CD-Rom edition (2001), CRC Press-Parthenon Publishers, ISBN: 185070368X, **http://www.amazon.com/exec/obidos/ASIN/185070368X/icongroupinterna**
- **Dorland's Illustrated Medical Dictionary (Standard Version)** by Dorland, et al, Hardcover - 2088 pages, 29th edition (2000), W B Saunders Co, ISBN: 0721662544, **http://www.amazon.com/exec/obidos/ASIN/0721662544/icongroupinterna**
- **Dorland's Electronic Medical Dictionary** by Dorland, et al, Software, 29th Book & CD-Rom edition (2000), Harcourt Health Sciences, ISBN: 0721694934, **http://www.amazon.com/exec/obidos/ASIN/0721694934/icongroupinterna**
- **Dorland's Pocket Medical Dictionary (Dorland's Pocket Medical Dictionary, 26th Ed)** Hardcover - 912 pages, 26th edition (2001), W B Saunders Co, ISBN: 0721682812, **http://www.amazon.com/exec/obidos/ASIN/0721682812/icongroupinterna/103-4193558-7304618**
- **Melloni's Illustrated Medical Dictionary (Melloni's Illustrated Medical Dictionary, 4th Ed)** by Melloni, Hardcover, 4th edition (2001), CRC Press-

Parthenon Publishers, ISBN: 85070094X,
http://www.amazon.com/exec/obidos/ASIN/85070094X/icongroupinterna

- **Stedman's Electronic Medical Dictionary Version 5.0 (CD-ROM for Windows and Macintosh, Individual)** by Stedmans, CD-ROM edition (2000), Lippincott Williams & Wilkins Publishers, ISBN: 0781726328, **http://www.amazon.com/exec/obidos/ASIN/0781726328/icongroupinterna**
- **Stedman's Medical Dictionary** by Thomas Lathrop Stedman, Hardcover - 2098 pages, 27th edition (2000), Lippincott, Williams & Wilkins, ISBN: 068340007X, **http://www.amazon.com/exec/obidos/ASIN/068340007X/icongroupinterna**
- **Tabers Cyclopedic Medical Dictionary (Thumb Index)** by Donald Venes (Editor), et al, Hardcover - 2439 pages, 19th edition (2001), F A Davis Co, ISBN: 0803606540, **http://www.amazon.com/exec/obidos/ASIN/0803606540/icongroupinterna**

INDEX

9 780497 110581

Lightning Source UK Ltd.
Milton Keynes UK
11 November 2010

162756UK00002B/3/A